Inequality in Immunization 2024

Inequality in Immunization 2024

Ahmad Reza Hosseinpoor
Devaki Nambiar
Nicole Bergen
M. Carolina Danovaro
Hope L. Johnson
Ciara Sugerman

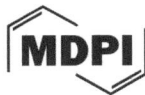

Basel • Beijing • Wuhan • Barcelona • Belgrade • Novi Sad • Cluj • Manchester

Editors

Ahmad Reza Hosseinpoor
Department of Data
and Analytics
World Health Organization
Geneva
Switzerland

Devaki Nambiar
Department of Data
and Analytics
World Health Organisation
Geneva
Switzerland

Nicole Bergen
Department of Data
and Analytics
World Health Organization
Geneva
Switzerland

M. Carolina Danovaro
Department of Immunization,
Vaccines, and Biologicals
World Health Organization
Geneva
Switzerland

Hope L. Johnson
Strategic Initiatives
Gavi, the Vaccine Alliance
Geneva
Switzerland

Ciara Sugerman
Global Immunization
Division
US Centres for Disease Control
Atlanta
United States

Editorial Office
MDPI AG
Grosspeteranlage 5
4052 Basel, Switzerland

This is a reprint of articles from the Special Issue published online in the open access journal *Vaccines* (ISSN 2076-393X) (available at: www.mdpi.com/journal/vaccines/special_issues/3DIMVZS00B).

For citation purposes, cite each article independently as indicated on the article page online and as indicated below:

Lastname, A.A.; Lastname, B.B. Article Title. *Journal Name* **Year**, *Volume Number*, Page Range.

ISBN 978-3-7258-2236-2 (Hbk)
ISBN 978-3-7258-2235-5 (PDF)
doi.org/10.3390/books978-3-7258-2235-5

Cover image courtesy of Conor Ashleigh/WHO, Geneva, Switzerland.

© 2024 by the authors. Articles in this book are Open Access and distributed under the Creative Commons Attribution license. The book as a whole is distributed by MDPI under the terms and conditions of the Creative Commons Attribution-NonCommercial-NoDerivs (CC BY-NC-ND) license.

Contents

About the Editors vii

Preface ix

Devaki Nambiar, Ahmad Reza Hosseinpoor, Nicole Bergen, M. Carolina Danovaro-Holliday, Ciara E. Sugerman and Hope L. Johnson
"Humanly Possible": Geographies, Metrics and Methods to Address Immunization Inequalities
Reprinted from: *Vaccines* 2024, 12, 1062, doi:10.3390/vaccines12091062 1

Nicole E. Johns, Cauane Blumenberg, Katherine Kirkby, Adrien Allorant, Francine Dos Santos Costa and M. Carolina Danovaro-Holliday et al.
Comparison of Wealth-Related Inequality in Tetanus Vaccination Coverage before and during Pregnancy: A Cross-Sectional Analysis of 72 Low- and Middle-Income Countries
Reprinted from: *Vaccines* 2024, 12, 431, doi:10.3390/vaccines12040431 5

Fulgence Niyibitegeka, Fiona M. Russell, Mark Jit and Natalie Carvalho
Inequitable Distribution of Global Economic Benefits from Pneumococcal Conjugate Vaccination
Reprinted from: *Vaccines* 2024, 12, 767, doi:10.3390/vaccines12070767 29

Carrie Lyons, Devaki Nambiar, Nicole E. Johns, Adrien Allorant, Nicole Bergen and Ahmad Reza Hosseinpoor
Inequality in Childhood Immunization Coverage: A Scoping Review of Data Sources, Analyses, and Reporting Methods
Reprinted from: *Vaccines* 2024, 12, 850, doi:10.3390/vaccines12080850 47

Ignacio E. Castro-Aguirre, Dan Alvarez, Marcela Contreras, Silas P. Trumbo, Oscar J. Mujica and Daniel Salas Peraza et al.
The Impact of the Coronavirus Pandemic on Vaccination Coverage in Latin America and the Caribbean
Reprinted from: *Vaccines* 2024, 12, 458, doi:10.3390/vaccines12050458 65

Kamal Fahmy, Quamrul Hasan, Md Sharifuzzaman and Yvan Hutin
Analyzing Subnational Immunization Coverage to Catch Up and Reach the Unreached in Seven High-Priority Countries in the Eastern Mediterranean Region, 2019–2021
Reprinted from: *Vaccines* 2024, 12, 285, doi:10.3390/vaccines12030285 75

Anna Kalbarczyk, Natasha Brownlee and Elizabeth Katz
Of Money and Men: A Scoping Review to Map Gender Barriers to Immunization Coverage in Low- and Middle-Income Countries
Reprinted from: *Vaccines* 2024, 12, 625, doi:10.3390/vaccines12060625 85

Gustavo C. Corrêa, Md. Jasim Uddin, Tasnuva Wahed, Elizabeth Oliveras, Christopher Morgan and Moses R. Kamya et al.
Measuring Zero-Dose Children: Reflections on Age Cohort Flexibilities for Targeted Immunization Surveys at the Local Level
Reprinted from: *Vaccines* 2024, 12, 195, doi:10.3390/vaccines12020195 100

Audrey Rachlin, Oluwasegun Joel Adegoke, Rajendra Bohara, Edson Rwagasore, Hassan Sibomana and Adeline Kabeja et al.
Building Data Triangulation Capacity for Routine Immunization and Vaccine Preventable Disease Surveillance Programs to Identify Immunization Coverage Inequities
Reprinted from: *Vaccines* 2024, 12, 646, doi:10.3390/vaccines12060646 111

Justice Moses K. Aheto, Iyanuloluwa Deborah Olowe, Ho Man Theophilus Chan, Adachi Ekeh, Boubacar Dieng and Biyi Fafunmi et al.
Geospatial Analyses of Recent Household Surveys to Assess Changes in the Distribution of Zero-Dose Children and Their Associated Factors before and during the COVID-19 Pandemic in Nigeria
Reprinted from: *Vaccines* **2023**, *11*, 1830, doi:10.3390/vaccines11121830 128

Branly Kilola Mbunga, Patrick Y. Liu, Freddy Bangelesa, Eric Mafuta, Nkamba Mukadi Dalau and Landry Egbende et al.
Zero-Dose Childhood Vaccination Status in Rural Democratic Republic of Congo: Quantifying the Relative Impact of Geographic Accessibility and Attitudes toward Vaccination
Reprinted from: *Vaccines* **2024**, *12*, 617, doi:10.3390/vaccines12060617 148

Pierre Muhoza, Monica P. Shah, Kwame Amponsa-Achiano, Hongjiang Gao, Pamela Quaye and William Opare et al.
Timeliness of Childhood Vaccinations Following Strengthening of the Second Year of Life (2YL) Immunization Platform and Introduction of Catch-Up Vaccination Policy in Ghana
Reprinted from: *Vaccines* **2024**, *12*, 716, doi:10.3390/vaccines12070716 162

Olufunto A. Olusanya, Nina B. Masters, Fan Zhang, David E. Sugerman, Rosalind J. Carter and Debora Weiss et al.
Sociodemographic Trends and Correlation between Parental Hesitancy towards Pediatric COVID-19 Vaccines and Routine Childhood Immunizations in the United States: 2021–2022 National Immunization Survey—Child COVID Module
Reprinted from: *Vaccines* **2024**, *12*, 495, doi:10.3390/vaccines12050495 181

Abyot Bekele Woyessa, Monica P. Shah, Binyam Moges Azmeraye, Jeff Pan, Leuel Lisanwork and Getnet Yimer et al.
Factors Associated with Uptake of Routine Measles-Containing Vaccine Doses among Young Children, Oromia Regional State, Ethiopia, 2021
Reprinted from: *Vaccines* **2024**, *12*, 762, doi:10.3390/vaccines12070762 202

Ankita Meghani, Manjula Sharma, Tanya Singh, Sourav Ghosh Dastidar, Veena Dhawan and Natasha Kanagat et al.
Enhancing COVID-19 Vaccine Uptake among Tribal Communities: A Case Study on Program Implementation Experiences from Jharkhand and Chhattisgarh States, India
Reprinted from: *Vaccines* **2024**, *12*, 463, doi:10.3390/vaccines12050463 219

About the Editors

Ahmad Reza Hosseinpoor

Ahmad Hosseinpoor is the Team Lead of the Health Inequality Monitoring team at the World Health Organization in Geneva. He has conceptualized and coordinated the development of resources and tools in this area, including the Health Inequality Monitor; the WHO global platform for disaggregated health data; the WHO Health Equity Assessment Toolkit (HEAT), a software application used to explore and compare health inequalities; and the WHO Handbook on Health Inequality Monitoring, a comprehensive resource used to strengthen and guide the development of health inequality monitoring. He is the lead author of a number of peer reviewed articles quantifying inequalities in health, both at the country level and the global level, as well as methodological articles such as health inequality decomposition. He has also been the Guest Editor of many Special Issues on the topic of health equity, including the 2023 and 2024 editions of Inequality in Immunization.

Devaki Nambiar

Devaki Nambiar is a Consultant with the World Health Organization and a Health Policy and Systems Researcher (HPSRer) with an interest in social inclusion, health equity, gender mainstreaming, and the right to health. Apart from research, she has provided technical inputs and co-facilitated regional and national courses and trainings across WHO regions on health equity, gender and health, as well as health inequality monitoring. She received her doctorate in Public Health from the Johns Hopkins Bloomberg School of Public Health in 2009 and received the 2018 Emerging Leader Award from the Royal Society for Tropical Medicine and Hygiene.

Nicole Bergen

Nicole Bergen is a Consultant with the Health Inequality Monitoring Team at the Department of Data and Analytics at the World Health Organization. With over 10 years of experience in health inequality monitoring, she has contributed to numerous peer reviewed journal articles, books, and scholarly reports on a range of topics, including childhood immunization, vaccine hesitancy, and COVID-19 vaccines. She has experience leading literature reviews on inequality topics and developing capacity-building resources for health inequality monitoring, including eLearning courses and instructional manuals and workbooks. Nicole received her PhD in Population Health from the University of Ottawa, where she now holds an Adjunct Professor appointment with the School of Epidemiology and Public Health.

M. Carolina Danovaro

Carolina Donovaro-Holliday has been working in different immunization-related activities in a variety of settings for over 20 years. She is part of the Global Immunization Monitoring team at the World Health Organization (WHO). In this role, she has supported the delivery of immunization programmes in a number of country contexts on a routine basis as well as in emergency contexts. She has co-authored over 100 articles in peer reviewed journals, book chapters, and technical documents. She is also involved in training and capacity strengthening through short courses and trainings with a particular interest in and passion to address health inequalities.

Hope L. Johnson

Dr Hope Johnson is a Special Advisor to the CEO, Strategic Initiatives, at Gavi, the Vaccine Alliance. She is responsible for overseeing Gavi's strategy, programmes, policies, and priority initiatives and the management of Gavi investments in immunisation data strengthening and research. An infectious disease epidemiologist with 25 years of experience in public health, including 18 years in vaccines and immunisation from country to global levels, Hope's previous work includes epidemiologic research and building an evidence base and capacity for data-driven decision-making to accelerate the development and implementation of maternal and child health interventions, with a specific focus on vaccine-preventable diseases.

Ciara Sugerman

Ciara Sugerman, PhD, is the lead of the Immunization Delivery Science Team in the Global Immunization Division (GID) at the US Centers for Disease Control and Prevention (CDC). She is an epidemiologist with over 20 years of experience in global public health. She was based in Addis Ababa, Ethiopia, for four years at the CDC-Ethiopia Country Office as the Immunization Program Director for GID where she worked on strengthening immunization systems in childhood and beyond. Her work focuses on increasing immunization coverage and equity, immunization recovery, strengthening the life course approach to immunizations, operational, and implementation research to inform improvements in immunization service delivery and the translation of evidence-based strategies into practice. She has published >70 peer reviewed scientific articles. She received her PhD from University College Cork, Ireland, along with a post-doctoral fellowship, and completed the Epidemic Intelligence Service Officer fellowship in applied field epidemiology at CDC.

Preface

Immunization coverage across the world and for people of all ages confronts a major challenge: inequality. Our understanding of the breadth, depth, and social patterning of immunization inequalities is incomplete. Aiming to fill this gap, the World Health Organization has partnered with Gavi, the Vaccine Alliance, and the US Centres for Disease Control to guest edit the 2024 edition of this Special Issue of *Vaccines* on Inequality in Immunization. This Special Issue showcases 14 research and review articles that deepen our understanding of immunization inequalities as well as highlight the entry points or modalities to reduce them.

On the 50th anniversary of the Expanded Programme on Immunization (EPI), the case we make is that it is "humanly possible" to understand inequalities in immunization, its drivers, as well as entry points for redressal.

This Special Issue is intended for technical experts, implementers, researchers, and scholars working in the areas of immunization and inequality monitoring.

Contributions address some of the important questions and methodological developments in the field. They represent the latest advancements in identifying where inequalities exist but also how they may be characterized with greater attention to root causes, complexities, and intent to act. Country analyses are drawn from India, the United States, the Democratic Republic of the Congo, Ethiopia, Ghana, and Nigeria, while aggregate analyses feature collaborations across Bangladesh, Mali, Nigeria, Uganda, and Rwanda. This Special Issue includes a global scoping review on childhood immunization as well as ecological analyses spanning Latin America and the Caribbean, as well as the Eastern Mediterranean region.

This Special Issue involves collaboration and coordination across scientists, learning hubs, and implementation groups spanning the globe, as well as premier academic and technical agencies. It demonstrates our shared commitment to tackling inequalities in immunization by marshalling science together.

Ahmad Reza Hosseinpoor, Devaki Nambiar, Nicole Bergen, M. Carolina Danovaro, Hope L. Johnson, and Ciara Sugerman
Editors

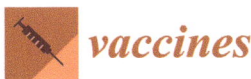

Editorial

"Humanly Possible": Geographies, Metrics and Methods to Address Immunization Inequalities

Devaki Nambiar [1], Ahmad Reza Hosseinpoor [1,*], Nicole Bergen [1], M. Carolina Danovaro-Holliday [2], Ciara E. Sugerman [3] and Hope L. Johnson [4]

[1] Department of Data and Analytics, World Health Organization, 20 Avenue Appia, 1211 Geneva, Switzerland; nambiard@who.int (D.N.); bergenn@who.int (N.B.)
[2] Department of Immunization, Vaccines, and Biologicals, World Health Organization, 20 Avenue Appia, 1211 Geneva, Switzerland; danovaroc@who.int
[3] Global Immunization Division, Global Health Center, Centers for Disease Control and Prevention, Atlanta, GA 30329, USA; bwf1@cdc.gov
[4] Measurement, Evaluation and Learning Department, Gavi, The Vaccine Alliance, 1218 Geneva, Switzerland; hjohnson@gavi.org
* Correspondence: hosseinpoora@who.int; Tel.: +41-22-791-3205

Citation: Nambiar, D.; Hosseinpoor, A.R.; Bergen, N.; Danovaro-Holliday, M.C.; Sugerman, C.E.; Johnson, H.L. "Humanly Possible": Geographies, Metrics and Methods to Address Immunization Inequalities. *Vaccines* **2024**, *12*, 1062. https://doi.org/10.3390/vaccines12091062

Received: 9 September 2024
Revised: 12 September 2024
Accepted: 12 September 2024
Published: 18 September 2024

Copyright: © World Health Organization 2024. Licensee MDPI. This article is distributed under the terms of the Creative Commons Attribution IGO License (https://creativecommons.org/licenses/by/3.0/igo/), which permits unrestricted use, distribution, and reproduction in any medium, provided the original work is properly cited. In any reproduction of this article, there should not be any suggestion that the WHO or this article endorse any specific organization or products. The use of the WHO logo is not permitted.

The year 2024 marks the 50th anniversary of the World Health Organization (WHO) Expanded Program on Immunization (EPI). WHO Director General Dr. Tedros Adhanom Ghebreyesus, acknowledging the incredible success of the EPI in showing what is "humanly possible", called for the continued support and funding of initiatives to ensure that life-saving vaccines are available to all [1]. This occasion has renewed attention on immunization as a critical component of primary health care. Immunization remains a continuing priority as countries seek to safeguard the health of populations, as well as strengthen their health systems.

However, the gains made in the last 50 years are not evenly distributed across all populations. The COVID-19 pandemic has exposed and exacerbated inequalities of immunization coverage in critical childhood and adolescent vaccines, such as the diphtheria–tetanus–pertussis-containing vaccine (DTP) and the Human Papillomavirus vaccine (HPV), with past progress being lost in some cases [2]. Equity-sensitive and action-oriented framing, including the identification of Zero Dose (ZD) children, namely those who do not receive even one dose of essential life-saving immunization in childhood, is increasingly applied for both research and programming addressing immunization inequities [3,4]. ZD framing draws attention to the intersections of different dimensions of inequality and is one way in which inequities may be made visible and understood.

The 2023 Special Issue of Inequality in Immunization highlighted various forms of inequalities, drivers of these inequalities, and the impact of equity-focused interventions [2]. We presented emerging evidence on a range of data sources and dimensions of inequality, as well as processes by which inequalities are emerging. We were pleased to reprise these themes and also go beyond them in the 2024 Special Issue of Inequality in Immunization. This Special Issue comprises 14 contributions including 10 research articles, 2 reviews, a project report and a perspective piece.

This Special Issue covers a wide scope of contexts where inequalities are arising and being addressed. Johns et al. and Kalbarczyk et al. carried out ecological analyses of low- and middle-income country contexts. At the regional level, Castro-Aguirre et al. explored immunization inequalities in Latin America and the Caribbean, and Fahmy et al. conducted an analysis of the Eastern Mediterranean region. A scoping review by Lyons et al. captured research on childhood immunization inequalities globally.

This Special Issue also features two method-focused papers. Rachlin et al. drew attention to data triangulation and linking of datasets and databases to enable inequality analysis in Bangladesh, Rwanda and Nigeria, and Corrêa et al. demonstrated the use of targeted local surveys to track ZD children in ZD Learning Hubs established by Gavi in Bangladesh, Mali, Nigeria, and Uganda. Niyibitegeka et al. explored pneumococcal conjugate vaccine inequalities in terms of the distribution of economic benefits.

A number of country-focused papers are also included, seeking to deepen our understanding of within-country inequalities for key vaccines. Aheto et al. assessed routine immunization and ZD prevalence in Nigeria, Muhoza et al. reported on the second year of life and catch-up vaccination in Ghana, Woyessa et al. looked at measles vaccine uptake and barriers in Ethiopia, Mbunga et al. addressed ZD status in the Democratic Republic of the Congo (DRC), Meghani et al. studied adult COVID vaccination in India, and Olusanya et al. analysed paediatric COVID-19 and routine immunization in the United States.

As aforementioned, ZD framing is important to identify and reach populations that have not received any vaccinations owing to experiences of diverse and multiple forms of disadvantage. Four papers in this Special Issue—authored by Fahmy et al., Corrêa et al., Aheto et al. and Mbunga et al.—covered inequalities in the prevalence of ZD, adopting different definitions for ZD to align with the study and country context. For example, Mbunga et al., in the context of DRC, and Fahmy et al., in the context of the Eastern Mediterranean Vaccine Action Plan countries, adopted the Immunization Agenda 2030 definition for ZD, namely children who have not received their first dose of the Pentavalent vaccine (DTP-Hib-HepB) by the age of 12 months. Aheto et al., in their article featuring Nigeria, defined ZD as non-receipt of DTP, measles-containing vaccine, oral polio vaccine, and BCG among children aged 12 to 23 months. While the conclusions drawn largely cohere, i.e., low levels of maternal education and utilisation of services, remoteness and distance from facility were associated with greater ZD prevalence, an argument is made for slightly variable measurement approaches to enable operational relevance. For instance, Corrêa et al. explore measuring the timeliness of immunization and including older age cohorts. As underscored in the paper by Lyons et al., having a range of indicator variations, some providing immediate operational input and others allowing broader analytical understanding of trends and gaps, enables analyses to reflect different contextual considerations, enhancing their use and relevance.

Wealth and maternal education levels were some of most explored dimensions of inequality in immunization at global and local levels, as well as those with the largest magnitudes and statistical significance, as evidenced by Johns et al., Aheto et al. and Lyons et al. Geographic accessibility is another major driver of inequalities explored in multiple studies in this Special Issue (including Fahmy et al., Aheto et al. and Mbunga et al.), largely through spatial analysis methods. One paper by Kalbarczyk et al. covered gender as an influence on immunization, finding that lack of time as well as cost constraints faced by women are major barriers to routine immunization coverage in sub-Saharan Africa and South Asia. The gender dimension in inequality research is still understudied, particularly in relation to other dimensions of inequality.

Attitudes and hesitancy towards vaccination represent another emerging theme that is closely connected to inequalities. Mbunga et al. and Olusanya et al., in contexts as variable as DRC and the United States, respectively, showed that parental/care-giver attitudes towards vaccination appeared to be highly correlated to under-vaccination and, in the case of DRC, to non-receipt of vaccination. In India, Meghani et al. identified engagement with community leaders, targeted counselling and door-to-door visits as important ways of addressing vaccine hesitancy and increasing awareness. Overall, this driver of inequalities warrants greater attention and further study across diverse country contexts.

This Special Issue has also explored inequality dimensions of the pneumococcal vaccine, which has been recommended for over two decades. The vaccine exists in surplus globally, but it is not equitably available across countries. Using 2021 birth cohort estimates, Niyibitegeka and colleagues developed a model of the total social welfare associated with the vaccine, demonstrating a 45-fold return on investment for manufacturers on the one hand, with 2.5–6.0% (per sensitivity analysis) of the total global surplus going to low-income countries, as compared to over a third of the surplus going to high-income countries. While more evidence related to the pneumococcal vaccine using an equity lens is needed, existing analyses suggest the need for redoubled efforts to increase vaccine access, reflecting the intention and spirit of EPI.

To conclude, this Special Issue provides evidence that transformation is "humanly possible" in two ways. First, the contributions show that immunization inequalities reflect structural factors like maternal education, gender inequality, societal norms, and global financing. And yet, these structural factors are remediable, suggesting on the one hand that these are inequities, but on the other that there is a possibility, and indeed a responsibility, for "human" intervention to mitigate them. Second, methodological insights related to measurement of ZD, standardization of indicators, use of various data sources and analytical approaches suggest that we are capable of refining our analyses, finding the gaps, and advancing on the path towards equity. The first fifty years of EPI have shown that it is possible to make vaccines accessible to large numbers of people around the world; in the coming 50 years, it is our responsibility to make immunization equity not merely possible or probable, but assured.

Funding: The Special Issue was funded in part by Gavi, The Vaccine Alliance. Beyond the individual contribution of H.L.J., who is a Gavi employee, the funder had no role in the writing of the Editorial.

Conflicts of Interest: The authors declare no conflicts of interest. The authors alone are responsible for the views expressed in this publication and they do not necessarily represent the views, decisions or policies of their institutions.

List of Contributions

1. Johns, N.; Blumenberg, C.; Kirkby, K.; Allorant, A.; Costa, F.; Danovaro-Holliday, M.C..; Lyons, C.; Yusuf, N.; Barros, A.; Hosseinpoor, A. Comparison of Wealth-Related Inequality in Tetanus Vaccination Coverage before and during Pregnancy: A Cross-Sectional Analysis of 72 Low- and Middle-Income Countries. *Vaccines* 2024, *12*, 431. https://doi.org/10.3390/vaccines12040431.
2. Kalbarczyk, A.; Brownlee, N.; Katz, E. Of Money and Men: A Scoping Review to Map Gender Barriers to Immunization Coverage in Low- and Middle-Income Countries. *Vaccines* 2024, *12*, 625. https://doi.org/10.3390/vaccines12060625.
3. Castro-Aguirre, I.; Alvarez, D.; Contreras, M.; Trumbo, S.; Mujica, O.; Salas Peraza, D.; Velandia-González, M. The Impact of the Coronavirus Pandemic on Vaccination Coverage in Latin America and the Caribbean. *Vaccines* 2024, *12*, 458. https://doi.org/10.3390/vaccines12050458.
4. Fahmy, K.; Hasan, Q.; Sharifuzzaman, M.; Hutin, Y. Analyzing Subnational Immunization Coverage to Catch up and Reach the Unreached in Seven High-Priority Countries in the Eastern Mediterranean Region, 2019–2021. *Vaccines* 2024, *12*, 285. https://doi.org/10.3390/vaccines12030285.
5. Lyons, C.; Nambiar, D.; Johns, N.; Allorant, A.; Bergen, N.; Hosseinpoor, A. Inequality in Childhood Immunization Coverage: A Scoping Review of Data Sources, Analyses, and Reporting Methods. *Vaccines* 2024, *12*, 850. https://doi.org/10.3390/vaccines12080850.
6. Rachlin, A.; Adegoke, O.; Bohara, R.; Rwagasore, E.; Sibomana, H.; Kabeja, A.; Itanga, I.; Rwunganira, S.; Mafende Mario, B.; Rosette, N.; et al. Building Data Triangulation Capacity for Routine Immunization and Vaccine Preventable Disease Surveillance Programs to Identify Immunization Coverage Inequities. *Vaccines* 2024, *12*, 646. https://doi.org/10.3390/vaccines12060646.
7. Corrêa, G.; Uddin, M.; Wahed, T.; Oliveras, E.; Morgan, C.; Kamya, M.; Kabatangare, P.; Namugaya, F.; Leab, D.; Adjakidje, D.; et al. Measuring Zero-Dose Children: Reflections on Age Cohort Flexibilities for Targeted Immunization Surveys at the Local Level. *Vaccines* 2024, *12*, 195. https://doi.org/10.3390/vaccines12020195.

8. Niyibitegeka, F.; Russell, F.; Jit, M.; Carvalho, N. Inequitable Distribution of Global Economic Benefits from Pneumococcal Conjugate Vaccination. *Vaccines* 2024, *12*, 767. https://doi.org/10.3390/vaccines12070767.
9. Aheto, J.; Olowe, I.; Chan, H.; Ekeh, A.; Dieng, B.; Fafunmi, B.; Setayesh, H.; Atuhaire, B.; Crawford, J.; Tatem, A.; et al. Geospatial Analyses of Recent Household Surveys to Assess Changes in the Distribution of Zero-Dose Children and Their Associated Factors before and during the COVID-19 Pandemic in Nigeria. *Vaccines* 2023, *11*, 1830. https://doi.org/10.3390/vaccines11121830.
10. Muhoza, P.; Shah, M.; Amponsa-Achiano, K.; Gao, H.; Quaye, P.; Opare, W.; Okae, C.; Aboyinga, P.; Opare, J.; Ehlman, D.; et al. Timeliness of Childhood Vaccinations Following Strengthening of the Second Year of Life (2YL) Immunization Platform and Introduction of Catch-Up Vaccination Policy in Ghana. *Vaccines* 2024, *12*, 716. https://doi.org/10.3390/vaccines12070716.
11. Woyessa, A.; Shah, M.; Azmeraye, B.; Pan, J.; Lisanwork, L.; Yimer, G.; Wang, S.; Nuorti, J.; Artama, M.; Matanock, A.; et al. Factors Associated with Uptake of Routine Measles-Containing Vaccine Doses among Young Children, Oromia Regional State, Ethiopia, 2021. *Vaccines* 2024, *12*, 762. https://doi.org/10.3390/vaccines12070762.
12. Mbunga, B.; Liu, P.; Bangelesa, F.; Mafuta, E.; Dalau, N.; Egbende, L.; Hoff, N.; Kasonga, J.; Lulebo, A.; Manirakiza, D.; et al. Zero-Dose Childhood Vaccination Status in Rural Democratic Republic of Congo: Quantifying the Relative Impact of Geographic Accessibility and Attitudes toward Vaccination. *Vaccines* 2024, *12*, 617. https://doi.org/10.3390/vaccines12060617.
13. Meghani, A.; Sharma, M.; Singh, T.; Dastidar, S.; Dhawan, V.; Kanagat, N.; Gupta, A.; Bhatnagar, A.; Singh, K.; Shearer, J.; et al. Enhancing COVID-19 Vaccine Uptake among Tribal Communities: A Case Study on Program Implementation Experiences from Jharkhand and Chhattisgarh States, India. *Vaccines* 2024, *12*, 463. https://doi.org/10.3390/vaccines12050463.
14. Olusanya, O.; Masters, N.; Zhang, F.; Sugerman, D.; Carter, R.; Weiss, D.; Singleton, J. Sociodemographic Trends and Correlation between Parental Hesitancy towards Pediatric COVID-19 Vaccines and Routine Childhood Immunizations in the United States: 2021–2022 National Immunization Survey—Child COVID Module. *Vaccines* 2024, *12*, 495. https://doi.org/10.3390/vaccines12050495.

References

1. World Health Organization. WHO Director-General's Opening Remarks at the Seventy-Seventh World Health Assembly Second Roundtable [Internet]. 2024. Available online: https://www.who.int/director-general/speeches/detail/who-director-general-s-opening-remarks-at-the-seventy-seventh-world-health-assembly-second-roundtable-29-may-2024 (accessed on 15 July 2024).
2. Nambiar, D.; Hosseinpoor, A.R.; Bergen, N.; Danovaro-Holliday, M.C.; Wallace, A.; Johnson, H.L. Inequality in Immunization: Holding on to Equity as We 'Catch Up'. *Vaccines* 2023, *11*, 913. [CrossRef] [PubMed]
3. Gavi, the Vaccine Alliance. New Funding Boosts Efforts to Vaccinate "Zero-Dose" Children in the Democratic Republic of Congo [Internet]. 2023. Available online: https://www.gavi.org/news/media-room/new-funding-boosts-efforts-vaccinate-zero-dose-children-democratic-republic-congo (accessed on 17 July 2024).
4. World Health Organization. Immunization Agenda 2030 [Internet]. 2020. Available online: https://www.who.int/publications/m/item/immunization-agenda-2030-a-global-strategy-to-leave-no-one-behind (accessed on 19 July 2024).

Disclaimer/Publisher's Note: The statements, opinions and data contained in all publications are solely those of the individual author(s) and contributor(s) and not of MDPI and/or the editor(s). MDPI and/or the editor(s) disclaim responsibility for any injury to people or property resulting from any ideas, methods, instructions or products referred to in the content.

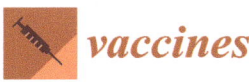

Article

Comparison of Wealth-Related Inequality in Tetanus Vaccination Coverage before and during Pregnancy: A Cross-Sectional Analysis of 72 Low- and Middle-Income Countries

Nicole E. Johns [1], Cauane Blumenberg [2,3], Katherine Kirkby [1], Adrien Allorant [1], Francine Dos Santos Costa [2], M. Carolina Danovaro-Holliday [4], Carrie Lyons [1], Nasir Yusuf [4], Aluísio J. D. Barros [2] and Ahmad Reza Hosseinpoor [1,*]

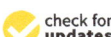

Citation: Johns, N.E.; Blumenberg, C.; Kirkby, K.; Allorant, A.; Costa, F.D.S.; Danovaro-Holliday, M.C.; Lyons, C.; Yusuf, N.; Barros, A.J.D.; Hosseinpoor, A.R. Comparison of Wealth-Related Inequality in Tetanus Vaccination Coverage before and during Pregnancy: A Cross-Sectional Analysis of 72 Low- and Middle-Income Countries. *Vaccines* **2024**, *12*, 431. https://doi.org/10.3390/vaccines12040431

Academic Editor: Kevin Coombs

Received: 29 February 2024
Revised: 21 March 2024
Accepted: 26 March 2024
Published: 17 April 2024

Correction Statement: This article has been republished with a minor change. The change does not affect the scientific content of the article and further details are available within the backmatter of the website version of this article.

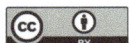

Copyright: © World Health Organization 2024. Licensee MDPI. This article is distributed under the terms of the Creative Commons Attribution IGO License. (https://creativecommons.org/licenses/by/3.0/igo/), which permits unrestricted use, distribution, and reproduction in any medium, provided the original work is properly cited. In any reproduction of this article there should not be any suggestion that WHO or this article endorse any specific organization or products. The use of the WHO logo is not permitted. This notice should be preserved along with the article's original URL.

[1] Department of Data and Analytics, World Health Organization, 20 Avenue Appia, 1211 Geneva, Switzerland; johnsn@who.int (N.E.J.)
[2] International Center for Equity in Health, Federal University of Pelotas, Rua Mal Deodoro 1160, Pelotas 96020-220, Brazil
[3] Causale Consulting, Avenida Adolfo Fetter 4331, Pelotas 96090-840, Brazil
[4] Department of Immunization, Vaccines, and Biologicals, World Health Organization, 20 Avenue Appia, 1211 Geneva, Switzerland
* Correspondence: hosseinpoora@who.int; Tel.: +41-22-791-3205

Abstract: Immunization of pregnant women against tetanus is a key strategy for reducing tetanus morbidity and mortality while also achieving the goal of maternal and neonatal tetanus elimination. Despite substantial progress in improving newborn protection from tetanus at birth through maternal immunization, umbilical cord practices and sterilized and safe deliveries, inequitable gaps in protection remain. Notably, an infant's tetanus protection at birth is comprised of immunization received by the mother during and before the pregnancy (e.g., through childhood vaccination, booster doses, mass vaccination campaigns, or during prior pregnancies). In this work, we examine wealth-related inequalities in maternal tetanus toxoid containing vaccination coverage before pregnancy, during pregnancy, and at birth for 72 low- and middle-income countries with a recent Demographic and Health Survey or Multiple Indicator Cluster Survey (between 2013 and 2022). We summarize coverage levels and absolute and relative inequalities at each time point; compare the relative contributions of inequalities before and during pregnancy to inequalities at birth; and examine associations between inequalities and coverage levels. We present the findings for countries individually and on aggregate, by World Bank country income grouping, as well as by maternal and neonatal tetanus elimination status, finding that most of the inequality in tetanus immunization coverage at birth is introduced during pregnancy. Inequalities in coverage during pregnancy are most pronounced in low- and lower-middle-income countries, and even more so in countries which have not achieved maternal and neonatal tetanus elimination. These findings suggest that pregnancy is a key time of opportunity for equity-oriented interventions to improve maternal tetanus immunization coverage.

Keywords: health inequality; maternal and neonatal tetanus; immunization; vaccination; health disparities

1. Introduction

Tetanus is a potentially life-threatening infection caused by the bacteria *Clostridium tetani*, often present in soil, manure, and agricultural waste. Maternal and neonatal tetanus (MNT) can be a consequence of deliveries and umbilical cord care practices in non-sterile and unsanitary conditions. When tetanus develops, the fatality rates are extremely high, especially when appropriate medical care is not available. Immunization against tetanus for women of reproductive age or during pregnancy is important for protecting both pregnant women and newborns. Maternal and neonatal tetanus elimination (MNTE) has been a goal of the World Health Organization (WHO) and global health partners since the 1980s, aiming to reduce MNT cases to such low levels that the disease is no longer a major public health concern (less than one case of neonatal tetanus per 1000 live births in every district in a country each year) [1]. While progress continues to be made, and MNTE has been achieved by 48 of 59 high-burden countries targeted for the global initiative since the turn of the century, 11 countries had still not reached MNTE status as of December 2023, all of which are low- or lower-middle- income countries [2]. Mali was validated for MNTE in August 2023; report forthcoming.

The burden of MNT is a health equity issue affecting those who experience disadvantage, poverty, and a lack of access to adequate health services [1]. A recent cross-sectional study of household survey data from 76 countries revealed that tetanus immunization protection at birth (PAB) of an infant was highest among mothers who were older, who had higher levels of education, who lived in urban (rather than rural) areas, and who had higher household wealth [3]. While the study found that inequalities had reduced in a ten-year period in six countries amid improvements in overall coverage, it also observed little change in inequalities on aggregate and substantially greater inequalities in coverage among countries which have not achieved MNTE. Reducing inequalities in immunization coverage is a key aim of MNTE programmes, as well as an overall target of global initiatives such as the Immunization Agenda 2030 (IA2030) [4].

Neonatal tetanus is preventable through safe delivery and umbilical cord care practices, as well as through tetanus toxoid-containing vaccines (TTCV), such as tetanus toxoid (TT) or tetanus-diphtheria (Td), which are included in routine immunization programmes globally and administered during antenatal care contacts in many countries. Tetanus protection at birth is a complex coverage metric composed of tetanus immunization during and before the most recent pregnancy (such as receipt of immunization through childhood diphtheria—tetanus—pertussis (DTP) vaccine, booster TTCV doses, mass immunization campaigns of women of reproductive age, or prior pregnancies) [5]. WHO tetanus immunization recommendations have evolved over time, going from targeting pregnant women to targeting women of reproductive age to now recommending a routine six-dose child and adolescent tetanus schedule. Pregnant women and their newborn infants are protected from birth-associated tetanus if the mother received either six doses during childhood or five doses during adolescence/adulthood [5]. However, national immunization schedules differ based on local epidemiology and various programmatic objectives and issues, meaning that they may not always be aligned with the latest WHO recommendations. Decomposing the inequalities in protection at birth to understand whether they are driven by inequalities in coverage before pregnancy, during pregnancy, or in both time periods has important policy and intervention implications. For instance, coverage inequalities that are related to inequalities that appear during pregnancy indicate gaps in antenatal care delivery, access, and utilization [6]. However, to date, there have been no multi-country analyses (nor even small-scale country-level analyses) that have explored this.

Inequalities by time of vaccination have been explored for other vaccination types to support the identification of potential health system gaps. For instance, inequalities in childhood receipt of the DTP vaccine can be broken down by receipt of the first DTP vaccine dose (DTP1) and the third DTP vaccine dose (DTP3) to provide insight into the performance of the vaccine delivery system. Inequalities in DTP1 coverage (recommended at around 6 to 8 weeks after birth) indicate systemic challenges with access to and utilization of child health services and the need for general health system strengthening, while inequalities in DTP3 coverage (recommended at around 14 weeks or 6 months of age, depending on the country) are a signal of health service quality and other barriers experienced by mothers or caregivers [7–9].

Data on the receipt of tetanus immunization during pregnancy and coverage at birth are available in Demographic and Health Surveys (DHS) and Multiple Indicator Cluster Surveys (MICS), which are nationally representative household surveys carried out in several low- and middle-income countries. In this study, we quantify the extent of wealth-related inequality in tetanus immunization coverage before pregnancy versus during pregnancy, summarizing the amount of inequality introduced or mitigated during pregnancy and exploring variation by country, country income level groupings, and MNTE status.

2. Materials and Methods

2.1. Data Sources

Data for this study come from recent DHS and MICS, which collect a wide range of information regarding health and other topics in low- and middle-income countries (extensive information on their methodologies has been published elsewhere) [10,11]. All publicly available surveys conducted within the prior 10 years at time of analysis (2013–2022) were considered for inclusion. Surveys were excluded if they did not contain the outcome measure of interest (defined below, resulting in exclusion of n = 21 countries), or if estimates stratified by the dimension of inequality could not be produced due to small numbers of respondents within one or more levels of the inequality dimension (defined as <25 individuals, resulting in exclusion of n = 4 countries). When multiple surveys from the same country were available within the study time range, the most recent survey was selected, as the aim of this research is to characterize the most recent state of inequality in maternal tetanus immunization coverage.

All data were processed by the International Center for Equity in Health (ICEH, www.equidade.org) at the Universidade Federal de Pelotas. All outcome measures used in analyses, detailed below, were calculated by the ICEH directly from raw survey data.

2.2. Outcome Measures

Maternal tetanus immunization coverage at the time of birth of the infant can be received either before or during pregnancy (or in the case of multiparous women, the most recent pregnancy). It, in turn, provides tetanus protection to the infant (i.e., coverage at birth):

Coverage before pregnancy + Coverage during pregnancy = Coverage at birth

Information about tetanus immunization coverage during pregnancy and coverage at birth was available directly in the survey data. Coverage before pregnancy was calculated as the arithmetic difference of these two measures:

Coverage at birth − Coverage during pregnancy = Coverage before pregnancy

Coverage of tetanus at birth: This indicator is defined as the proportion of women aged 15–49 years who had a live birth within the five years (for DHS) or two years (for MICS) preceding the survey and who received one of the following: (a) Two tetanus toxoid-containing vaccine (TTCV, tetanus toxoid—TT or tetanus-diphtheria—Td) doses during the pregnancy for her most recent live birth; (b) two or more TTCV doses before the last pregnancy (the last within 3 years of the most recent live birth); (c) three or more TTCV doses before the last pregnancy (the last within 5 years of the most recent live birth); (d) four or more TTCV doses before the last pregnancy (the last within 10 years of the most recent live birth); or (e) five or more TTCV doses at any time prior to the most recent live birth.

Coverage of tetanus during pregnancy: This indicator is defined as the proportion of women aged 15–49 years who had a live birth within the five years (for DHS) or two years (for MICS) preceding the survey and who received two or more TTCV doses during pregnancy.

Data collection for these indicators is restricted to the lastborn child in both DHS and MICS surveys. Data is obtained by maternal recall for both surveys, though both ask to see vaccination cards where available.

This analysis was limited to women who had only one live birth (i.e., for whom the birth reported in the survey was their first live birth). In women who have had multiple pregnancies, coverage before the current pregnancy could have occurred (a) in childhood, (b) through other adolescent/adult immunization outside of pregnancy, or (c) during prior pregnancies. We chose to limit the analyses to women for whom the survey data related to a first birth to aid in interpretation of the coverage before the pregnancy time period, as this population restriction largely eliminates the possibility of vaccination occurring during previous pregnancies.

2.3. Dimension of Inequality

We assess wealth-related inequality in tetanus immunization coverage using country-specific household wealth quintiles. Household wealth is derived from household asset indices and is directly provided in DHS and MICS datasets [12]. The households, weighted by size, are divided into five equal groups, or wealth quintiles, each representing 20% of the population.

2.4. Statistical Analyses

We start by summarizing tetanus immunization coverage at the three time points of interest (before pregnancy, during pregnancy, and at birth) for the study sample overall. We then present the percentage of coverage occurring during pregnancy, overall and by country World Bank income grouping at time of survey (low income, lower-middle income, and upper-middle income) [13]. Population-weighted mean values and corresponding 95% confidence intervals are presented for aggregate group estimates.

We measure absolute wealth-related inequalities in tetanus immunization coverage at each time point using the slope index of inequality (SII) and relative inequality using the relative index of inequality (RII) [14]. The SII is calculated via population-weighted logistic regression of coverage across five wealth quintiles ranked from the least to most wealthy, ultimately indicating the absolute difference in the predicted coverage between the wealthiest and least wealthy subgroups. We multiplied the SII by 100 to facilitate interpretation in percentage points, and thus the SII values presented here range from −100 to 100. A positive SII value indicates that coverage is higher among the wealthiest, while a negative SII indicates the opposite; a value of 0 for SII represents equity. The RII is calculated similarly and represents the ratio of the coverage predicted for the wealthiest quintile divided by the coverage predicted for the least wealthy quintile. A RII value greater than 1 suggests that coverage is higher among the wealthiest, while a RII value less than 1 suggests that coverage is higher among the least wealthy and a value of 1 for RII represents equity.

For both absolute and relative inequality, and for both before pregnancy and during pregnancy time periods, we summarize countries with inequality favoring the wealthiest quintile (statistically significant SII > 0, RII > 1), relatively equitable coverage (SII with 95% confidence interval including 0; RII with 95% confidence interval including 1), or inequality favoring the least wealthy quintile (statistically significant SII < 0, RII < 1). We then test the association between inequality before versus during pregnancy via Pearson correlation coefficients.

Next, we summarize the SII during pregnancy to show the amount of absolute inequality introduced or mitigated during pregnancy. We present SII by country, as well as weighted mean estimates for the sample overall and by country income grouping. We characterized countries as having a meaningful increase in absolute inequality favoring the wealthiest (statistically significant SII during pregnancy > 0), similar inequality (SII during pregnancy statically equivalent to 0), or a meaningful decrease in inequality favoring the wealthiest (statistically significant SII during pregnancy < 0). However, because inequality is bimodal in SII (−100 = total inequality favoring the least wealthy on one end, 100 = total inequality favoring the wealthiest on the other), a negative value for a SII during pregnancy could actually reflect an increase in inequality favoring the least wealthy. Thus, we stratify by the nature of inequality before pregnancy to additionally categorize countries with inequality favoring the least wealthy before pregnancy and a negative SII during pregnancy as 'a meaningful increase in inequality favoring the least wealthy'.

We then assess whether there is an association between SII during pregnancy with the level of tetanus immunization coverage at birth, summarizing the patterns of coverage and inequality.

Finally, we summarize inequality for countries which have and have not achieved maternal and neonatal tetanus elimination at the time of survey.

As a post hoc sensitivity analysis, we examine whether key findings are sensitive to the recency of data availability, summarizing coverage and inequality separately for countries with data available within the past five years (2019–2022) and countries with data greater than five years old (2013–2018).

Statistical analyses were conducted using Stata Statistical Software version 18.0, College Station, TX [15]. All country-level point estimates and uncertainty estimates took into account relevant survey sampling design and survey weights using the *svy* command; for calculation of standard errors, strata with a single primary sampling unit were centered at the grand mean via *singleunit (centered)* specifications. Multi-country average estimates were weighted based on the national population of women of reproductive age (15–49) from UN World Population Prospects 2022 data [16]. Significance was set at $p = 0.05$ for all comparisons; 95% confidence intervals (CIs) are reported throughout.

Ethical clearance for surveys analyzed in this study was obtained through the responsible institutions that administered the surveys. Each of the 72 included surveys underwent individual review from a relevant in-country ethical review board, and additional detail can be found in individual survey final reports. In addition, all DHS surveys were reviewed and approved by the institutional review board of ICF, the organization which oversees DHS implementation [17]. All analyses presented here were conducted using anonymized databases, ensuring the protection of privacy and confidentiality.

3. Results

3.1. Sample Characteristics

The final analytic sample included 72 low- and middle-income countries with a recent DHS or MICS (2013–2022) containing measures of tetanus immunization coverage and wealth quintiles. The total sample included 158,753 women who had their first live birth in the five (for DHS) or two (for MICS) years prior to the survey. Our sample included 21 low-income countries, 33 lower-middle-income countries, and 18 upper-middle-income countries at time of survey. Additionally, all tetanus protection occurred during pregnancy in one country (Chad). As this means that coverage before pregnancy was 0% for all wealth quintiles, the SII and RII before pregnancy could not be calculated; thus, the sample for all analyses involving measures of inequality before pregnancy is 71 countries.

Tetanus immunization schedules vary widely across settings. The WHO recommends a six-dose schedule, including three doses in infancy and one dose each at 12–23 months, 4–7 years, and 9–15 years. At the time of survey, all countries' immunization schedules included a three-dose TTCV series in infancy (see Supplementary Table S1). Only a third of countries (26 of 72) included a booster dose at age 12–23 months, 29 countries included a booster dose at age 4–7 years, and 19 countries included a booster dose at age 9–15 years. About half of countries (37 of 72) did not include any boosters between the infant series and pregnancy. Only a fifth of countries (15 of 72) included the full recommended six-dose TTCV series in their immunization schedule at time of survey. Note, however, that women of reproductive age at time of survey would have received these recommended booster doses based on prior schedules in place during their childhood and adolescence, or through mass vaccination campaigns happening outside of the standard schedule.

3.2. Tetanus Immunization Coverage before Pregnancy, during Pregnancy, and at Birth

Tetanus coverage at each time point varied widely across countries (See Table 1, Supplementary Figures S1–S3). Coverage before pregnancy was 10% [95% CI 7–12%] on average in our study population, ranging from 0% in Chad to 51% in Bangladesh. Coverage during pregnancy was higher at 67% [95% CI 62–72%] on average, ranging from 9% in

Suriname to 88% in India. Coverage at birth, the sum of these two coverages, averaged 76% [95% CI 72–80%] and ranged from 15% in Suriname to 93% in India (See Figures 1 and 2).

Table 1. Tetanus immunization coverage at birth, before pregnancy, and during pregnancy among first births; most recent DHS or MICS estimates 2013–2022 for 72 included study countries.

Geography	Survey Year	Year of MNTE	Coverage at Birth %	Coverage before Pregnancy %	Coverage during Pregnancy %
All Countries (median)			67.5	8.6	56.7
All Countries (mean *)			76.3	9.6	66.7
Low-Income Countries (median)			67.3	7.9	60.6
Low-Income Countries (mean *)			63.7	8.5	55.2
Afghanistan	2015	NA	59.2	17.8	41.5
Benin	2017	2010	67.3	3.0	64.2
Burundi	2016	2009	69.1	19.5	49.6
Central African Republic	2018	NA	58.7	10.2	48.5
Chad	2019	2019	52.8	0.0	52.8
Democratic Republic of the Congo	2017	2019	55.7	10.4	45.3
Ethiopia	2016	2017	56.5	8.6	48.0
Gambia	2019	<2000	54.8	3.7	51.1
Guinea	2018	NA	60.2	8.6	51.6
Guinea-Bissau	2018	2012	77.9	9.9	68.0
Haiti	2016	2017	74.7	6.0	68.7
Liberia	2019	2011	82.0	1.9	80.1
Madagascar	2021	2014	71.7	2.4	69.3
Malawi	2019	2002	83.5	2.7	80.8
Mali	2018	2023	48.6	8.9	39.7
Niger	2021	2016	49.2	5.0	44.3
Rwanda	2019	2004	62.5	2.0	60.6
Sierra Leone	2019	2013	84.4	6.3	78.1
Togo	2017	2005	77.5	7.9	69.6
Uganda	2016	2011	75.4	13.3	62.0
United Republic of Tanzania	2015	2012	77.6	8.4	69.2
Lower-Middle-Income Countries (median)			67.9	7.2	61.4
Lower-Middle-Income Countries (mean *)			79.7	9.0	70.7
Angola	2015	NA	68.6	10.8	57.8
Bangladesh	2019	2008	87.6	50.9	36.7
Cambodia	2021	2015	63.6	6.9	56.7
Cameroon	2018	2012	69.2	4.2	65.1
Congo	2014	2009	75.3	11.0	64.3
Côte d'Ivoire	2016	2013	67.9	5.5	62.4
Egypt	2014	2007	76.8	0.6	76.2
El Salvador	2014	<2000	81.3	13.7	67.6
Eswatini	2014	<2000	79.5	1.1	78.4
Ghana	2017	2011	66.7	9.2	57.5
Guatemala	2014	<2000	78.0	7.2	70.7
Honduras	2019	<2000	65.9	11.5	54.4
India	2019	2015	92.7	4.4	88.3
Indonesia	2017	2016	56.8	20.4	36.4
Kenya	2022	2018	53.0	4.6	48.4
Kiribati	2018	<2000	53.5	2.4	51.1
Lao People's Democratic Republic	2017	2013	54.7	21.9	32.8
Lesotho	2018	<2000	77.6	0.9	76.7
Mauritania	2019	2015	46.9	8.9	38.0
Myanmar	2015	2010	75.2	1.7	73.5
Nepal	2022	2005	64.6	1.8	62.8
Nigeria	2021	NA	71.6	4.2	67.4
Pakistan	2017	NA	72.7	1.3	71.3
Papua New Guinea	2016	NA	40.8	7.3	33.5

Table 1. Cont.

Geography	Survey Year	Year of MNTE	Coverage at Birth %	Coverage before Pregnancy %	Coverage during Pregnancy %
Philippines	2022	2017	55.1	6.3	48.8
Senegal	2019	2011	84.9	2.0	82.9
Sudan	2014	NA	66.0	4.5	61.4
Timor-Leste	2016	2012	77.5	15.3	62.2
Tunisia	2018	<2000	38.8	12.6	26.2
Viet Nam	2020	2005	79.9	8.7	71.2
Yemen	2013	NA	28.3	15.7	12.6
Zambia	2018	2007	67.2	33.3	33.9
Zimbabwe	2019	2000	45.6	13.6	32.1
Upper-Middle-Income Countries (median)			67.0	13.8	46.9
Upper-Middle-Income Countries (mean *)			64.7	15.2	49.6
Belize	2015	<2000	63.5	4.3	59.2
Costa Rica	2018	<2000	44.6	35.5	9.1
Cuba	2019	<2000	66.3	20.3	46.0
Dominican Republic	2019	<2000	86.7	6.3	80.4
Fiji	2021	<2000	49.1	32.8	16.2
Gabon	2019	2013	69.7	3.4	66.4
Guyana	2019	<2000	22.4	13.0	9.4
Iraq	2018	2013	67.6	11.5	56.2
Jordan	2017	<2000	25.6	14.6	11.0
Maldives	2016	<2000	74.2	26.3	47.9
Mexico	2015	<2000	71.2	18.6	52.6
Namibia	2013	2001	67.7	25.7	42.1
Paraguay	2016	<2000	79.6	11.1	68.5
Peru	2019	<2000	70.0	13.4	56.6
Samoa	2019	<2000	33.9	14.1	19.8
South Africa	2016	2002	35.2	5.7	29.6
Suriname	2018	<2000	14.5	5.5	9.0
Thailand	2019	<2000	77.6	19.6	58.0

* Means are population weighted and use female population age 15–49 with *aweight* specifications in Stata. MNTE: Maternal and neonatal tetanus elimination; NA: Not achieved. Note that, in some cases, coverage at birth may differ by 0.1 from the sum of coverage before and during pregnancy due to rounding.

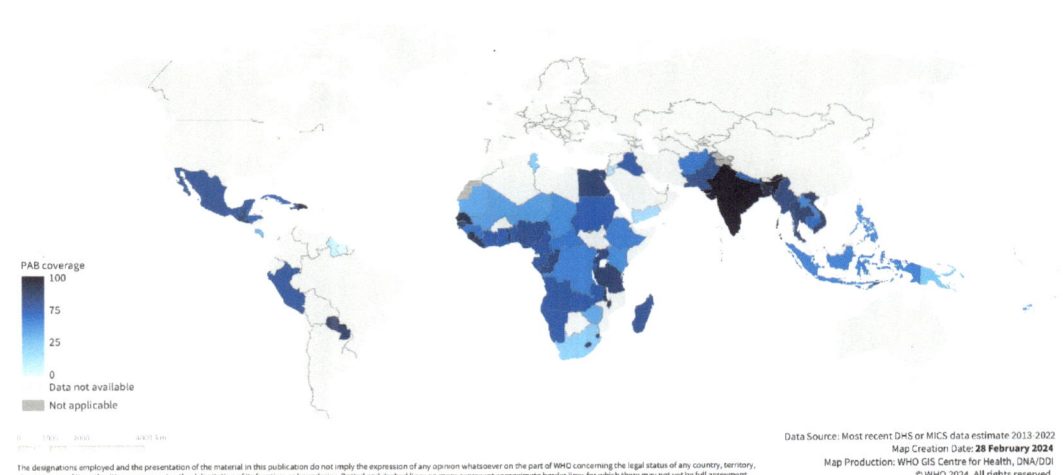

Figure 1. National maternal tetanus immunization coverage at birth among first births; most recent DHS or MICS estimates 2013–2022 for 72 included study countries.

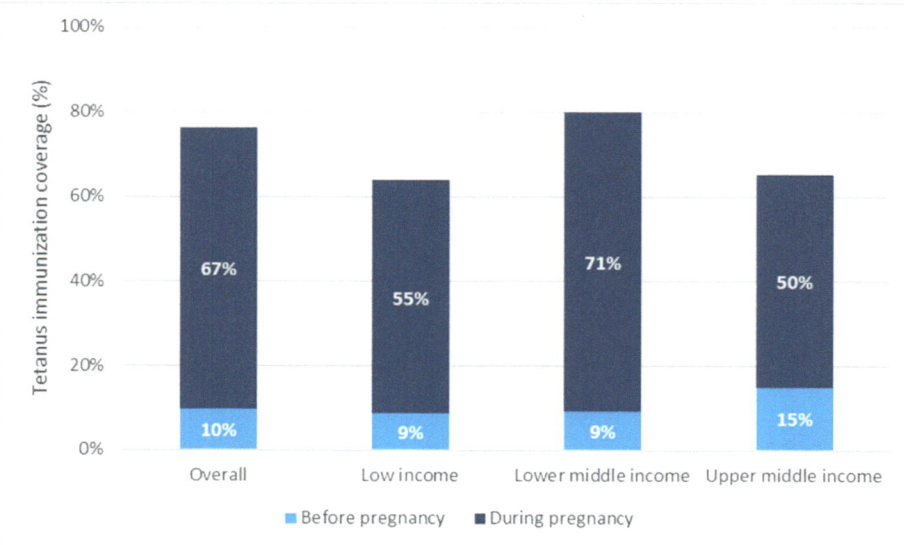

Figure 2. Maternal tetanus immunization coverage by country income grouping, weighted mean coverage level.

Immunization coverage at birth increased monotonically with increasing wealth overall and for low- and lower-middle-income countries. This is due largely to increases in coverage during pregnancy with increasing wealth (See Figure 3).

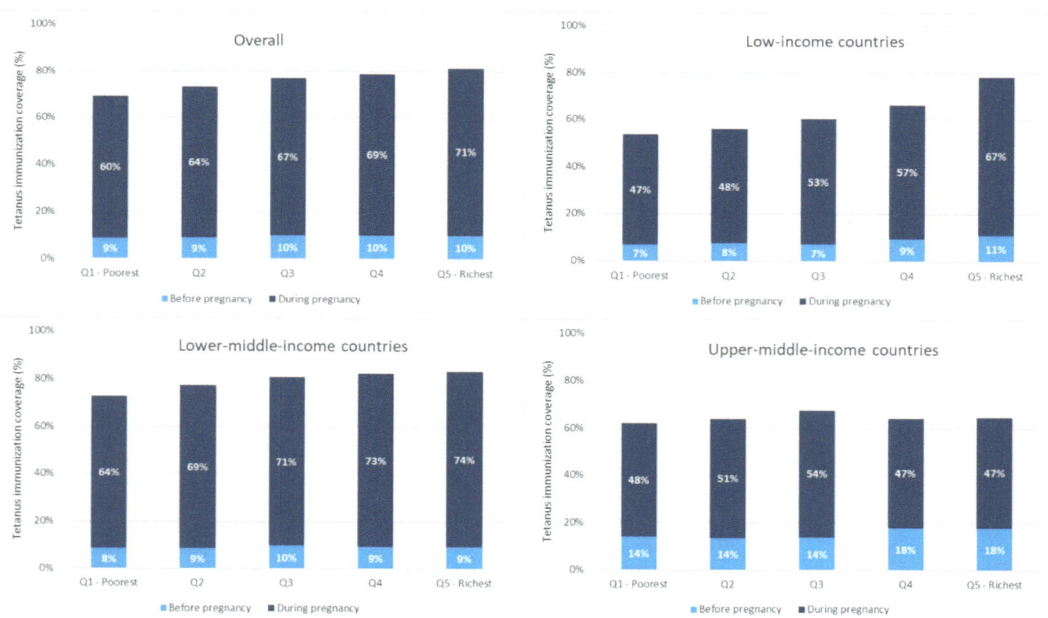

Figure 3. Maternal tetanus immunization coverage by wealth quintile, weighted mean, overall, and by country income grouping.

Overall, tetanus coverage at birth is comprised mostly of coverage during the recent pregnancy. In 66 of 72 countries, the majority of coverage (more than 50%) occurred in pregnancy. Across countries, the average percentage of PAB coverage occurring in pregnancy was 86% [95% CI 83–90%], ranging from 20% of total PAB coverage occurring in pregnancy in Costa Rica to 100% of total PAB coverage occurring in pregnancy in Chad. The percentage of coverage occurring during pregnancy was significantly higher among low- and lower-middle-income relative to upper-middle-income countries: low-income countries had an average 86% [95% CI 83–89%] of coverage occur during pregnancy; lower-middle-income countries had 88% [95% CI 82–93%] of coverage during pregnancy; while upper-middle-income countries had 76% [95% CI 71–81%] of coverage during pregnancy.

3.3. Inequality in Tetanus Immunization Coverage before Pregnancy, during Pregnancy, and at Birth

On the whole, there was greater absolute inequality in tetanus immunization coverage (measured via SII) favoring the wealthiest quintile during pregnancy compared to before pregnancy (See Table 2). The SII before pregnancy averaged 2.4 percentage points [95% CI 1.0–3.7], ranging from −17.5 percentage points in Suriname to 35.1 percentage points in Zambia; the SII during pregnancy averaged 10.5 percentage points [95% CI 5.3–15.6], ranging from −24.9 percentage points in Iraq to 64.3 percentage points in Nigeria; and the SII at birth averaged 12.8 percentage points [95% CI 7.7–17.9], ranging from −24.4 percentage points in Suriname to 66.3 percentage points in Nigeria.

Table 2. Absolute wealth-related inequality in tetanus immunization coverage at birth, before pregnancy, and during pregnancy; most recent DHS or MICS estimates 2013–2022 for 72 included study countries.

Geography	Survey Year	SII at Birth			SII before Pregnancy			SII during Pregnancy		
		Estimate	LL	UL	Estimate	LL	UL	Estimate	LL	UL
All Countries (median)		13.3	9.0	19.5	2.4	0.3	4.2	10.6	3.4	15.6
*All Countries (mean *)*		12.8	7.7	17.9	2.4	1.0	3.7	10.5	5.3	15.6
Low-Income Countries (median)		19.6	11.2	33.7	1.7	−0.1	5.8	18.4	10.6	30.4
*Low-Income Countries (mean *)*		30.5	23.8	37.2	5.8	1.8	9.8	25.4	19.8	31.0
Afghanistan	2015	19.6	−0.5	39.8	20.9	−5.6	47.3	−1.0	−13.7	11.8
Benin	2017	34.8	28.6	41.0	0.3	−2.6	3.3	34.5	30.6	38.4
Burundi	2016	16.0	5.0	27.1	−3.5	−15.9	8.9	19.4	3.5	35.4
Central African Republic	2018	54.8	35.2	74.4	3.4	−2.7	9.5	51.8	30.2	73.5
Chad	2019	32.5	23.9	41.1	--	--	--	32.5	23.9	41.1
Democratic Republic of the Congo	2017	44.6	32.1	57.0	15.3	−0.8	31.4	30.6	6.4	54.9
Ethiopia	2016	48.0	27.7	68.4	8.4	2.2	14.7	40.6	25.3	55.9
Gambia	2019	−2.6	−5.4	0.1	−0.1	−2.9	2.7	−2.6	−6.5	1.4
Guinea	2018	34.7	19.2	50.3	2.3	−2.4	6.9	32.6	19.4	45.7
Guinea-Bissau	2018	19.4	13.4	25.3	6.1	−5.1	17.2	13.3	−2.2	28.8
Haiti	2016	13.1	5.4	20.8	2.4	1.2	3.5	10.7	2.1	19.4
Liberia	2019	3.1	−7.9	14.2	−1.1	−4.3	2.0	4.3	−6.5	15.0
Madagascar	2021	22.1	13.7	30.6	3.3	1.8	4.8	19.0	9.4	28.7
Malawi	2019	10.6	0.9	20.3	0.2	−2.6	2.9	10.4	−1.7	22.5
Mali	2018	39.6	28.0	51.2	16.1	12.5	19.7	25.1	13.3	36.9
Niger	2021	21.9	4.0	39.8	8.2	−0.1	16.4	14.2	4.7	23.8
Rwanda	2019	10.6	5.7	15.4	0.3	−1.6	2.1	10.3	3.9	16.7
Sierra Leone	2019	9.4	5.4	13.4	1.2	−4.0	6.4	8.2	1.2	15.2
Togo	2017	12.0	2.0	22.0	−6.3	−11.9	−0.6	18.2	9.8	26.5
Uganda	2016	6.3	−0.7	13.3	−12.2	−13.5	−10.9	18.4	12.4	24.4
United Republic of Tanzania	2015	28.7	20.5	37.0	−1.5	−8.7	5.7	30.1	18.9	41.2
Lower-Middle-Income Countries (median)		18.6	2.5	30.0	1.4	−0.3	5.9	13.4	−1.3	19.4
*Lower-Middle-Income Countries (mean *)*		11.4	3.6	19.2	1.4	−0.2	3.0	10.0	2.1	17.8

Table 2. Cont.

Geography	Survey Year	SII at Birth			SII before Pregnancy			SII during Pregnancy		
		Estimate	LL	UL	Estimate	LL	UL	Estimate	LL	UL
Angola	2015	53.5	43.6	63.4	3.0	−3.2	9.3	50.6	42.6	58.6
Bangladesh	2019	3.1	1.7	4.6	10.8	6.5	15.1	−7.7	−10.5	−4.8
Cambodia	2021	2.1	−9.2	13.5	−2.2	−4.5	0.2	4.3	−5.0	13.6
Cameroon	2018	40.3	33.1	47.6	6.4	5.1	7.7	34.5	25.7	43.2
Congo	2014	28.6	9.6	47.6	15.6	8.9	22.4	13.4	−10.5	37.4
Côte d'Ivoire	2016	20.5	−2.9	43.9	6.0	3.9	8.1	14.7	−10.4	39.8
Egypt	2014	−20.1	−29.5	−10.7	0.0	−1.3	1.3	−20.1	−30.7	−9.5
El Salvador	2014	−10.6	−18.1	−3.0	−7.5	−15.3	0.3	−3.1	−10.8	4.6
Eswatini	2014	17.4	−8.2	43.0	−1.6	−5.5	2.3	19.0	−5.2	43.1
Ghana	2017	31.5	20.6	42.4	0.2	−4.0	4.3	31.3	21.5	41.0
Guatemala	2014	−8.4	−29.6	12.9	8.2	7.1	9.4	−16.4	−38.8	6.0
Honduras	2019	21.1	7.7	34.5	−0.9	−3.5	1.7	22.0	9.7	34.2
India	2019	1.8	0.6	2.9	−1.1	−1.7	−0.6	2.9	1.3	4.5
Indonesia	2017	−0.6	−12.3	11.1	5.5	0.0	11.0	−6.1	−13.7	1.4
Kenya	2022	1.4	−3.0	5.9	−1.0	−2.9	0.9	2.4	−1.0	5.8
Kiribati	2018	8.9	−2.9	20.7	−3.2	−9.9	3.6	12.0	3.2	20.8
Lao People's Democratic Republic	2017	32.9	17.0	48.8	17.7	10.5	24.9	15.8	4.7	26.9
Lesotho	2018	−5.8	−22.8	11.3	−0.4	−2.0	1.2	−5.4	−22.3	11.6
Mauritania	2019	14.1	9.8	18.5	8.6	7.0	10.3	5.7	−0.1	11.4
Myanmar	2015	18.6	8.5	28.7	0.2	−0.8	1.2	18.4	9.1	27.7
Nepal	2022	−5.9	−12.5	0.7	1.7	0.5	2.9	−7.6	−14.2	−1.0
Nigeria	2021	66.3	63.4	69.2	1.4	−1.9	4.8	64.3	60.9	67.7
Pakistan	2017	47.0	35.4	58.6	0.4	−0.6	1.5	46.5	33.6	59.4
Papua New Guinea	2016	48.4	45.1	51.7	2.9	−0.5	6.4	46.0	42.5	49.4
Philippines	2022	−14.1	−21.9	−6.3	5.8	−3.6	15.1	−19.7	−31.6	−7.8
Senegal	2019	19.6	10.2	29.0	−0.2	−1.4	1.1	19.7	9.3	30.0
Sudan	2014	48.0	40.8	55.2	−2.1	−6.4	2.3	49.7	46.6	52.8
Timor-Leste	2016	25.2	16.4	33.9	8.3	−1.3	17.9	17.0	12.4	21.5
Tunisia	2018	−23.3	−36.6	−10.0	−3.9	−8.6	0.9	−19.5	−35.7	−3.3
Viet Nam	2020	38.1	18.3	57.9	−2.9	−10.7	5.0	40.1	25.9	54.2
Yemen	2013	33.9	31.0	36.8	7.7	2.2	13.2	27.8	22.5	33.2
Zambia	2018	30.3	23.2	37.4	35.1	30.0	40.3	−4.9	−13.0	3.1
Zimbabwe	2019	11.6	7.8	15.4	16.7	11.3	22.0	−4.9	−15.0	5.3
Upper-Middle-Income Countries (median)		2.6	−6.9	10.5	3.5	0.7	7.2	−2.0	−13.1	5.8
Upper-Middle-Income Countries (mean *)		1.9	−1.9	5.7	5.8	2.8	8.8	−3.8	−8.7	1.0
Belize	2015	−7.1	−11.5	−2.6	−2.0	−15.3	11.4	−5.1	−16.2	6.0
Costa Rica	2018	13.6	−8.1	35.3	29.5	1.6	57.5	−17.1	−21.1	−13.2
Cuba	2019	−11.4	−23.8	1.1	7.5	−0.3	15.4	−18.8	−25.2	−12.4
Dominican Republic	2019	2.1	−4.8	9.0	2.7	−2.0	7.4	−0.6	−11.0	9.9
Fiji	2021	−3.1	−25.9	19.7	3.9	−6.5	14.3	−7.0	−25.5	11.5
Gabon	2019	20.8	16.0	25.6	0.1	−0.2	0.5	20.7	15.5	25.8
Guyana	2019	16.7	−1.2	34.7	5.0	−12.1	22.1	11.9	8.3	15.5
Iraq	2018	−6.6	−22.9	9.8	19.1	9.7	28.5	−24.9	−44.0	−5.9
Jordan	2017	−5.5	−8.0	−3.0	−8.7	−15.8	−1.6	3.2	−4.6	11.0
Maldives	2016	10.7	−25.8	47.2	0.6	−4.4	5.5	10.2	−24.5	44.8
Mexico	2015	4.2	−0.4	8.7	6.4	0.0	12.9	−2.3	−12.4	7.8
Namibia	2013	−9.9	−27.3	7.4	10.9	−8.7	30.5	−20.7	−22.8	−18.7
Paraguay	2016	17.0	8.3	25.7	5.4	−0.5	11.3	11.6	1.2	22.0
Peru	2019	−14.1	−29.3	1.1	0.8	−3.6	5.3	−14.9	−34.7	4.8
Samoa	2019	7.3	−17.4	32.0	9.0	−6.0	24.1	−1.7	−16.2	12.8
South Africa	2016	3.1	−2.0	8.3	2.6	−6.4	11.7	0.5	−6.3	7.3
Suriname	2018	−24.4	−38.4	−10.4	−17.5	−26.1	−9.0	−8.7	−19.1	1.7
Thailand	2019	9.9	2.3	17.6	3.1	−0.5	6.7	6.9	−3.5	17.2

* Means are population weighted and use female population age 15–49 with *aweight* specifications in Stata. SII: Slope index of inequality; LL: Lower 95% confidence interval of estimate; UL: Upper 95% confidence interval of estimate.

Relative inequality (measured via RII) was equivalent with regard to the direction of inequalities at each time point. In contrast to absolute inequality, however, we observed similar magnitudes of relative inequality before versus during pregnancy (See Table 3). The RII before pregnancy averaged 1.4 [95% CI 1.1–1.6], ranging from 0.04 in Suriname to 6.4 in Mali; the RII during pregnancy averaged 1.4 [95% CI 1.1–1.6], ranging from 0.14 in Costa Rica to 10.2 in Yemen; and the RII at birth averaged 1.3 [95% CI 1.2–1.5], ranging from 0.18 in Suriname to 3.7 in Papua New Guinea.

Table 3. Relative wealth-related inequality in tetanus immunization coverage at birth, before pregnancy, and during pregnancy; most recent DHS or MICS estimates 2013–2022 for 72 included study countries.

Geography	Survey Year	RII at Birth			RII before Pregnancy			RII during Pregnancy		
		Estimate	LL	UL	Estimate	LL	UL	Estimate	LL	UL
All Countries (median)		1.25	1.14	1.36	1.31	1.10	1.49	1.20	1.06	1.30
All Countries (mean *)		1.35	1.19	1.50	1.38	1.14	1.62	1.36	1.13	1.59
Low-Income Countries (median)		1.37	1.18	1.78	1.26	0.99	2.60	1.35	1.18	1.83
Low-Income Countries (mean *)		1.82	1.57	2.08	2.61	1.85	3.37	1.74	1.51	1.97
Afghanistan	2015	1.40	0.89	1.91	3.32	0.00	8.35	0.98	0.68	1.28
Benin	2017	1.72	1.52	1.92	1.12	0.02	2.21	1.75	1.62	1.89
Burundi	2016	1.26	1.06	1.47	0.84	0.32	1.35	1.49	1.02	1.96
Central African Republic	2018	2.86	1.57	4.16	1.39	0.62	2.16	3.27	1.50	5.03
Chad	2019	1.89	1.51	2.28	--	--	--	1.89	1.51	2.28
Democratic Republic of the Congo	2017	2.36	1.81	2.92	4.45	0.00	9.17	2.01	1.03	2.99
Ethiopia	2016	2.53	1.29	3.77	2.70	1.09	4.31	2.45	1.39	3.52
Gambia	2019	0.95	0.91	1.00	0.98	0.24	1.71	0.95	0.88	1.02
Guinea	2018	1.83	1.21	2.45	1.30	0.60	2.01	1.93	1.28	2.57
Guinea-Bissau	2018	1.29	1.19	1.39	1.85	0.10	3.60	1.22	0.95	1.49
Haiti	2016	1.19	1.07	1.32	1.49	1.17	1.80	1.17	1.02	1.32
Liberia	2019	1.04	0.90	1.18	0.54	0.00	1.52	1.05	0.91	1.20
Madagascar	2021	1.37	1.20	1.55	3.78	1.45	6.12	1.32	1.13	1.51
Malawi	2019	1.14	1.00	1.27	1.06	0.00	2.17	1.14	0.97	1.31
Mali	2018	2.37	1.59	3.15	6.40	2.26	10.53	1.91	1.22	2.60
Niger	2021	1.57	1.00	2.16	5.27	0.00	15.18	1.38	1.09	1.68
Rwanda	2019	1.18	1.10	1.27	1.14	0.10	2.17	1.19	1.07	1.31
Sierra Leone	2019	1.12	1.06	1.17	1.21	0.24	2.18	1.11	1.01	1.21
Togo	2017	1.17	1.01	1.32	0.45	0.18	0.73	1.30	1.15	1.46
Uganda	2016	1.09	0.98	1.19	0.40	0.35	0.44	1.35	1.21	1.49
United Republic of Tanzania	2015	1.47	1.30	1.64	0.83	0.13	1.54	1.57	1.30	1.84
Lower-Middle-Income Countries (median)		1.29	1.03	1.56	1.31	0.92	1.70	1.27	0.98	1.44
Lower-Middle-Income Countries (mean *)		1.31	1.08	1.55	1.14	0.92	1.37	1.35	0.98	1.72
Angola	2015	2.43	1.81	3.05	1.32	0.56	2.09	2.63	2.01	3.24
Bangladesh	2019	1.04	1.02	1.05	1.24	1.13	1.35	0.81	0.75	0.87
Cambodia	2021	1.03	0.85	1.22	0.73	0.49	1.00	1.08	0.90	1.26
Cameroon	2018	1.87	1.60	2.13	4.65	2.58	6.71	1.74	1.46	2.03
Congo	2014	1.48	1.06	1.91	4.23	0.51	7.95	1.23	0.76	1.71
Côte d'Ivoire	2016	1.36	0.88	1.84	3.00	1.37	4.63	1.27	0.76	1.78
Egypt	2014	0.77	0.66	0.87	1.05	0.00	3.22	0.76	0.65	0.88
El Salvador	2014	0.88	0.80	0.96	0.58	0.19	0.96	0.96	0.85	1.06
Eswatini	2014	1.25	0.82	1.68	0.23	0.00	1.14	1.28	0.86	1.70
Ghana	2017	1.63	1.33	1.94	1.02	0.56	1.48	1.76	1.41	2.10
Guatemala	2014	0.90	0.65	1.15	3.15	2.54	3.76	0.79	0.53	1.06
Honduras	2019	1.38	1.11	1.66	0.92	0.71	1.14	1.51	1.17	1.85
India	2019	1.02	1.01	1.03	0.77	0.67	0.87	1.03	1.01	1.05
Indonesia	2017	0.99	0.79	1.19	1.31	0.96	1.66	0.84	0.66	1.03
Kenya	2022	1.03	0.94	1.11	0.81	0.49	1.12	1.05	0.98	1.12
Kiribati	2018	1.18	0.92	1.45	0.27	0.00	0.90	1.27	1.06	1.47

Table 3. Cont.

Geography	Survey Year	RII at Birth			RII before Pregnancy			RII during Pregnancy		
		Estimate	LL	UL	Estimate	LL	UL	Estimate	LL	UL
Lao People's Democratic Republic	2017	1.87	1.19	2.54	2.27	1.35	3.19	1.62	1.01	2.24
Lesotho	2018	0.93	0.72	1.14	0.66	0.00	1.68	0.93	0.72	1.14
Mauritania	2019	1.35	1.22	1.49	2.65	1.99	3.32	1.16	0.98	1.34
Myanmar	2015	1.29	1.11	1.46	1.14	0.49	1.80	1.29	1.12	1.46
Nepal	2022	0.91	0.82	1.01	2.55	0.67	4.44	0.89	0.79	0.98
Nigeria	2021	3.21	2.92	3.50	1.40	0.40	2.39	3.20	2.88	3.51
Pakistan	2017	2.05	1.56	2.55	1.39	0.26	2.52	2.05	1.50	2.61
Papua New Guinea	2016	3.66	3.25	4.07	1.50	0.73	2.27	4.47	3.96	4.97
Philippines	2022	0.77	0.67	0.88	2.52	0.00	5.46	0.66	0.49	0.83
Senegal	2019	1.27	1.11	1.42	0.93	0.37	1.48	1.27	1.10	1.45
Sudan	2014	2.23	1.92	2.54	0.63	0.02	1.25	2.44	2.29	2.60
Timor-Leste	2016	1.40	1.23	1.57	1.72	0.65	2.80	1.32	1.21	1.42
Tunisia	2018	0.54	0.36	0.73	0.73	0.47	1.00	0.47	0.19	0.75
Viet Nam	2020	1.68	1.14	2.21	0.72	0.06	1.37	1.83	1.36	2.30
Yemen	2013	3.51	3.04	3.98	1.64	1.10	2.18	10.23	5.03	15.42
Zambia	2018	1.60	1.41	1.78	3.03	2.47	3.59	0.86	0.66	1.07
Zimbabwe	2019	1.29	1.18	1.40	3.49	1.83	5.15	0.86	0.59	1.13
Upper-Middle-Income Countries (median)		*1.04*	*0.87*	*1.22*	*1.43*	*1.04*	*1.57*	*0.94*	*0.65*	*1.17*
Upper-Middle-Income Countries (mean *)		*1.04*	*0.97*	*1.10*	*1.78*	*1.16*	*2.41*	*0.95*	*0.84*	*1.06*
Belize	2015	0.89	0.83	0.96	0.63	0.00	2.44	0.92	0.75	1.09
Costa Rica	2018	1.36	0.65	2.07	2.36	0.06	4.66	0.14	0.05	0.24
Cuba	2019	0.84	0.68	1.00	1.45	0.89	2.01	0.66	0.57	0.75
Dominican Republic	2019	1.02	0.94	1.11	1.54	0.30	2.77	0.99	0.86	1.12
Fiji	2021	0.94	0.51	1.37	1.13	0.78	1.48	0.65	0.00	1.34
Gabon	2019	1.35	1.26	1.45	1.04	0.92	1.16	1.37	1.26	1.48
Guyana	2019	2.13	0.20	4.05	1.47	0.00	3.51	3.63	2.03	5.23
Iraq	2018	0.91	0.69	1.12	5.50	1.91	9.09	0.64	0.42	0.85
Jordan	2017	0.81	0.73	0.88	0.55	0.30	0.80	1.34	0.32	2.36
Maldives	2016	1.16	0.59	1.72	1.02	0.83	1.21	1.24	0.36	2.12
Mexico	2015	1.06	0.99	1.13	1.41	0.93	1.90	0.96	0.77	1.14
Namibia	2013	0.86	0.63	1.09	1.53	0.43	2.64	0.61	0.57	0.64
Paraguay	2016	1.24	1.10	1.38	1.63	0.70	2.56	1.19	1.00	1.37
Peru	2019	0.82	0.64	1.00	1.07	0.71	1.42	0.77	0.49	1.04
Samoa	2019	1.24	0.33	2.15	1.90	0.00	3.83	0.92	0.26	1.58
South Africa	2016	1.09	0.94	1.25	1.59	0.00	4.16	1.02	0.78	1.25
Suriname	2018	0.18	0.00	0.39	0.04	0.00	0.09	0.38	0.00	0.91
Thailand	2019	1.14	1.02	1.25	1.17	0.95	1.39	1.13	0.92	1.33

* Means are population weighted and use female population age 15–49 with *aweight* specifications in Stata. RII: Relative index of inequality; LL: Lower 95% confidence interval of estimate; UL: Upper 95% confidence interval of estimate.

The distribution of countries by presence and direction of absolute inequalities at each time point is summarized in Figure 4.

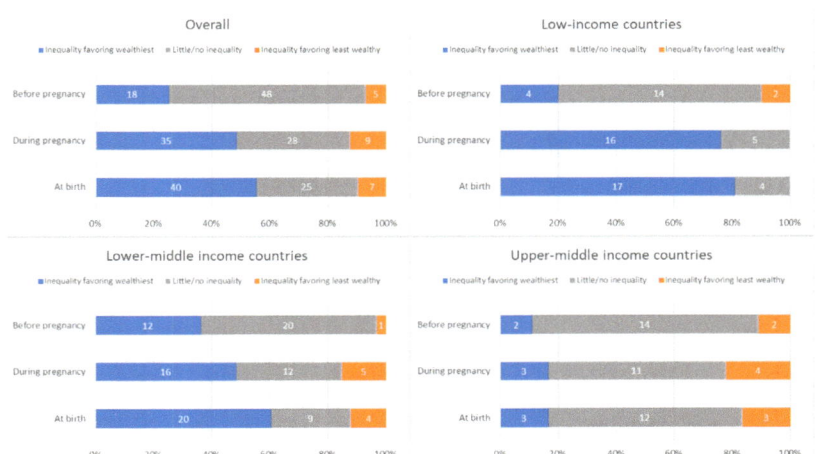

Figure 4. Distribution of countries' absolute inequality in tetanus immunization coverage before pregnancy, during pregnancy, and at birth; overall and by country income grouping.

3.4. Inequalities in Coverage before Versus during Pregnancy

There is no clear single pattern of the relationship between absolute inequalities in coverage before versus during pregnancy (See Figure 5). There was not a significant correlation between SII before vs. SII during pregnancy, for the sample overall, nor by country income group (overall r = −0.18, p = 0.14). A third of countries (24 out of 71) had little to no inequality in coverage before pregnancy and inequality favoring the wealthiest quintile during pregnancy. A quarter of countries (19 out of 71) had little to no inequality at both time points. Ten percent (7 of 71) had inequality favoring the wealthiest at both time points. Patterns of inequality before and during pregnancy are similar when examining relative rather than absolute inequality (See Supplementary Figure S4).

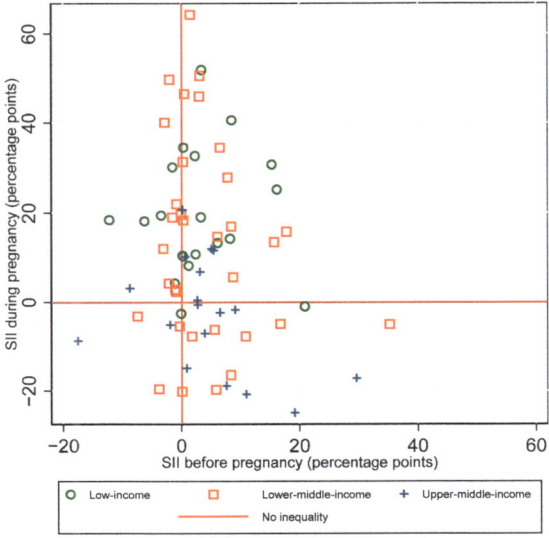

Figure 5. Absolute inequality (SII) in maternal tetanus immunization coverage by wealth quintile, before versus during pregnancy.

3.5. Change in Absolute Inequality from before Pregnancy to Birth

The value of the SII during pregnancy reflects the change in absolute inequality that was introduced or mitigated during pregnancy (See Figure 6). Half of countries (35) had a meaningful increase in inequality favoring the wealthiest in tetanus immunization coverage during pregnancy; 28 countries had similar inequality, eight countries had a meaningful decrease in inequality favoring the wealthiest, and only one country had a meaningful increase in inequality favoring the least wealthy.

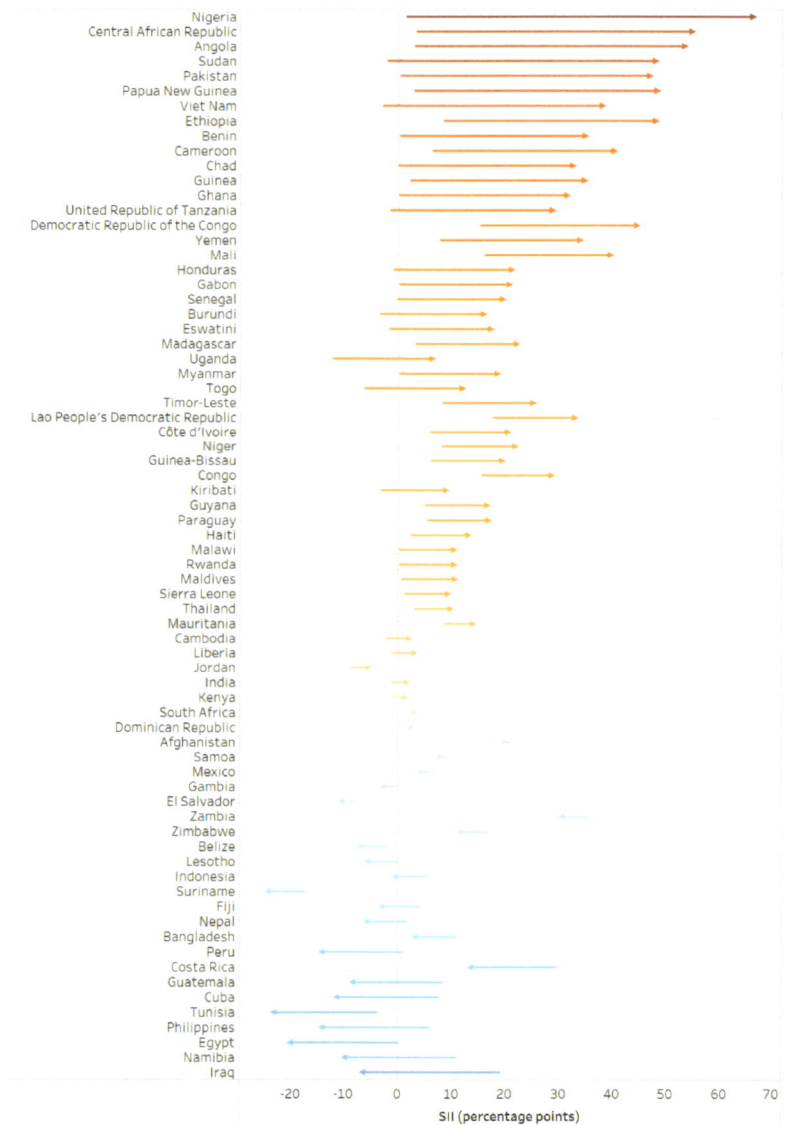

Figure 6. Change in absolute inequality in tetanus immunization coverage before pregnancy versus at birth.

Overall, we observe inequality favoring the wealthiest during the pregnancy time period, with the largest increases in inequality in low-income countries. Upper-middle-income countries, in contrast, had no collective change in inequality during the pregnancy time period. The average SII in pregnancy for the overall sample was 10.5 percentage points [95% CI 5.3–15.6], 25.4 [95% CI 19.8–31.0] for low-income countries, 10.0 [95% CI 2.1–17.8] for lower-middle-income countries, and −3.8 [95% CI −8.7–1.0] for upper-middle-income countries.

Observed increases in absolute inequality favoring the wealthiest during pregnancy were coupled with increases in tetanus immunization coverage during this period, both overall and in low- and lower-middle-income countries (See Figures 7 and 8). However, absolute inequality in pregnancy was not significantly associated with coverage in pregnancy for the sample overall, nor by country income groupings (overall r = 0.21, p = 0.07). Furthermore, several countries had meaningful decreases in absolute inequality and increases in coverage during pregnancy, despite the overall trend. Eight countries—Bangladesh, Costa Rica, Cuba, Egypt, Iraq, Namibia, Nepal, and the Philippines—all had statistically significant decreases in absolute inequality favoring the wealthiest during pregnancy of five percentage points or more, coupled with increases in immunization coverage.

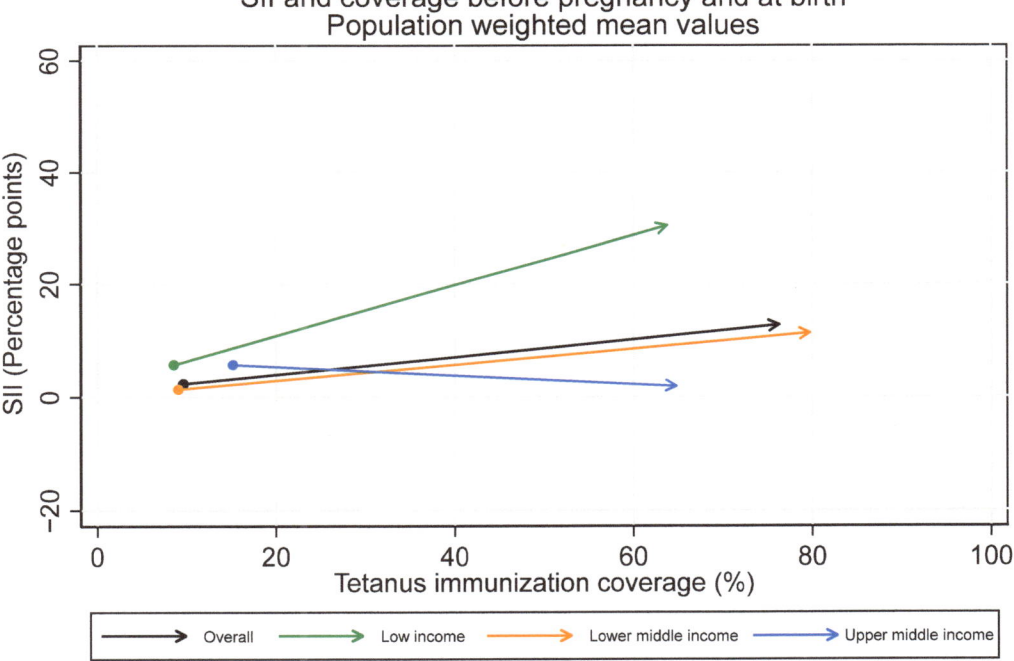

Figure 7. Absolute inequality in maternal tetanus immunization coverage and average coverage level, before pregnancy and at birth. (Dot represents coverage level and SII in tetanus immunization coverage before pregnancy; arrowhead represents coverage and SII at birth).

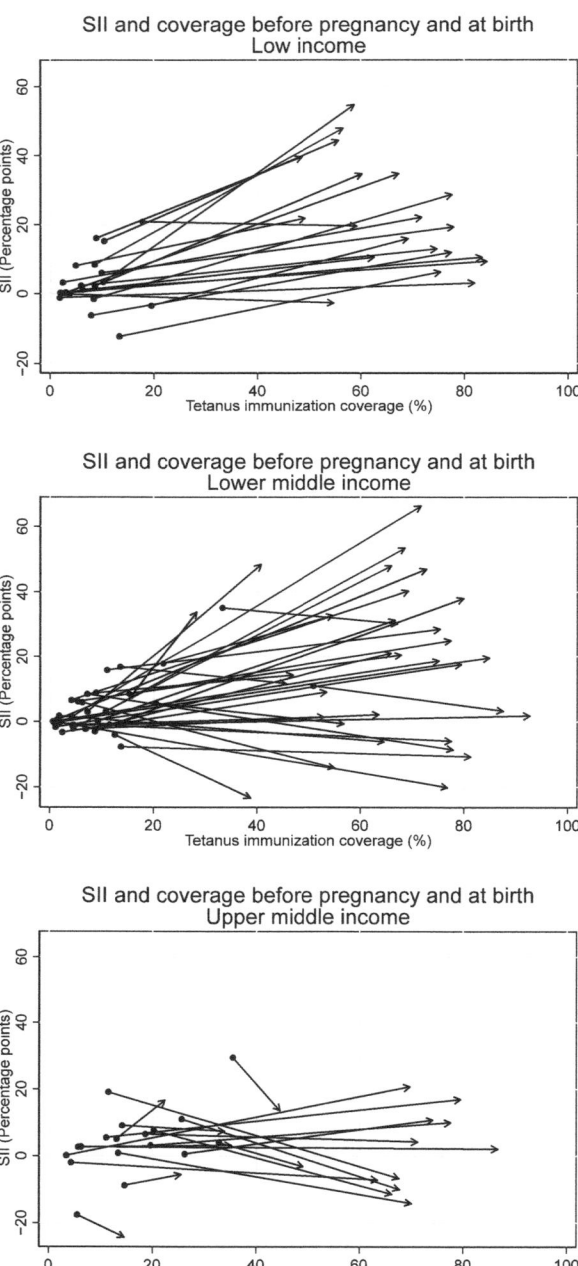

Figure 8. Absolute inequality in maternal tetanus immunization coverage and average coverage level, before pregnancy and at birth, by country income grouping. (Dot represents coverage level and SII in tetanus immunization coverage before pregnancy; arrowhead represents coverage and SII at birth).

3.6. Absolute Inequality and Maternal and Neonatal Tetanus Elimination Status

Coverage and equity in tetanus immunization is of particular relevance for those countries which have not yet achieved maternal and neonatal tetanus elimination (MNTE) (defined as less than one case per 1000 live births in every district of a country); we therefore examine differences in absolute inequality between countries that had achieved or had not achieved MNTE at time of survey. We have data from nine countries which had not achieved MNTE as of 2023 (Afghanistan, Angola, Central African Republic, Guinea, Nigeria, Pakistan, Papua New Guinea, Sudan, and Yemen), as well as data from five countries where MNTE was achieved after the most recent available survey (Chad, Democratic Republic of the Congo, Ethiopia, Haiti, and Mali). Average TTCV coverage was significantly lower among countries which had not achieved MNTE relative to countries which had achieved MNTE before pregnancy (6.0% vs. 10.5%, $p = 0.03$), during pregnancy (58.6% vs. 68.7%, $p = 0.04$), and at birth (64.6% vs. 79.1%, $p < 0.001$).

Absolute inequality in tetanus immunization coverage during pregnancy was significantly higher among countries which had not achieved MNTE compared to those which had achieved elimination (See Figure 9). The average SII before pregnancy was 4.8 percentage points [95% CI 1.3–8.3] in countries that had not achieved MNTE compared to 1.8 percentage points [95% CI 0.3–3.2] in countries that had achieved MNTE ($p = 0.12$). The average SII during pregnancy was 45.0 percentage points [95% CI 36.3–53.7] in countries that had not achieved MNTE compared to 2.1 percentage points [95% CI −1.3—5.5] in countries which had achieved MNTE ($p < 0.001$). Nearly all countries which had not achieved MNTE (13 of 14) had significant inequality of favoring the wealthiest during pregnancy.

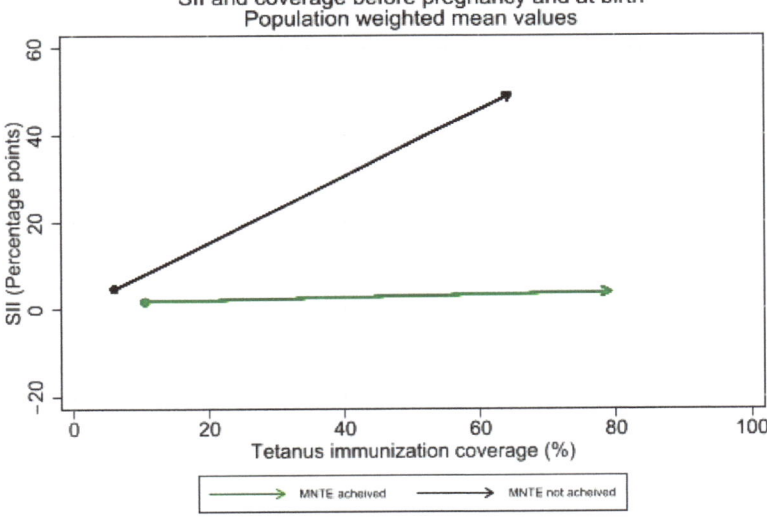

Figure 9. Inequality in maternal tetanus immunization coverage and average coverage level, before pregnancy and at birth, by whether countries had or had not achieved MNTE at time of survey. (Dot represents coverage level and SII in tetanus immunization coverage before pregnancy; arrowhead represents coverage and SII at birth).

3.7. Sensitivity Analysis—Recency of Data Availability

To examine whether findings from this study were sensitive to the recency of data availability, we replicate key analyses separately for countries with data available from the past five years (2019–2022, $n = 28$) and countries with data greater than five years old (2013–2018, $n = 44$). The results indicate that the majority of tetanus immunization coverage at birth occurs during pregnancy in most countries with recent data (25/28, 89%) as well as in most countries with older data (41/44, 93%). We find significantly lower average absolute wealth-related inequality in the more recent data before pregnancy (average SII for recent data 0.8 vs. 4.9 for older data, $p = 0.003$) and significantly lower average inequality at birth (average SII for recent data 8.7 vs. 19.3 for older data, $p = 0.04$), though we find no significant difference in average inequality during pregnancy ($p = 0.20$). We find consistent patterns of inequality whereby a similar proportion of countries have statistically significant inequalities before pregnancy, during pregnancy, and at birth (See Figure 10).

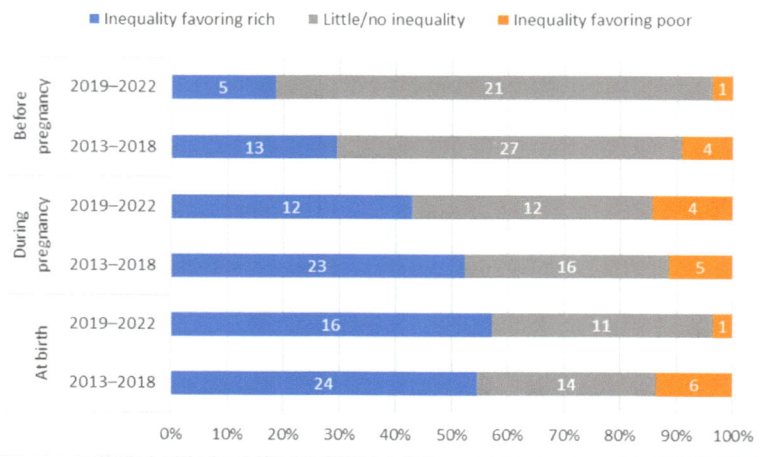

Figure 10. Distribution of countries' absolute inequality in tetanus immunization coverage before pregnancy, during pregnancy, and at birth; by recency of data collection.

In both the more recent and older data, we observe significant average inequality favoring the wealthiest during the pregnancy time period (average SII for recent data 7.9, 95% CI 0.3–15.5; average SII for older data 14.6, 95% CI 7.4–21.8). Note that these findings should not imply temporal trends, as each time period contains a unique group of countries. However, consistent findings of significant inequality during pregnancy and consistent evidence of greater inequality during pregnancy compared to before pregnancy suggest that the overall conclusions of the study are not sensitive to a 5-year rather than 10-year analysis time frame.

4. Discussion

Findings from this study of 72 low- and middle-income countries suggest that the majority of tetanus immunization PAB for first births is the result of TTCV doses received during pregnancy. This study also highlights absolute wealth-related inequality in tetanus immunization PAB, finding that the majority of this inequality is introduced during pregnancy rather than before it. This is particularly evident in low- and lower-middle-income countries.

In 92% of countries examined in this study (66 of 72), PAB appears to be driven by immunizations received during pregnancy, with limited coverage pre-pregnancy. The World Health Organization formally recommends coverage of six doses of TTCV for all people, including the 3-dose primary series received in childhood and three boosters given at 12–23 months, 4–7 years, and 9–15 years of age [5]. Adherence to this schedule would result in all women of reproductive age having PAB prior to any pregnancies. However, only 21% of examined countries had adopted this schedule at the time of survey, and it's likely that even fewer had this schedule in place at the time the women surveyed were children/adolescents and eligible for these booster doses. This ultimately results in a reliance on the pregnancy time period to provide sufficient TTCV doses to protect the neonate and mother by the time of birth. As more countries shift to the six-dose schedule, the relative contributions of coverage before and during pregnancy will likely shift. However, the data examined here suggest that coverage in pregnancy remains the primary input to PAB as of these recent surveys, and thus warrants ongoing attention.

Though tetanus immunization before pregnancy was low overall, and TTCV doses received in pregnancy increased PAB coverage, this increase in coverage was accompanied by increased inequality in coverage in half of the countries we examined. Thirty-five out of 71 countries had a meaningful increase in inequality favoring the wealthiest in tetanus immunization coverage from pre-pregnancy to birth. Absolute inequality was markedly larger during pregnancy compared to pre-pregnancy for the overall sample (SII 10 versus 2 percentage points). Though countries have the same statistically significant inequalities at each time point when using a relative rather than absolute measure of inequality, the relative inequality measure suggests a similar magnitude of inequality before versus during pregnancy. This indicates that the large differences in absolute inequality during versus before pregnancy are driven in part by the large amount of coverage occurring in pregnancy.

Inequalities in TTCV receipt during pregnancy are likely driven in part by inequalities in antenatal care (ANC) access and utilization [18,19]. Other studies have observed increases in uptake of ANC services alongside increased inequalities in service utilization favoring the wealthiest in low-income settings [20]. However, higher coverage of ANC visits relative to coverage of TTCVs, particularly in settings which have not achieved MNTE, suggests ongoing missed opportunities for vaccination within routine pregnancy care [21–24]. Other studies have shown inconsistent trends in the utilization of tetanus vaccination among pregnant women in the context of antenatal care over time [25]. Additionally, inequalities in healthcare utilization may result in inequalities in tetanus protection beyond that conveyed by vaccination alone; specifically, facility delivery and skilled birth attendance are associated with greater use of safe and sterile delivery and umbilical cord care practices, as well as subsequent reductions in tetanus mortality [26]. As such, inequalities in healthcare utilization during pregnancy and birth may contribute to inequalities in tetanus protection beyond inequalities in immunization alone. Importantly, inequalities in ANC uptake among pregnant women also signal adverse outcomes for early childhood among their children. For example, lower levels of ANC visits among pregnant women have also been shown to be associated with incomplete vaccination among their children in early childhood [27]. Findings from our study support equity-oriented interventions and policies targeted towards pregnant women both within and outside of routine healthcare, such as additional education for healthcare providers on the importance of screening for, providing, and recording TTCV doses during ANC visits, or supplemental immunization activities (SIAs) focused on geographic areas at greatest disadvantage [21,28].

In low-income countries in particular, inequalities in coverage at birth were introduced during pregnancy. While only 4 of 21 examined low-income countries had significant inequality favoring the wealthiest in tetanus immunization coverage before pregnancy, 16 of 21 had significant inequality during pregnancy. On aggregate, the average absolute inequality among low-income countries was notably higher during pregnancy (SII 25 percentage points) compared to before pregnancy (SII six percentage points). Conversely, the majority of upper-middle-income countries in our study had negligible inequality during pregnancy (11 of 18), and, on average, had a decrease in inequality during pregnancy (SII-4 percentage points). Upper-middle-income countries also had notably different patterns of tetanus PAB coverage relative to low- and lower-middle-income countries. A significantly greater proportion of PAB coverage occurred before pregnancy, or, in other words, significantly less PAB coverage occurred during pregnancy. Additionally, PAB coverage was highest among middle-wealth mothers (3rd quintile), with lower coverage among both the least and most wealthy quintiles, while in low- and lower-middle-income countries, PAB coverage increased monotonically with increasing wealth.

The divergent patterns of coverage and inequality observed in this study among upper-middle-income countries are likely driven by several factors. First, the greater coverage before pregnancy highlights better access to and implementation of immunization services throughout the life course prior to pregnancy [29], likely reflecting better documentation of immunizations, as discussed in further detail below. The pattern of highest PAB coverage among middle-wealth women, driven by higher levels of coverage in pregnancy, might be explained by an indirect relationship between tetanus vaccination and better birth and antenatal care conditions. As the coverage of institutional delivery increases and the structure of services also increase, less attention might be applied to tetanus immunization, as safe birth and umbilical cord care conditions are present. Meanwhile, the wealthiest women are likely accessing the highest quality of birth care, where prevention of neonatal tetanus may no longer be a priority concern. Such findings align with previous work examining institutional deliveries [30]. Analyses which jointly consider tetanus immunization and measures of care utilization such as institutional delivery are beyond the current study's scope but would help in further understanding this potential relationship.

In addition to differences across country income groupings, we see striking differences in inequalities between countries that had and had not achieved MNTE. Countries which had not achieved MNTE at time of survey had a 20 times higher average absolute inequality in coverage compared to countries which had achieved MNTE (SII 45 vs. 2 percentage points). The large amount of absolute inequality in coverage within countries that had not achieved MNTE is expected, as the ongoing presence of neonates who develop NT requires a substantial population of mothers who lack immunization coverage and who face exposure to tetanus through unsafe birth or umbilical cord care practices. MNTE efforts that seek to identify these populations routinely find that areas with greatest risk are rural, remote, and economically unstable [31]. MNTE strategies typically include supplemental immunization activities (SIAs) aiming to serve these groups, which may quickly improve coverage and reduce inequality in coverage before pregnancy but will not reduce during-pregnancy inequalities [32]. All countries which had not achieved MNTE were classified as low or lower-middle income countries at time of survey; some of the trends in coverage and inequality observed may have thus been driven by trends in country income level and related factors, such as existing health system structure, rather than MNTE achievement status specifically. However, if we limit the comparison to low- and lower-middle income countries which have achieved MNTE, we find the same significant results, in that the average SII during pregnancy was 45 percentage points in countries that had not achieved MNTE compared to three percentage points in low- and lower-middle-income countries which had achieved MNTE, $p < 0.001$ (results not shown).

Despite overall trends, several countries reduced inequality or kept it low during pregnancy, which can yield important lessons. Eight countries—Bangladesh, Costa Rica, Cuba, Egypt, Iraq, Namibia, Nepal, and the Philippines—all had statistically significant decreases in absolute inequality favoring the wealthiest during pregnancy of five percentage points or more. In Nepal, for example, the Safe Delivery Incentive Programme was implemented in 2005 to include reimbursement for delivery travel costs for all Nepali women and free delivery care and healthcare facility delivery cost reimbursement for women in lower-income districts; this program was shown to significantly improve prenatal care visit and tetanus vaccination uptake while reducing wealth-based inequalities in coverage at the district level [33,34]. In Bangladesh, the use of antenatal services has been steadily increasing [35], and women across socioeconomic groups have shown similar patterns in the utilization of public and private health facilities throughout pregnancy [36]. Better understanding of the country-specific contexts, including tetanus immunization schedules, standards of care for pregnancy and childbirth, as well as other related policies and interventions, could be leveraged to inform efforts to improve tetanus immunization coverage and simultaneously reduce inequality during pregnancy.

Findings from this study should be viewed in light of several limitations. First, though we have limited analyses to first births, a small number of women may have received tetanus vaccines during a prior pregnancy which ended in a miscarriage or abortion, so some caution should be exercised with interpretation of the before-pregnancy coverage time period. However, most miscarriages and abortions occur during the first trimester (Week 12 or earlier) [37,38], before women in pregnancy would typically receive tetanus toxoid (national schedules vary, but generally in weeks 13+), so the number of women this applies to is likely small. Additionally, limiting the sample to first births likely underestimates PAB for births as a whole, as each pregnancy event provides an opportunity for interaction with the health system and an opportunity to receive any necessary or missing TTCV doses. Indeed, an analysis using a similar set of country years of data found a slightly higher median PAB (69.1% vs. 67.5% observed in this study); PAB estimates should thus be considered reflective of first births only [3].

Second, PAB from TTCV doses received prior to pregnancy may be derived from a number of immunization sources. TTCVs received prior to pregnancy include standard childhood vaccine doses, adolescent and adult boosters, women of reproductive age-specific boosters, and doses received as part of SIAs. MNTE initiatives in particular have historically included SIA campaigns targeted at women of reproductive age. For the analyses presented here, we grouped all these sources of pre-pregnancy immunization. As childhood tetanus vaccination coverage differs widely across the examined settings, the relative contributions of these pre-pregnancy immunization sources will also differ substantially by country. Additionally, average age at first birth also varies substantially across countries, affecting how long women have the opportunity to receive needed adult boosters prior to pregnancy and the length of time since early childhood and adolescent doses most subject to recall bias. Any country-specific application of findings should take into consideration the broader fertility and immunization system context in that country, inclusive of childhood immunization coverage and evolving tetanus vaccination strategies and schedules, to generate the most appropriate conclusions for that setting. The limitations in recording and maintaining records of immunization during the life course may also have resulted in misclassification of vaccination status and the contribution of each immunization delivery strategy [39,40]. Future work that disentangles the relative contribution to PAB of each of these sources would be necessary to inform more specific targets to improve PAB coverage and equity prior to pregnancy.

Third, where immunization monitoring and tracking systems are not reliably available at the individual level, women may receive additional and ultimately unnecessary doses of TTCV in pregnancy as a result of poor documentation and recall rather than true need for immunity. The World Health Organization recommends that countries which have not achieved MNTE provide two doses of TTCV to any pregnant women "for whom reliable information on previous tetanus vaccinations is not available" [5]. Conversely, women who do not require additional doses at birth because they were fully immunized before delivery might have this information inaccurately recorded in their home-based or hospital records, or may report it incorrectly in surveys [39]. Consequently, these women could be mistakenly classified as lacking PAB despite the absence of birth doses being justified. Issues of recall also differentially affect TTCV doses received prior to and during pregnancy; as pregnancy doses are more recent, they are by definition less subject to recall bias, as well as more likely to be captured by electronic records and immunization documentation, which are improving over time in most settings. Findings suggesting greater TTCV coverage during pregnancy compared to before pregnancy must be viewed in light of this limitation, though findings regarding inequality within each time frame are less sensitive to this recall bias. Increasing use of electronic records and better immunization documentation and monitoring should lead to a decrease in use of extraneous pregnancy TTCV doses and an increase in accurate reporting of coverage received prior to birth.

Fourth, this research is subject to the limits of the available data, including only a sample of low- and middle-income countries with nationally representative surveys and data which may be up to 10 years old. The coverage and timing of TTCV dose receipts are also subject to immunization card ownership or recall. Patterns of coverage and inequality may have changed since the time of survey, and survey estimates may under-represent true coverage. The sensitivity analyses conducted to examine data collected within five years and greater than five years ago suggest that the conclusions of these analyses are not sensitive to a five-year rather than ten-year analysis time frame; however, findings may still be changing over time. In particular, the COVID-19 pandemic has had large impacts on immunization systems and healthcare service delivery generally, and children, adolescents, and women who missed TTCV doses due to the pandemic or resultant health system impacts should be targeted for catch-up doses to sustain coverage and minimize inequality. Studies which replicate these analyses using the most up-to-date data in a given context will be most valuable for elucidating the current state of inequality.

Finally, the analyses presented here are cross-sectional and limited to the examination of a single dimension of inequality, namely household wealth. Other dimensions, such as maternal age, maternal education, or urban/rural residence, may also be meaningful determinants of tetanus immunization coverage and, when considered jointly, may in fact be greater drivers of inequality than wealth alone. It is beyond the scope of these analyses to examine additional determinants of coverage, dimensions of inequality, or the relative contribution of multiple dimensions of inequality, and future work in these areas would allow for greater understanding of the full complexities of inequalities in immunization coverage.

5. Conclusions

In this study of first births among women in 72 low- and middle-income countries, we find that most tetanus PAB coverage is the result of TTCV doses received during pregnancy. We present evidence of significant inequality favoring the wealthiest in PAB coverage, finding that most of this inequality is introduced during pregnancy rather than before it. This is particularly evident in low- and lower-middle-income countries, whereas upper-middle-income countries have greater wealth-related inequality in tetanus immunization coverage during pregnancy. Efforts to ensure high PAB coverage levels at the population level, particularly those taking place during pregnancy, should also consider equity in coverage as a key goal and outcome.

Supplementary Materials: The following supporting information can be downloaded at: https://www.mdpi.com/article/10.3390/vaccines12040431/s1, Table S1: TTCV schedule for 72 study countries at time of survey; Figure S1: Tetanus immunization coverage before pregnancy, during pregnancy, and at birth in the wealthiest and least wealthy wealth quintiles in 21 low-income countries; Figure S2: Tetanus immunization coverage before pregnancy, during pregnancy, and at birth in the wealthiest and least wealthy wealth quintiles in 33 lower-middle income countries; Figure S3: Tetanus immunization coverage before pregnancy, during pregnancy, and at birth in the wealthiest and least wealthy wealth quintiles in 18 upper-middle income countries; Figure S4: Relative inequality (RII) in maternal tetanus immunization coverage by wealth quintile before versus during pregnancy.

Author Contributions: A.R.H. led the conceptualization of the study and interpretation of results. N.E.J. led data analysis and manuscript development. C.B. and F.D.S.C. led data preparation; K.K. and A.A. contributed to data visualization. All authors had full access to the data in the study; C.B., F.D.S.C. and A.J.D.B. had direct access to and verified the underlying data reported in the manuscript. A.R.H., C.B., K.K., A.A., F.D.S.C., M.C.D.-H., C.L., N.Y. and A.J.D.B. provided interpretation, text, and review of findings specific to inequalities and immunization. All authors have read and agreed to the published version of the manuscript.

Funding: This research was funded by Gavi, the Vaccine Alliance. The funders had no role in the design of the study; in the collection, analyses, or interpretation of data; in the writing of the manuscript; or in the decision to publish the results.

Institutional Review Board Statement: Not applicable.

Informed Consent Statement: Not applicable.

Data Availability Statement: All analyses were carried out using publicly available datasets that can be obtained directly from the DHS (dhsprogram.com (accessed on 29 September 2023)) and the MICS (mics.unicef.org (accessed on 29 September 2023)) websites. Datasets are continuously sourced and updated by the International Center for Equity in Health (equidade.org) as they are released. Analyses used the latest available dataset versions as of 29 September 2023.

Conflicts of Interest: Author Cauane Blumenberg was employed by the company Causale Consulting. The remaining authors declare that they have no conflict of interest. The authors alone are responsible for the views expressed in this publication and do not necessarily represent the views, decisions, or policies of their institutions.

References

1. World Health Organization. *Protecting All against Tetanus: Guide to Sustaining Maternal and Neonatal Tetanus Elimination (MNTE) and Broadening Tetanus Protection for All Populations*; World Health Organization: Geneva, Switzerland, 2019.
2. World Health Organization. Maternal and Neonatal Tetanus Elimination. Available online: https://www.who.int/initiatives/maternal-and-neonatal-tetanus-elimination-(mnte) (accessed on 22 September 2022).
3. Johns, N.E.; Cata-Preta, B.O.; Kirkby, K.; Arroyave, L.; Bergen, N.; Danovaro-Holliday, M.C.; Santos, T.M.; Yusuf, N.; Barros, A.J.; Hosseinpoor, A.R. Inequalities in Immunization against Maternal and Neonatal Tetanus: A Cross-Sectional Analysis of Protection at Birth Coverage Using Household Health Survey Data from 76 Countries. *Vaccines* **2023**, *11*, 752. [CrossRef] [PubMed]
4. World Health Organization. *Immunization Agenda 2030: A Global Strategy to Leave No One Behind*; WHO: Geneva, Switzerland, 2020.
5. World Health Organization. Tetanus vaccines: WHO position paper—February 2017. *Wkly. Epidemiol. Rec.* **2017**, *92*, 53–76.
6. Pathirana, J.; Nkambule, J.; Black, S. Determinants of maternal immunization in developing countries. *Vaccine* **2015**, *33*, 2971–2977. [CrossRef] [PubMed]
7. Ghosh, A.; Laxminarayan, R. Demand-and supply-side determinants of diphtheria-pertussis-tetanus nonvaccination and dropout in rural India. *Vaccine* **2017**, *35*, 1087–1093. [CrossRef] [PubMed]
8. Wiysonge, C.S.; Uthman, O.A.; Ndumbe, P.M.; Hussey, G.D. Individual and contextual factors associated with low childhood immunisation coverage in sub-Saharan Africa: A multilevel analysis. *PLoS ONE* **2012**, *7*, e37905. [CrossRef]
9. Suprenant, M.P.; Nyankesha, E.; Moreno-Garcia, R.; Buj, V.; Yakubu, A.; Shafique, F.; Zaman, M.H. Assessing the relationship between operationally defined zero-dose communities and access to selected primary healthcare services for children and pregnant women in emergency settings. *PLoS ONE* **2023**, *18*, e0281764. [CrossRef]
10. Khan, S.; Hancioglu, A. Multiple indicator cluster surveys: Delivering robust data on children and women across the globe. *Stud. Fam. Plan.* **2019**, *50*, 279–286. [CrossRef]
11. Corsi, D.J.; Neuman, M.; Finlay, J.E.; Subramanian, S. Demographic and health surveys: A profile. *Int. J. Epidemiol.* **2012**, *41*, 1602–1613. [CrossRef]
12. Filmer, D.; Pritchett, L.H. Estimating wealth effects without expenditure data—Or tears: An application to educational enrollments in states of India. *Demography* **2001**, *38*, 115–132.
13. The World Bank. World Bank Country and Lending Groups. Available online: https://datahelpdesk.worldbank.org/knowledgebase/articles/906519-world-bank-country-and-lending-groups (accessed on 18 January 2023).
14. Regidor, E. Measures of health inequalities: Part 2. *J. Epidemiol. Community Health* **2004**, *58*, 900. [CrossRef]
15. StataCorp. *Stata Statistical Software, Release 18*; StataCorp LLC: College Station, TX, USA, 2023.
16. United Nations Department of Economics and Social Affairs. World Population Prospects 2022. Available online: https://population.un.org/wpp/ (accessed on 10 March 2023).
17. The DHS Program. Protecting the Privacy of DHS Survey Respondents. Available online: https://dhsprogram.com/Methodology/Protecting-the-Privacy-of-DHS-Survey-Respondents.cfm (accessed on 14 March 2024).
18. Arroyave, L.; Saad, G.E.; Victora, C.G.; Barros, A.J. Inequalities in antenatal care coverage and quality: An analysis from 63 low and middle-income countries using the ANCq content-qualified coverage indicator. *Int. J. Equity Health* **2021**, *20*, 102. [CrossRef] [PubMed]
19. Downe, S.; Finlayson, K.; Tunçalp, Ö.; Gülmezoglu, A.M. Provision and uptake of routine antenatal services: A qualitative evidence synthesis. *Cochrane Database Syst. Rev.* **2019**, *6*, 1–69. [CrossRef] [PubMed]
20. Mezmur, M.; Navaneetham, K.; Letamo, G.; Bariagaber, H. Socioeconomic inequalities in the uptake of maternal healthcare services in Ethiopia. *BMC Health Serv. Res.* **2017**, *17*, 367. [CrossRef] [PubMed]
21. Yusuf, N.; Raza, A.A.; Chang-Blanc, D.; Ahmed, B.; Hailegebriel, T.; Luce, R.R.; Tanifum, P.; Masresha, B.; Faton, M.; Omer, M.D. Progress and barriers towards maternal and neonatal tetanus elimination in the remaining 12 countries. *Lancet Glob. Health* **2021**, *9*, e1610–e1617. [CrossRef] [PubMed]
22. Davies, B.; Olivier, J.; Amponsah-Dacosta, E. Health Systems Determinants of Delivery and Uptake of Maternal Vaccines in Low-and Middle-Income Countries: A Qualitative Systematic Review. *Vaccines* **2023**, *11*, 869. [CrossRef] [PubMed]
23. Ayouni, I.; Amponsah-Dacosta, E.; Noll, S.; Kagina, B.M.; Muloiwa, R. Interventions to Improve Knowledge, Attitudes, and Uptake of Recommended Vaccines during Pregnancy and Postpartum: A Scoping Review. *Vaccines* **2023**, *11*, 1733. [CrossRef] [PubMed]

24. Bergin, N.; Murtagh, J.; Philip, R.K. Maternal vaccination as an essential component of life-course immunization and its contribution to preventive neonatology. *Int. J. Environ. Res. Public Health* **2018**, *15*, 847. [CrossRef] [PubMed]
25. Tikmani, S.S.; Ali, S.A.; Saleem, S.; Bann, C.M.; Mwenechanya, M.; Carlo, W.A.; Figueroa, L.; Garces, A.L.; Krebs, N.F.; Patel, A. Trends of antenatal care during pregnancy in low-and middle-income countries: Findings from the global network maternal and newborn health registry. In *Seminars in Perinatology*; Elsevier: Amsterdam, The Netherlands, 2019; pp. 297–307.
26. Blencowe, H.; Cousens, S.; Mullany, L.C.; Lee, A.C.; Kerber, K.; Wall, S.; Darmstadt, G.L.; Lawn, J.E. Clean birth and postnatal care practices to reduce neonatal deaths from sepsis and tetanus: A systematic review and Delphi estimation of mortality effect. *BMC Public Health* **2011**, *11*, S11. [CrossRef] [PubMed]
27. Ndwandwe, D.; Nnaji, C.A.; Mashunye, T.; Uthman, O.A.; Wiysonge, C.S. Incomplete vaccination and associated factors among children aged 12–23 months in South Africa: An analysis of the South African demographic and health survey 2016. *Hum. Vaccines Immunother.* **2021**, *17*, 247–254. [CrossRef]
28. Dhir, S.K.; Dewan, P.; Gupta, P. Maternal and Neonatal Tetanus Elimination: Where are We Now? *Res. Rep. Trop Med.* **2021**, *12*, 247–261. [CrossRef]
29. Wallace, A.; Ryman, T.; Privor-Dumm, L.; Morgan, C.; Fields, R.; Garcia, C.; Sodha, S.; Lindstrand, A.; Lochlainn, L.N. Leaving no one behind: Defining and implementing an integrated life course approach to vaccination across the next decade as part of the immunization Agenda 2030. *Vaccine* **2022**, in press. [CrossRef] [PubMed]
30. Victora, C.G.; Joseph, G.; Silva, I.C.; Maia, F.S.; Vaughan, J.P.; Barros, F.C.; Barros, A.J. The inverse equity hypothesis: Analyses of institutional deliveries in 286 national surveys. *Am. J. Public Health* **2018**, *108*, 464–471. [CrossRef] [PubMed]
31. Roper, M.H.; Vandelaer, J.H.; Gasse, F.L. Maternal and neonatal tetanus. *Lancet* **2007**, *370*, 1947–1959. [CrossRef] [PubMed]
32. Yusuf, N.; Steinglass, R.; Gasse, F.; Raza, A.; Ahmed, B.; Blanc, D.C.; Yakubu, A.; Gregory, C.; Tohme, R.A. Sustaining Maternal and Neonatal Tetanus Elimination (MNTE) in countries that have been validated for elimination—Progress and challenges. *BMC Public Health* **2022**, *22*, 691. [CrossRef] [PubMed]
33. Lamichhane, P.; Sharma, A.; Mahal, A. Impact evaluation of free delivery care on maternal health service utilisation and neonatal health in Nepal. *Health Policy Plan.* **2017**, *32*, 1427–1436. [CrossRef] [PubMed]
34. Pandey, S.; Daley, A. Free delivery care and supply-side incentives in Nepal's poorest districts: The effect on prenatal care and neonatal tetanus vaccinations. *J. Dev. Eff.* **2021**, *13*, 100–115. [CrossRef]
35. National Institute of Population Research and Training (NIPORT) and ICF. *Bangladesh Demographic and Health Survey 2017-18*; NIPORT and ICF: Dhaka, Bangladesh; Rockville, MD, USA, 2020.
36. Pervin, J.; Venkateswaran, M.; Nu, U.T.; Rahman, M.; O'Donnell, B.F.; Friberg, I.K.; Rahman, A.; Frøen, J.F. Determinants of utilization of antenatal and delivery care at the community level in rural Bangladesh. *PLoS ONE* **2021**, *16*, e0257782. [CrossRef] [PubMed]
37. Dugas, C.; Slane, V.H. *Miscarriage*; StatPearls Publishing: Treasure Island, FL, USA, 2018.
38. Henkel, A.; Shaw, K.A. First trimester abortion care in low-and middle-income countries. *Clin. Obstet. Gynecol.* **2021**, *64*, 449–459. [CrossRef]
39. Dansereau, E.; Brown, D.; Stashko, L.; Danovaro-Holliday, M.C. A systematic review of the agreement of recall, home-based records, facility records, BCG scar, and serology for ascertaining vaccination status in low and middle-income countries. *Gates Open Res.* **2019**, *3*, 923. [CrossRef]
40. World Health Organization. *WHO Recommendations on Home-Based Records for Maternal, Newborn and Child Health*; World Health Organization: Geneva, Switzerland, 2018.

Disclaimer/Publisher's Note: The statements, opinions and data contained in all publications are solely those of the individual author(s) and contributor(s) and not of MDPI and/or the editor(s). MDPI and/or the editor(s) disclaim responsibility for any injury to people or property resulting from any ideas, methods, instructions or products referred to in the content.

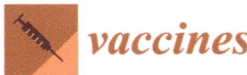 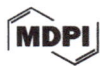

Article

Inequitable Distribution of Global Economic Benefits from Pneumococcal Conjugate Vaccination

Fulgence Niyibitegeka [1,*], Fiona M. Russell [2,3], Mark Jit [4] and Natalie Carvalho [1,2]

1. Centre for Health Policy, Melbourne School of Population and Global Health, The University of Melbourne, Carlton, VIC 3053, Australia; natalie.carvalho@unimelb.edu.au
2. Asia-Pacific Health, Murdoch Children's Research Institute, Melbourne, VIC 3052, Australia; fmruss@unimelb.edu.au
3. Centre for International Child Health, Department of Paediatrics, The University of Melbourne, Parkville, VIC 3052, Australia
4. Department of Infectious Disease Epidemiology, London School of Hygiene and Tropical Medicine, London WC1H 9SH, UK; mark.jit@lshtm.ac.uk
* Correspondence: fulgence.niyibitegeka@student.unimelb.edu.au

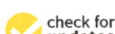

Citation: Niyibitegeka, F.; Russell, F.M.; Jit, M.; Carvalho, N. Inequitable Distribution of Global Economic Benefits from Pneumococcal Conjugate Vaccination. *Vaccines* **2024**, *12*, 767. https://doi.org/10.3390/vaccines12070767

Academic Editors: Ahmad Reza Hosseinpoor, M. Carolina Danovaro, Devaki Nambiar, Hope L. Johnson, Ciara Sugerman and Nicole Bergen

Received: 5 June 2024
Revised: 27 June 2024
Accepted: 4 July 2024
Published: 12 July 2024

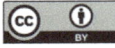

Copyright: © 2024 by the authors. Licensee MDPI, Basel, Switzerland. This article is an open access article distributed under the terms and conditions of the Creative Commons Attribution (CC BY) license (https://creativecommons.org/licenses/by/4.0/).

Abstract: Many low- and middle-income countries have been slow to introduce the pneumococcal conjugate vaccine (PCV) into their routine childhood immunization schedules despite a high burden of disease. We estimated the global economic surplus of PCV, defined as the sum of the net value to 194 countries (i.e., monetized health benefits minus net costs) and to vaccine manufacturers (i.e., profits). We further explored the distribution of global economic surplus across country income groups and manufacturers and the effect of different pricing strategies based on cross-subsidization, pooled procurement, and various tiered pricing mechanisms. We found that current PCV pricing policies disproportionately benefit high-income countries and manufacturers. Based on the 2021 birth cohort, high-income countries and manufacturers combined received 76.5% of the net economic benefits generated by the vaccine. Over the two decades of PCV availability, low- and middle-income countries have not received the full economic benefits of PCV. Cross-subsidization of the vaccine price for low- and middle-income countries and pooled procurement policies that would relate the vaccine price to the value of economic benefits generated for each country could reduce these inequalities. This analysis offers important considerations that may improve the equitable introduction and use of new and under-utilized vaccines.

Keywords: vaccine pricing; inequitable vaccine uptake; fair prices; pricing policy

1. Introduction

Pneumonia remains one of the leading causes of childhood mortality, responsible for over 700,000 childhood deaths in 2021, with more than 50% of these deaths occurring in sub-Saharan Africa and south-east Asia [1–4]. While pneumococcal conjugate vaccine (PCV) has substantially reduced childhood morbidity and mortality [4], adoption into Expanded Programs on Immunization (EPI) around the world has been uneven and country income-dependent [5]. PCV was first introduced in high-income countries (HICs) in the early 2000s [5,6]. In 2007, the World Health Organization (WHO) issued a recommendation for all countries to include PCV in their EPI [7]. With financial support from Gavi, the Vaccine Alliance, many low-income countries (LICs) have introduced PCV. Similarly, many countries in Latin America have introduced PCV with support for negotiated prices through the Pan American Health Organization (PAHO). However, by the end of 2021, only 148 out of 194 WHO member states had included PCV in national or subnational immunization programs [8,9], and approximately half (49%) of the global birth cohort had not received all recommended PCV doses by age 5, with the majority of these under-vaccinated children living in low- and middle-income countries [9]. In particular, middle-income countries

(MICs) that lack support from Gavi or PAHO and self-procure vaccines have lagged furthest in terms of vaccine introduction despite bearing the majority of the global pneumococcal disease burden [5].

PCV has been found to be cost-effective or cost-saving in most countries [10–12]. Nevertheless, alongside cost-effectiveness, considerations around vaccine price, affordability, financing, and financial sustainability are key drivers in decision making regarding the introduction of and sustaining new vaccines into the EPI [13]. Unlike childhood vaccines that have been included as part of the EPI for decades, PCV is an expensive vaccine. A recent report from the WHO's Market Information for Access to Vaccines (MI4A) initiative reported that the high price of PCV was mentioned by respondents in many MICs as a major barrier to introduction [14]. An affordability analysis conducted by the WHO in 32 non-Gavi, non-PAHO MICs found that adding PCV to the vaccine schedule may be financially challenging in 6 of these countries, where introduction would require an estimated 53–87% increase to the existing immunization budget [14].

To achieve the WHO's Immunization Agenda 2030 (IA2030) [15], there is an increasing need for strategic pricing policies to ensure vaccine affordability in every country, regardless of income. Current formal pooled procurement policies are available through Gavi, which negotiates the lowest prices in the world for the poorest countries and further subsidizes vaccine purchase costs, and PAHO's Revolving Fund, which allows countries in the PAHO region to access the second lowest prices. However, self-procuring MICs outside the PAHO region and those ineligible or that have transitioned from Gavi support [16] do not have recourse to these mechanisms. Some still access discounted (but higher) prices through the United Nations Children's Fund (UNICEF), while other countries self-procure vaccines at prices similar to or sometimes higher than HICs [17].

The inequitable PCV uptake across countries is well-known as UNICEF and the WHO publish global vaccine coverage data every year [9]. However, the inequality in net societal value produced by PCV across countries and the extent to which the distribution of this value is influenced by current pricing and procurement policies remain less understood. To our knowledge, no study has explored the economic surplus of PCV. The economic surplus of a new technology or vaccine (which can also be referred to as the net societal value or total social welfare) is the sum of the consumer surplus (net economic benefits retained by consumers, in this case, countries, after paying for the vaccine) and the producer surplus (profits made by producers/manufacturers after recovering the cost of production) [18]. The aims of this analysis were to estimate the global economic surplus of PCV and its distribution using an approach that has been utilized previously for the human papillomavirus (HPV) vaccine [19]. Furthermore, we describe the effect of different pricing strategies on the distribution of economic surplus across country income groups and vaccine manufacturers.

2. Methods

2.1. Study Design

We used a previously defined framework to estimate the net societal value, total social welfare, or global economic surplus of PCV [19]. As illustrated in Figure 1, the global economic surplus consisted of the sum of the net economic benefits to countries as consumers of PCV and the net economic benefits to manufacturers as producers and sellers. The net economic benefit to countries (consumer surplus) was made up of the monetized health benefits of vaccination minus the costs of the vaccination program, while the net benefits to vaccine manufacturers (producer surplus) were calculated as the revenue from PCV sales minus the cost of developing, manufacturing, marketing, and distributing the vaccine.

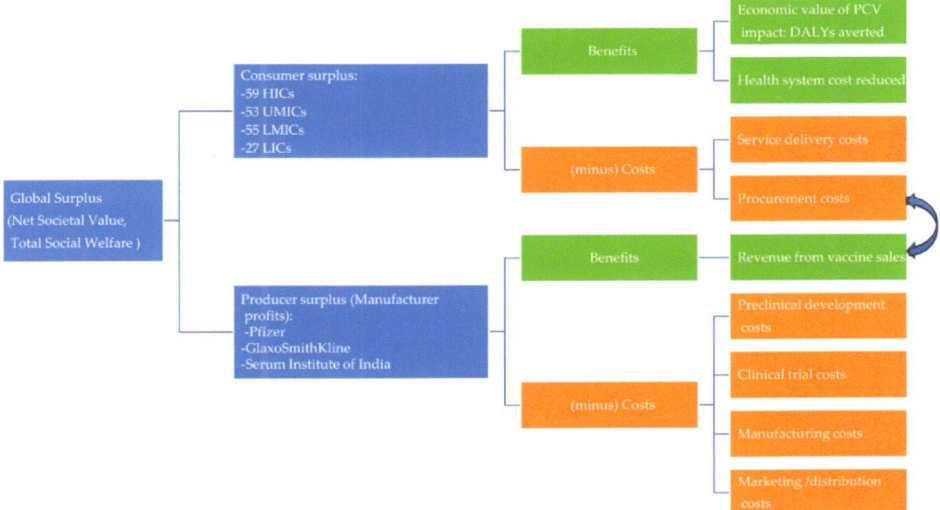

Figure 1. Conceptual framework showing how the global economic surplus for PCV is calculated. **1.** Note: Green boxes indicate benefits and orange boxes indicate costs. **2.** Abbreviations: LICs, low-income countries; LMICs, lower-middle-income countries; UMICs, upper-middle-income countries; HICs, high-income countries; DALYs, disability-adjusted life years.

To estimate the consumer surplus, we valued benefits and costs for 194 countries and territories grouped by income category—high-income countries (HICs), upper-middle-income countries (UMICs), lower-middle-income countries (LMICs), and low-income countries (LICs)—based on World Bank classification for the year 2021 [20]. For the producer component of economic surplus, we valued benefits and costs for all 3 manufacturers of PCV already prequalified by the WHO [21], i.e., 13-valent PCV manufactured by Pfizer (PCV-13, Prev(e)nar 13®), a 10-valent PCV manufactured by GlaxoSmithKline (PCV-10 GSK, Synflorix®), and a 10-valent PCV manufactured by Serum Institute of India (PCV-10 SII, Pneumosil®), acknowledging that there are other PCVs under development and nationally being licensed for use [21,22].

2.1.1. Consumer Surplus

Benefits: Benefits of PCV to the consumer included the monetized value of health benefits measured in terms of disability-adjusted life years (DALYs) averted and healthcare system cost savings resulting from reduced disease burden. To estimate the disease burden reduction by PCV, we used a previously validated model that estimated vaccine effectiveness in terms of incidence rate ratio (IRR) for four clinical outcomes of pneumococcal disease: meningitis (with and without sequelae), pneumonia (invasive and non-invasive), invasive non-pneumonia non-meningitis (NPNM) pneumococcal disease, and acute otitis media (AOM) [10]. We further estimated the total health system cost consisting of the diagnosis, treatment, and services cost to manage each clinical presentation in both the scenario with and without the PCV program. Briefly, the model used a population-based approach and incorporated both the carriage and serotypes coverage data to predict the incidence rate ratios of different clinical presentations of pneumococcal diseases. By using a variety of assumptions, the model condensed the long-term impact projections from more complex susceptible–infectious–susceptible-type dynamic transmission models into a single predictive equation, including serotype replacement and herd immunity. The number of cases of pneumococcal disease and the deaths were estimated by multiplying the expected disease events rate by the IRR adjusted by immunization coverage. The model predictions were based on PCV13-specific serotypes and carriage data. We used interchangeably the PCV impact for both PCV10 and PCV13 and for any dosing schedule assuming non-inferiority across PCVs and dosing schedules, as a recent systematic review found that long-term PCV impact (5 years after PCV10/13 introduction) on pneumococcal disease was similar for PCV10 and PCV13 [23,24].

Overall, model input parameters were derived from various sources, including global meta-analysis studies [4,10,25,26], systematic reviews [27–29], and electronic databases [30,31] (Table 1). To allow the comparison of the health benefits across countries with different timelines of vaccine introduction, benefits were based on vaccine impact from baseline prior to PCV introduction using country-specific epidemiological disease burden [26]. For simplicity, this analysis was restricted to children under five years; we did not consider the indirect impacts of childhood PCV programs on older age groups or adult vaccination programs. More details about the model, input parameters, and methodological assumptions are provided in the Supplementary Materials. Total DALYs averted were converted into monetary values using country-specific opportunity cost-based thresholds [32]. This approach assumes that PCV programs are government-funded, and funds spent on PCV could have alternatively been directed toward other healthcare programs capable of preventing an equivalent number of DALYs within each country. Other approaches to convert health benefits into economic value were explored in sensitivity analysis, as described below.

Cost of PCV program: The cost of the vaccination program to the consumer was estimated from the provider's perspective and included the cost of vaccine acquisition and administration. The costs of vaccine acquisition, which included the vaccine purchasing cost and freight cost as well as the cost of injection supplies, were estimated from various sources, including a UNICEF database [33], PAHO database [34], and WHO Market information for access to vaccines (MI4A) database [31]. The delivery cost per dose for any individual country was derived from a recent global modeling study estimating immunization delivery costs across 194 countries [35]. Key model inputs are shown in Table 1, and further details are provided in the Supplementary Materials.

Table 1. Model input parameters and sources.

Parameter Description	HICs	UMICs	LMICs	LICs	Source
2021 Birth cohort (million)	12.6	27	70.7	24.2	UN Population Division [30]
Baseline pre-PCV introduction disease burden incidence rate (per 100,0000 children)					
Meningitis	9	13	21	33	O'Brien et al., 2009 [26]
IPD NPNM	52	73	108	166	O'Brien et al., 2009 [26]
Pneumonia	975	1305	2339	3169	O'Brien et al., 2009 [26]
AOM	8984	12,031	14,085	22,330	Monasta et al., 2012 [25]
Mortality rate (per 100,000 children)					
Meningitis	4	8	13	24	O'Brien et al., 2009 [26]
IPD NPNM	3	4	5	7	O'Brien et al., 2009 [26]
Pneumonia	44	77	166	312	O'Brien et al., 2009 [26]
Vaccine impact and effectiveness estimates					
Vaccine impact on IPD < 1 year after vaccination (IRR)	0.63	0.65	0.71	0.74	Chen et al., 2019 [10]
Vaccine impact on IPD > 1 year after vaccination (IRR)	0.53	0.56	0.63	0.67	Chen et al., 2019 [10]
Vaccine impact on non-invasive pneumonia (IRR)	0.80	0.80	0.80	0.80	Canevari et al., 2024 [36]
Vaccine effectiveness against AOM (RR)	0.90	0.90	0.90	0.90	Wannarong et al., 2023 [37]
PCV coverage (2021)	87	39	45	64	WHO/UNICEF [38]
PCV program costs (USD 2021)					
Vaccine delivery cost	18.86	5.94	3.28	1.39	Sriudomporn et al., 2023 [35]
Vaccine price per dose	30.83	16.62	8.99	2.92	UNICEF [33], PAHO Revolving Fund [34], WHO MI4A [31]
Wastage rate (%)	5	5	5	5	UNICEF [33]
Buffer stock (%)	25	25	25	25	UNICEF [33]
Disease management costs (USD 2021)					
Health system cost of pneumonia	3305	1072	481	80	Portnoy et al., 2015; the World Bank; WHO [27–29]

Table 1. Cont.

Parameter Description	HICs	UMICs	LMICs	LICs	Source
Health system cost of meningitis	12,730	6646	2938	668	Portnoy et al., 2015 [27], Chen et al., 2019 [10]
Health system cost IPD NPNM	6111	3497	1417	329	Chen et al., 2019 [10]
Health system cost of AOM	141	51	21	6	Chen et al., 2019 [10]
Health service utilization (%)					
Meningitis	100	100	100	100	Chen et al., 2019 [10]
IPD NPNM	100	100	100	100	Chen et al., 2019 [10]
Pneumonia	100	72	63	53	UNICEF [3]
AOM	85	66	59	54	Chen et al., 2019 [10]
Disability weights					
Pneumonia	0.28	0.28	0.28	0.28	Neonatal pneumonia" in GBD "Mathers et al. 2006 [39]
Meningitis	0.62	0.62	0.62	0.62	Meningitis, S. pneumonia in GBD—Mathers et al. 2006 [39]
IPD NPNM	0.15	0.15	0.15	0.15	Meningococcaemia without meningitis in GBD—Mathers et al. 2006 [39]
AOM	0.013	0.013	0.013	0.013	Otitis media in GBD—Mathers 2006 [39]
Meningitis sequelae	0.06	0.06	0.06	0.06	Meningitis sequelae in GBD—Mathers et al., 2006 (43)
Duration of morbidity (days)					
Pneumonia	7	7	7	7	Ojal et al. [40]
Meningitis	15	15	15	15	Ojal et al. [40]
Meningitis sequelae	Lifetime	Lifetime	Lifetime	Lifetime	Edmond et al. [41], Lucas et al. [42]
IPD NPNM	15	15	15	15	Ojal et al. [40]
AOM	3	3	3	3	Little et al., 2001 [43]

1. Abbreviations: AOM, acute otitis media; IPD, invasive pneumococcal disease; NPNM, non-pneumonia non-meningitis; GBD, global burden of disease; LICs, low-income countries; LMICs, lower-middle-income countries; UMICs, upper-middle-income countries; HICs, high-income countries; IRR, incidence rate ratio; RR, relative ratio; PCV, pneumococcal conjugate vaccine. 2. Note: The parameters in the table are for comparison purposes between the income groups and are aggregated across country-specific estimates used in the model (except vaccine characteristics, wastage, risk of meningitis sequelae, disability weights, and duration of morbidity). Aggregation per income group was performed using the average weighted by the under-five population size except for per capita GDP, where the average was weighted by the total population size in 2021. Effectiveness data for IPD presented by income group is a breakdown of the original predictions, which were presented by regions (see Table S1 of Supplementary Materials).

2.1.2. Manufacturer Surplus

Manufacturer benefits: Data on vaccine sales were collected using publicly available annual reports released by each vaccine manufacturer in the United States Securities and Exchange Commission databases or vaccine manufacturers' companies' websites [44,45]. We extracted all the revenue made by each vaccine manufacturer from 2000 to 2021. For Pneumosil®, we extracted vaccine sales from the WHO MI4A database [17] as it was not reported to SEC.

Cost to manufacturers: The cost of research and development (R&D), including the cost of failure for products that failed to reach market approval, was estimated over the entire development period from preclinical development to post-marketing evaluation based on an approach recently used in previous papers [19,46,47]. The cost of clinical trials was estimated based on the number and size of all clinical trials conducted for each vaccine. A literature review was conducted to identify all PCV-related phase I, II, III, and IV clinical trials funded/sponsored by each manufacturer or subsidiary (see details in the Supplementary Materials). Estimated total R&D cost was later compared with the total revenues made from the first year (2000) of PCV entry to the market up to 2021 to evaluate the manufacturer's return on investment [45]. A positive return on investment indicated a profitable investment in vaccine development. We further annualized the development cost, assuming a gradual and progressive recovery of the investment over the entire period of patent protection expiring in 2026 [45]. The total cost to manufacturers was therefore estimated as the sum of annual R&D cost and the cost of manufacturing, marketing, and distributing the total number of PCV doses required to vaccinate the 2021 birth cohort in each scenario of the analysis. Further details of the methods to estimate each cost component from the manufacturer's perspective are provided in the Supplementary Materials.

2.2. Analysis

All cost estimates were converted to 2021 US dollars (USD). Estimated revenues were inflated to 2021 USD using the respective consumer price indexes. In the base case analysis, a discount rate of 3% was applied to future costs and health outcomes as per WHO vaccine evaluation guidelines [48]. We relied on coverage rates achieved by individual countries in 2021 to estimate the current global social welfare and distribution of economic surplus across country income groups and manufacturers. Additionally, we conducted a hypothetical scenario analysis to explore the potential outcomes if at least 90% of the birth cohort across all countries was vaccinated to align with the Immunization Agenda 2030 (IA 2030) global target [15]. Finally, we explored the impact of various alternative pricing scenarios (described below) on the distribution of economic surplus, assuming the IA 2030 coverage target was met.

2.2.1. Sensitivity Analysis

We explored the effect of changes to base case parameters and assumptions. First, we explored the effect of different approaches to monetize health benefits: using a human capital-based approach (1xGDP per capita per DALY averted) and the full income approach, adopted in 2013 by a Lancet Commission in "Global Health 2035" (2.3 times GDP per capita per DALY averted) [49]. The human capital approach is based on the impact of improved health on productivity and earnings and quantifies the economic value of health by considering increased lifespan, reduced medical costs, and higher work productivity. The full income approach extends beyond basic assessments of health relative to per capita gross domestic product (GDP) or foregone earnings and values health by considering both monetary and non-monetary aspects of well-being, acknowledging that health contributes to overall quality of life. More details on the economic valuation of health benefits were previously explored by Herlihy [19]. Second, we looked at how discounting affects our findings. The recent WHO update guide on discounting rates recommends presenting results with two scenarios: one applying a 3% discount rate for both health benefits and costs (which is applied in our base case analysis) and an alternative applying a zero-discount rate to health benefits and a 3% discount rate to costs [50]. We then considered a scenario using a zero-discount rate for health benefits, valuing them the same as present benefits while applying a 3% discount rate to costs. Further, we considered a scenario where future costs and benefits were discounted at a higher rate (5%) each year to reflect values considered in some countries (e.g., Australia) [51]. Third, we explored the effect of uncertainty in vaccine impact estimates as reported in the global modeling study to account for the sparsity of carriage data and heterogeneity of serotype distribution across regions [10]. Hence, we varied vaccine impact on pneumococcal diseases by using the 95% uncertainty interval (lower and upper bounds) from Chen's study to account for uncertainty related to modeled IRR estimates for vaccine effectiveness [10].

2.2.2. Alternative Pricing Scenario Analysis

We considered the effect of different pricing strategies, including pooled procurement mechanisms, subsidization, and value-based tiered pricing. First, we considered a scenario where all UMICs, LMICs, and LICs access PCV at the Pneumosil® price (USD 1.5) offered to Gavi-eligible countries. Second, we explored a scenario where all Gavi-ineligible MICs would receive the vaccine at the PAHO price (USD 14.14). Third, we explored a scenario based on cross-subsidization of vaccine prices for LICs and LMICs either by HICs or manufacturers. To explore the greatest extent to which this policy could affect the distribution of economic surplus, we explore the most generous but unlikely scenario of zero procurement cost for these countries, either at the cost of HICs or manufacturers. Fourth, we applied the US private market price to self-procurement HICs and UMICs. Finally, we kept the manufacturer's revenue unchanged and assumed all countries accessed the vaccine at the same price in the absence of any tiered pricing arrangements.

3. Results

3.1. Manufacturer Return on Investment

From 2000 to 2021, the total manufacturer revenue from PCV sales was USD 91.74 billion (Table 2). Pfizer received the greatest revenue (USD 66 billion) from the sales of Prevnar 13®, while its subsidiary Wyeth received the second largest share (USD 17.77 billion) from the sales of Prevnar 7® followed by GSK with revenue of USD 7.88 billion from the sales of Synflorix®. Serum Institute of India (SII) received the least revenue of USD 0.09 billion from the sales of Pneumosil®.

Table 2. Manufacturer revenue (million 2021 USD).

Year	Prevnar 7® (Wyeth)	Prevnar13® (Wyeth-Pfizer)	Synflorix® (GSK)	Pneumosil® (SII)
2021	n/a	5272.00	491.02	86.91
2020	n/a	6124.83	539.60	6.12
2019	n/a	6197.22	633.14	n/a
2018	n/a	6260.95	610.43	n/a
2017	n/a	6191.67	724.19	n/a
2016	n/a	6455.67	768.29	n/a
2015	n/a	7139.60	665.47	n/a
2014	n/a	5109.53	749.60	n/a
2013	n/a	4622.46	736.46	n/a
2012	n/a	4858.94	717.77	n/a
2011	n/a	4405.36	675.53	n/a
2010	n/a	3002.27	424.35	n/a
2009	n/a	362.49	143.64	n/a
2009	1942.56	n/a	n/a	n/a
2008	3429.80	n/a	n/a	n/a
2007	3080.69	n/a	n/a	n/a
2006	2477.21	n/a	n/a	n/a
2005	1905.05	n/a	n/a	n/a
2004	1330.74	n/a	n/a	n/a
2003	1194.34	n/a	n/a	n/a
2002	817.82	n/a	n/a	n/a
2001	1008.16	n/a	n/a	n/a
2000	581.76	n/a	n/a	n/a
Total revenue by brand	17,768.15	66,003.01	7879.47	93.02
Total revenue for all PCVs	91,743.65			

Abbreviations: GSK, GlaxoSmithKline; SII, Serum Institute of India; n/a, not applicable; PCV, pneumococcal conjugate vaccine.

As for the cost of PCVs to manufacturers, the results indicate that the total clinical development cost of all pre-qualified PCVs, accounting for the probability of failure in vaccine development, was estimated to be USD 1.4 billion. The cost of the preclinical phase of vaccine development was estimated to be approximately USD 0.6 billion (see Supplementary Table S2). Assuming the total preclinical cost was funded by the vaccine manufacturers, we estimated the total R&D cost to be about USD 2.035 billion. Specifically, the cost of development of PCV was USD 0.50 billion for Prevnar 7®, USD 0.77 billion for Prevnar 13®, USD 0.73 billion for Synflorix®, and USD 0.04 billion for Pneumosil®. For the purpose of comparison, from 2000 to 2015, the amount of public funding that was invested in pneumococcal vaccine-related research from preclinical development to public health research was estimated to be USD 857.5 million [52]. This amount represents 339 individual grants awarded to diverse institutions across the globe [52].

Compared with the total R&D cost, manufacturers altogether would have made a return on investment of about 45 times. Similarly to previous studies [19], these findings indicate that the high research and development expenditures can be quickly fully recovered by high revenues from the vaccine sales, particularly to HICs like the United States, where the price of PCV was listed as USD 150.83 per dose in 2021 [53].

3.2. Economic Surplus per Vaccinated Cohort

A total of 133.47 million live births were included in the analysis. LICs and LMICs combined represented 71% of the global birth cohort. A total of approximately 5.9 million DALYs were averted in 2021 due to PCVs. The largest share of DALYs averted was in LICs (36.6%) and LMICs (50.0%). PCV was cost-effective in all country income groups when comparing assumed vaccine prices to the average threshold cost in each country income group. The cost per DALY avoided was lowest in LICs and LMICs. Based on the 2021 vaccine uptake, the global economic surplus generated from PCV was estimated to be USD 15.9 billion. HICs and manufacturers received the largest share of the economic surplus at 47.9% and 28.7%, respectively. Of the total manufacturers' economic surplus, Pfizer received more than 96%. The economic surplus per vaccinated child was estimated to be USD 752 in HICs as compared to USD 120 in UMICs, USD 62 in LMICs, and USD 31 in LICs (Table 3).

Table 3. Calculation of share of global economic surplus of PCV accrued to different actors, based on 2021 PCV coverage.

Outcome	Global	Consumer				Manufacturer		
		HICs	UMICs	LMICs	LICs	Pfizer	GSK	SII
Birth cohort (2021) (million)	133.47	11.59	26.99	70.65	24.24	n/a	n/a	n/a
Share of birth cohort (%)	100%	9%	20%	53%	18%	n/a	n/a	n/a
DALYs averted (million)	5.90	0.34	0.45	2.95	2.16	n/a	n/a	n/a
Share of DALYs averted	100.0%	5.8%	7.6%	50.0%	36.6%	n/a	n/a	n/a
Healthcare cost savings (million)	518.59	392.95	68.08	48.04	9.52	n/a	n/a	n/a
Cost of PCV program (million)	7202.62	4991.89	968.90	996.49	245.35	880.78	347.73	66.03
Benefits of the vaccine (million)	18,026.90	12,210.21	2168.96	2933.21	714.51	5272.00	491.02	86.91
Cost per DALY averted	1132.76	13,347.13	2015.87	321.68	109.14	n/a	n/a	n/a
Average threshold (USD/DALY averted)	7601	31,816	6829	1317	326	n/a	n/a	n/a
Economic surplus (million)	15,898.25	7611.28	1268.14	1984.77	478.69	4391.22	143.28	20.87
Share of global surplus (%)	100%	47.9%	8.0%	12.5%	3.0%	27.6%	0.9%	0.1%
Economic surplus per immunized child	232	752	120	62	31	97	6	2

1. Note: Costs, economic benefits, and surpluses are in 2021 USD; n/a: not applicable. 2. Abbreviations: LICs, low-income countries; LMICs, lower-middle-income countries; UMICs, upper-middle-income countries; HICs, high-income countries; DALYs, disability-adjusted life years; GSK, GlaxoSmithKline; SII, Serum Institute of India; PCV, pneumococcal conjugate vaccine.

3.2.1. Distribution of Economic Surplus and Sensitivity Analysis

The distribution of the economic surplus among countries and manufacturers varied across different sensitivity analyses. Overall, the share of economic surplus going to LICs remained relatively small, under 6% of the total global surplus (Table 4). This share did not change much when a different monetization rate of DALYs averted was used (either 1 or 2.3 times GDP per capita), with a slightly larger portion of the surplus going to consumers, particularly HICs. Unlike the situation without any discounting, the increased discounting rate reduced the global net consumer benefit to the benefit of the manufacturer. However, the inequitable distribution among consumers (countries' income groups) remained substantial, disproportionately benefiting HICs. The greatest change in the distribution of economic surplus was observed in the sensitivity analysis on vaccine impact on different serotypes. When the estimated vaccine impact was reduced to the lower bound of its 95% confidence interval, a greater portion of the economic surplus went to manufacturers to the detriment of consumers, particularly those in LMICs; the share of the economic surplus received by LICs was less than 1% in this sensitivity analysis.

Table 4. Distribution of economic surplus and sensitivity analysis.

Analyses	Global Value	HICs Value	HICs Share	UMICs Value	UMICs Share	LMICs Value	LMICs Share	LICs Value	LICs Share	Manufacturer Value	Manufacturer Share
Birth cohort (2021) (million)	133	12	8.7%	27	20.2%	71	52.9%	24	18.2%	n/a	n/a
Base case	15,898	7611	47.9%	1268	8.0%	1985	12.5%	479	3.0%	4555	28.7%
Sensitivity analysis											
Valuation of health at 1XGDP per capita	26,451	12,932	48.9%	2665	10.1%	5010	18.9%	1288	4.9%	4555	17.2%
Valuation of health at 2.3XGDP per capita	63,603	35,722	56.2%	7301	11.5%	12,756	20.1%	3269	5.1%	4555	7.2%
0% discount rate to health benefits and 3% discount rate to costs	43,314	27,305	63.0%	4253	9.8%	5825	13.4%	1375	3.2%	4555	10.5%
5% discount rate to health benefits and costs	9638	3290	34.1%	536	5.6%	1012	10.5%	244	2.5%	4555	47.3%
Vaccine impact increased (95% CI)	21,080	9854	46.7%	2018	9.6%	3736	17.7%	917	4.3%	4555	21.6%
Vaccine impact reduced (95% CI)	10,511	5136	48.9%	513	4.9%	245	2.3%	61	0.6%	4555	43.3%

1. Note: Values of economic surpluses are in million 2021 USD. 2. Abbreviations: LICs, low-income countries; LMICs, lower-middle-income countries; UMICs, upper-middle-income countries; HICs, high-income countries; GDP, gross domestic product; n/a, not applicable.

3.2.2. Distribution of Economic Surplus under IA2030 Aspirational Coverage Scenario

With the IA2030 coverage target, about 9.1 million DALYs would have been averted in 2021, compared to 5.9 million DALYs using actual 2021 coverage, an additional 3.2 million DALYs averted. Overall, scaling up global PCV coverage to at least 90% would roughly increase the economic surplus to both the manufacturers and consumers, particularly middle-income countries, and would almost double the economic surplus. Globally, the total economic surplus would roughly increase from USD 15.9 billion to USD 20.9 billion. However, HICs and manufacturers would still share more than 68% of the surplus generated by the vaccination (Table 5). This indicates that increasing vaccine coverage without changing vaccine price would have little impact on the inequitable distribution of the economic surplus across country income groups and manufacturers.

Table 5. Calculation of share of economic surplus of PCV based on IA2030 aspirational coverage.

Outcome	Global	HICs	UMICs	LMICs	LICs	Manufacturer
Birth cohort (2021) (million)	133.47	11.59	26.99	70.65	24.24	133
Share of birth cohort	100%	9%	20%	53%	18%	n/a
DALYs averted (million)	9.12	0.36	0.87	4.94	2.94	n/a
Share of DALYs averted	100.0%	4.0%	9.6%	54.2%	32.3%	n/a
Healthcare cost savings (million)	704.73	418.90	144.38	128.28	13.17	n/a
Cost of PCV program (million)	10,505.22	5346.39	2399.24	2418.27	341.32	2000.76
Benefits of the vaccine (million)	24,511.80	13,059.80	4834.17	5643.33	974.50	8231.69
Cost per DALY averted	1074.64	13,532.34	2581.88	463.62	111.50	n/a
Average threshold (USD/DALY averted)	7601	31,816	6829	1317	326	n/a
Economic surplus (million)	20,942.24	8132.31	2579.31	3353.34	646.35	6230.93
Share of global surplus (%)	100%	38.8%	12.3%	16.0%	3.1%	29.8%
Economic surplus per immunized child	173	763	106	52	30	52

1. Note: Costs, economic benefits, and surpluses are in 2021 USD. 2. Abbreviations: LICs, low-income countries; LMICs, lower-middle-income countries; UMICs, upper-middle-income countries; HICs, high-income countries; DALYs, disability-adjusted life years; n/a, not applicable; PCV, pneumococcal conjugate vaccine.

3.2.3. Effect of Pricing Scenarios on the Distribution of Economic Surplus

Overall, the greatest change across alternative pricing scenarios was seen when the full retail price was applied to all self-procurement countries (Table 6). This scenario would dramatically reduce the consumer surplus and increase the manufacturer surplus, with many middle-income countries paying more for vaccination than the value they received in return. If tiered pricing was not used at all, then low-income countries' share of the surplus would drop. Allocating explicit subsidies to lower-middle- and low-income countries resulted in a notable increase in the surplus for these countries, either at the expense of high-income countries or manufacturers. We found that even with the most generous subsidies, which effectively would eliminate vaccine procurement costs for low- and lower-middle-income countries, the economic surplus captured by high-income countries would only decrease from 47.9% to 27.5%, or by manufacturers from 28.7% to 19.9%. Additionally, if HICs subsidized vaccine costs for LICs and LMICs, then HICs would need to pay up to USD 117.20 per dose, assuming the manufacturer surplus is unchanged.

Table 6. Effect of pricing scenarios on the distribution of economic surplus.

Analyses	Global	HICs Value	HICs Share	UMICs Value	UMICs Share	LMICs Value	LMICs Share	LICs Value	LICs Share	Manufacturer Value	Manufacturer Share
Birth cohort (2021) (million)	133	12	8.7%	27	20.2%	71	52.9%	24	18.2%	n/a	n/a
Economic surplus (million USD)											
Base case	15,898	7611	47.9%	1268	8.0%	1985	12.5%	479	3.0%	4555	28.7%
Hypothetical IA2030 coverage achieved	20,942	8132	38.8%	2579	12.3%	3353	16.0%	646	3.1%	6231	29.8%
Pricing scenario analysis on top of IA2030 coverage											
1. All LMICs and LICs pay the tail Gavi price for Pneumosil® (USD 1.5)	21,590	8132	37.7%	4596	21.3%	5044	23.4%	780	3.6%	3038	14.1%
2. All MICs Gavi-ineligible pay the PAHO price (USD 14.14)	21,077	8132	38.6%	3252	15.4%	3476	16.5%	646	3.1%	5570	26.4%
3a. LICs and LMICs fully subsidized by HICs	20,939	5750	27.5%	2579	12.3%	5459	26.1%	920	4.4%	6231	29.8%
3b. LICs and LMICs fully subsidized by manufacturers	21,342	8132	38.1%	2579	12.1%	5459	25.6%	920	4.3%	4251	19.9%
4. Retail price to all self-procurement HICs and UMICs (USD 211.86)	17,445	1621	9.3%	−11,610	−66.5%	3353	19.2%	646	3.7%	23,434	134.3%
5. All countries pay the same price to maintain constant manufacturer surplus (USD 17.02)	20,956	11,689	55.8%	2950	14.1%	748	3.6%	−662	−3.2%	6231	29.8%

1. Note: Values of economic surpluses are in 2021 USD. 2. Abbreviations: LICs, low-income countries; LMICs, lower-middle-income countries; MICs, middle-income countries; UMICs, upper-middle-income countries; HICs, high-income countries; IA2030, Immunization Agenda 2030; n/a, not applicable; PAHO, Pan American Health Organization.

4. Discussion

Our findings indicate that at current PCV pricing and uptake, HICs and manufacturers receive the largest share of the economic surplus generated by PCV. Even at 90% coverage, at current prices, low- and middle-income countries would still receive the lowest share of the economic surplus. These findings are consistent with previous findings for the HPV vaccine [19]. One explanation for this similarity may be that the market supply for both vaccines has been dominated by only two manufacturers (Pfizer and GSK for the PCV and GSK and Merck for the HPV vaccine) based in HICs until recently. Due to a lack of competition, higher prices were set throughout the initial life cycle of the first generation of vaccines before the recent entry into the market of new suppliers based in low- and middle-income countries, such as Pneumosil. Furthermore, even though PCV13 was based on its precursor, PCV7, it came to the market at an even higher price [45].

We found even higher levels of inequality in the distribution of economic surplus across country income groups compared to what was estimated for the HPV vaccine. Based on 2015 prices, Herlihy found that per child vaccinated, HICs received two times, four times, and five times the HPV vaccine economic surplus of UMICs, LMICs, and LICs, respectively [19]. Our findings indicate that, based on 2021 PCV prices, HICs received 6 times, 12 times, and 24 times the PCV economic surplus of UMICs, LMICs, and LICs, respectively.

To reduce this inequity, innovative pricing policies, among other strategies, are required if the full benefits of PCV are to be achieved globally and, in particular, for those with the highest burden. An affordable vaccine price can be achieved through buyer-led (for example, pooled procurement mechanisms or joint efforts to subsidize vaccine purchase cost) or manufacturer-driven (for example, greater tiered pricing) initiatives [54]. In an effort to address the high cost of vaccines and crowding of the current EPI schedule, clinical trials have been completed for PCV10 and PCV13 to evaluate the potential for using two rather than three PCV doses and the use of fractional doses for PCV [55–58]. These trials have been funded by philanthropy or public funds. Additionally, over the past two decades, there have been several developments in fair vaccine pricing policies and mechanisms, such as Gavi negotiating lower prices for eligible countries via its advance market commitment (AMC) [59], an innovative financing mechanism intended to guarantee a market for pharmaceutical companies for the development of new vaccines. Another example includes the new Gavi MICs strategy adopted in December 2020 to address some key issues related to new vaccine introduction with a focus on PCV, rotavirus vaccine, and HPV in some former Gavi-eligible countries [60]. However, there remains a large, unaddressed gap in providing solutions for equitable pricing and procurement [61] for MICs, some of which have been paying even higher vaccine prices than HICs [17,61]. Despite calls by organizations including Médecins Sans Frontières (MSF) for price reductions [62], median PCV prices increased by 43% from 2019 to 2021 for self-procurement MICs, according to the WHO MI4A report [17]. In recognition of this, the World Society for Pediatric Infectious Diseases has launched a Call to Action for fairer vaccine prices [61].

While existing PCV 10 and PCV 13 with WHO prequalification remain underutilized in low- and middle-income countries, HICs are already transitioning to higher-valency PCVs [63,64]. As the use of these higher-valency PCVs increases, the incremental cost-effectiveness of the vaccines will change. Consequently, the model inputs will need to be updated based on the effectiveness of these new vaccines. These extended valency PCVs that are currently in the market in HICs or under development will provide additional protection for up to 25 serotypes. Although the vaccine costs for these are not known, it is highly likely they will be even more expensive, and therefore, the adoption of these vaccines by low- and middle-income countries will be delayed, and this will further drive inequity.

Our results indicate that the distribution of consumer surplus is more equitable if prices are tiered compared to scenarios without tiered pricing. We found that if all countries paid the same (high) price for PCV, the total consumer surplus would shrink, and many countries, particularly low- and middle-income countries, would be paying more than the value of the vaccine benefits. Our analysis based on 2021 tiered prices indicates that the majority of benefits still favor HICs and manufacturers, highlighting the insufficiency of current tiered pricing to fully address the existing inequitable distribution of social welfare from PCV across countries and manufacturers. Additionally, the mechanism by which prices are set for self-procuring countries is unclear [65]. This study implies that one potential solution to achieve equitable distribution of social welfare from PCV is to explicitly set vaccine prices based on the net societal value of the vaccine to different countries.

Furthermore, results indicate that even the tiered pricing offered to LICs by multinational companies was inferior to competitive prices from developing country manufacturers (DMCs). The economic surplus accrued to low- and middle-income countries substantially increased when applying the Pneumosil® price. This suggests that lowering the intellectual property and technological barriers that LMICs to develop and manufacture vaccines may enable lower prices [66]. The recent WHO prequalification of Pneumosil®, a 10-valent pneumococcal conjugate vaccine developed by SII in partnership with PATH and the Bill and Melinda Gates Foundation, has resulted in LMICs being able to access lower PCV prices [67]. In 2023, Pneumosil® was available for LICs at a price of USD 1.5, compared to USD 2.75 for Prevnar 13® and USD 2.9 for Synflorix® after both being available on the market for more than 13 years [33].

Nevertheless, recent years have seen progress in reducing vaccine prices, leading many countries to introduce PCV into routine schedules [33]. Additionally, prices of PCV are anticipated to drop further after the entry of new manufacturers based in developing countries into the market and the expiration of patents in 2026 [68]. However, even though generic vaccines and developing country-based vaccines tend to be less expensive [33], their adoption into routine schedules might be delayed due to insufficiency of real-world data to support decision making into EPI, particularly as their counterparts HICs are already moving to high valent vaccines. Delays in adopting affordable PCVs can cause preventable deaths and disabilities. A more steeply tiered pricing policy for already existing vaccines would improve the distribution of the net societal value across countries faster rather than relying solely on new market dynamics.

Findings from this study highlight the importance of cross-subsidies in removing or alleviating the financial barriers to accessing PCV. We found that increasing subsidies to LICs and LMICs could contribute to achieving equitable prices that could accelerate vaccine uptake in these countries while maintaining high consumer surpluses for HICs and positive surpluses for manufacturers. However, implementing this policy would be challenging as it requires an increase in vaccine prices to wealthier countries and/or a reduction in manufacturer revenues with a potential negative impact on the R&D products pipeline. For example, if HICs subsidized vaccine costs for LICs and LMICs, HICs would need to pay up to USD 117.20 per dose, assuming no change in manufacturer profits. While this price is lower than the price USA was paying in 2021 (~USD 150.83 per dose), it is likely to be higher than many other HICs were paying in the same year.

Our findings emphasize the value of pooled procurement mechanisms for MICs; if Gavi-ineligible non-PAHO MICs accessed PCV at PAHO prices, the economic surplus to these countries would more than double. This policy scenario would also result in an increased surplus for manufacturers. There has been some success in regional pooled procurement outside of Gavi pooled procurement through UNICEF and PAHO's Revolving Fund [54,69]. For example, in May 2012, three Baltic countries (Estonia, Lithuania, and Latvia) initiated a partnership agreement aimed at pooling pharmaceutical and vaccine procurement [69]. The group was able to secure a reduction in price by 17–25% per immunization course compared to what each individual country had previously spent. Data extracted from the MI4A database [31] indicated that countries involved in pooled procurement mechanisms were able to achieve 42% lower prices than self-procurement for 18 widely used vaccines in MICs in 2022, though savings varied across specific vaccines.

Hence, international organizations and governments should explore alternative procurement strategies and promote regional cooperation to encourage these pooled procurement mechanisms [61].

There are several limitations of the analysis to note. First, the indirect benefits of childhood PCV on the adult population were not captured, which may lead to an underestimation of the consumer surplus of PCV, particularly in HICs with older populations. Another source of underestimation of the surplus is the use of a healthcare system perspective to estimate healthcare cost savings rather than a societal perspective due to a lack of data to inform the latter. Furthermore, the unknown but potentially beneficial impact of PCV on antimicrobial resistance was not considered. Second, the model used in this analysis assumed that the PCV serotype carriage would be eliminated after immunization, but this has not been observed in many low- and middle-income countries [70–73]. This may lead to overestimation of vaccine impact and thus economic surplus, especially in low- and middle-income countries with a high force of infection [72]. However, we found that even for the lowest vaccine impact, the distribution of economic benefits across country income groups remained the same, and if a lower vaccine impact was selectively considered in low- and middle-income settings, their share of the global economic surplus of PCV would be even lower than currently estimated. Third, this analysis attributed the entire producer surplus to vaccine manufacturers, but some of these profits might be shared with distributors like wholesalers. Fourth, the cost of research and development borne by manufacturers may have been offset by research grants, funds, and loans from public institutions. This might have led to an underestimation of the manufacturers' economic surplus. Fifth, due to insufficient data on the cost of adverse events following PCV administration, our analysis did not include these events. This may result in an overestimation of the consumer surplus. However, even if our model could account for these adverse effects, it is unlikely that the results regarding current inequality would change. Sixth, data on disease burden and the economic costs of pneumococcal disease are limited in many parts of the world; hence, our results should be interpreted in the context of the sensitivity analyses we conducted around key parameters. Furthermore, private healthcare in low- and middle-income countries is often unmonitored, complicating accurate calculations of vaccine impact and cost-effectiveness. While these limitations may influence the overall magnitude of the estimated global economic surplus, they are unlikely to have a major impact on the distribution of economic surplus across country groupings and producers, nor influence this study's conclusions with respect to the impact of different pricing policies.

5. Conclusions

In conclusion, this study provides clear evidence that current vaccine pricing policies disproportionately benefit HICs and manufacturers, who receive the highest share of the economic surplus generated by PCV. Unaffordable prices due to limited health budgets and competing healthcare needs, and lack of transparency in price setting have negatively impacted vaccine uptake in MICs. This study offers important lessons for other new vaccines and technologies coming to market. It has taken over two decades before PCV has seen widespread introduction in MICs. Early adoption of appropriate pooled procurement mechanisms, promoting vaccine manufacturing in LMICs and more steeply tiered prices, especially in MICs, could promote greater vaccine access outside Gavi and PAHO members. Evidence from this study can be used to inform pricing policies that facilitate equitable dissemination of new and existing vaccines.

Supplementary Materials: The following supporting information can be downloaded at: https://www.mdpi.com/article/10.3390/vaccines12070767/s1, Table S1: PCV impact for invasive pneumococcal diseases per region; Table S2: Estimated research and development cost of PCV. References [3–5,7,10,19,21–35,37,38,40,41,43,47,65,74–93] are cited in the Supplementary Materials.

Author Contributions: Conceptualization, F.N., F.M.R., M.J. and N.C.; methodology, F.N., F.M.R., M.J. and N.C.; validation, F.M.R., M.J. and N.C.; formal analysis, F.N.; investigation, F.N.; resources, F.N.; data curation, F.N.; writing—original draft preparation, F.N.; writing—review and editing, F.N., F.M.R., M.J. and N.C., visualization, F.N.; supervision, F.M.R., M.J. and N.C.; project administration, N.C.; funding acquisition, F.N., F.M.R., M.J. and N.C. All authors have read and agreed to the published version of the manuscript.

Funding: F.N. receives a Melbourne Research Scholarship. F.N and N.C. receive funding from the Australian National Health and Medical Research Council (NHMRC) Centre of Research Excellence for Pneumococcal Disease Control in the Asia-Pacific (GN1196415). MCRI is supported by the Victorian Government's Operational Infrastructure Support Project. F.M.R. has a NHMRC Investigator grant (GN1177245).

Institutional Review Board Statement: Not applicable.

Informed Consent Statement: Not applicable.

Data Availability Statement: The data supporting the findings of this study are available within the article/Supplementary Materials. Further inquiries can be directed to the corresponding author.

Acknowledgments: F.N. acknowledges the financial support from the Melbourne Research Scholarship and NHMRC Centre of Research Excellence for Pneumococcal Disease Control in the Asia-Pacific.

Conflicts of Interest: The authors declare no conflicts of interest.

References

1. Troeger, C.; Blacker, B.; Khalil, I.A.; Rao, P.C.; Cao, J.; Zimsen, S.R.M.; Albertson, S.B.; Deshpande, A.; Farag, T.; Abebe, Z.; et al. Estimates of the global, regional, and national morbidity, mortality, and aetiologies of lower respiratory infections in 195 countries, 1990–2016: A systematic analysis for the Global Burden of Disease Study 2016. *Lancet Infect. Dis.* **2018**, *18*, 1191–1210. [CrossRef] [PubMed]
2. The World Health Organization. Pneumonia in Children 2022. Available online: https://www.who.int/news-room/fact-sheets/detail/pneumonia (accessed on 22 November 2022).
3. Unicef. Pneumonia. Available online: https://data.unicef.org/topic/child-health/pneumonia/ (accessed on 20 March 2023).
4. Wahl, B.; O'Brien, K.L.; Greenbaum, A.; Majumder, A.; Liu, L.; Chu, Y.; Lukšić, I.; Nair, H.; McAllister, D.A.; Campbell, H.; et al. Burden of Streptococcus pneumoniae and Haemophilus influenzae type b disease in children in the era of conjugate vaccines: Global, regional, and national estimates for 2000-15. *Lancet Glob. Health* **2018**, *6*, e744–e757. [CrossRef] [PubMed]
5. International Vaccine Access Center (IVAC); Johns Hopkins Bloomberg School of Public Health. Vaccine Introduction: PCV Current Vaccine Intro Status. Available online: https://view-hub.org/vaccine/pcv (accessed on 25 January 2023).
6. Centers for Disease Control and Prevention. Progress in Introduction of Pneumococcal Conjugate Vaccine-Worldwide, 2000--2008. Available online: https://www.cdc.gov/mmwr/preview/mmwrhtml/mm5742a2.htm (accessed on 16 May 2023).
7. World Health Organization. Pneumococcal conjugate vaccine for childhood immunization—WHO position paper = Vaccin antipneumococcique conjugué pour la vaccination infantile—note d'information de l'OMS. *Wkly. Epidemiol. Rec. = Relev. Épidémiol. Hebd.* **2007**, *82*, 93–104.
8. Centers for Disease Control and Prevention. Global Pneumococcal Disease and Vaccine. Available online: https://www.cdc.gov/pneumococcal/?CDC_AAref_Val=https://www.cdc.gov/pneumococcal/global.html (accessed on 18 February 2023).
9. World Health Organization. WHO/UNICEF Estimates of National Immunization Coverage (WUENIC). Available online: https://www.who.int/publications/m/item/progress-and-challenges (accessed on 1 October 2023).
10. Chen, C.; Cervero Liceras, F.; Flasche, S.; Sidharta, S.; Yoong, J.; Sundaram, N.; Jit, M. Effect and cost-effectiveness of pneumococcal conjugate vaccination: A global modelling analysis. *Lancet Glob. Health* **2019**, *7*, e58–e67. [CrossRef] [PubMed]
11. Zakiyah, N.; Insani, W.N.; Suwantika, A.A.; van der Schans, J.; Postma, M.J. Pneumococcal Vaccination for Children in Asian Countries: A Systematic Review of Economic Evaluation Studies. *Vaccines* **2020**, *8*, 426. [CrossRef] [PubMed]
12. Saokaew, S.; Rayanakorn, A.; Wu, D.B.; Chaiyakunapruk, N. Cost Effectiveness of Pneumococcal Vaccination in Children in Low- and Middle-Income Countries: A Systematic Review. *Pharmacoeconomics* **2016**, *34*, 1211–1225. [CrossRef]
13. Guillaume, D.; Meyer, D.; Waheed, D.-e.-N.; Schlieff, M.; Muralidharan, K.; Chou, V.B.; Limaye, R. Factors influencing the prioritization of vaccines by policymakers in low- and middle-income countries: A scoping review. *Health Policy Plan.* **2022**, *38*, 363–376. [CrossRef]
14. World Health Organization. WHO Pneumococcal Vaccines Global Market Study June 2020. Available online: https://www.who.int/publications/m/item/who-pneumococcal-vaccines-global-market-study-june-2020 (accessed on 17 February 2023).
15. World Health Organization. Immunization Agenda 2030: A Global Strategy to Leave No One Behind. Available online: https://www.who.int/teams/immunization-vaccines-and-biologicals/strategies/ia2030 (accessed on 3 February 2023).

16. The Pan American Health Organization. Operating Procedures of the PAHO Revolving Fund for the Purchase of Vaccines, Syringes, and Other Related Supplies. Available online: https://www3.paho.org/English/AD/FCH/IM/RF_OperatingProcedures_e.pdf (accessed on 6 March 2023).
17. World Health Organization. Market Information for Access to Vaccines. Available online: https://www.who.int/teams/immunization-vaccines-and-biologicals/vaccine-access/mi4a (accessed on 17 February 2023).
18. Zweifel, P.; Breyer, F.; Kifmann, M. *Health Economics*; Springer: New York, NY, USA, 2009.
19. Herlihy, N.; Hutubessy, R.; Jit, M. Current Global Pricing For Human Papillomavirus Vaccines Brings The Greatest Economic Benefits To Rich Countries. *Health Aff.* **2016**, *35*, 227–234. [CrossRef] [PubMed]
20. The World Bank. The World by Income and Region. Available online: https://datatopics.worldbank.org/world-development-indicators/the-world-by-income-and-region.html (accessed on 9 August 2023).
21. The World Health Organization. Considerations for Pneumococcal Conjugate Vaccine (PCV) Product Choice. Available online: https://www.who.int/publications/i/item/considerations-for-pneumococcal-conjugate-vaccine-(pcv)-product-choice (accessed on 23 November 2022).
22. CGTN. First China-Made 13-Valent Pneumonia Vaccine to Hit the Market. Available online: https://news.cgtn.com/news/2020-01-02/First-China-made-13-valent-pneumonia-vaccine-to-hit-the-market-MVR3v4QTle/index.html#:~:text=The%20approved%20China-made%20pneumococcal,dollars)%20for%20all%20four%20doses (accessed on 11 March 2023).
23. Izurieta, P.; Scherbakov, M.; Nieto Guevara, J.; Vetter, V.; Soumahoro, L. Systematic review of the efficacy, effectiveness and impact of high-valency pneumococcal conjugate vaccines on otitis media. *Hum. Vaccin. Immunother.* **2022**, *18*, 2013693. [CrossRef]
24. Bennett, J.C.; Knoll, M.D. Changes in Invasive Pneumococcal Disease Incidence following Introduction of PCV10 and PCV13 among Children <5 Years: The PSERENADE Project. *Open Forum. Infect. Dis.* **2021**, *8*, S677–S678. [CrossRef]
25. Monasta, L.; Ronfani, L.; Marchetti, F.; Montico, M.; Vecchi Brumatti, L.; Bavcar, A.; Grasso, D.; Barbiero, C.; Tamburlini, G. Burden of disease caused by otitis media: Systematic review and global estimates. *PLoS ONE* **2012**, *7*, e36226. [CrossRef]
26. O'Brien, K.L.; Wolfson, L.J.; Watt, J.P.; Henkle, E.; Deloria-Knoll, M.; McCall, N.; Lee, E.; Mulholland, K.; Levine, O.S.; Cherian, T. Burden of disease caused by Streptococcus pneumoniae in children younger than 5 years: Global estimates. *Lancet* **2009**, *374*, 893–902. [CrossRef] [PubMed]
27. Portnoy, A.; Jit, M.; Lauer, J.; Blommaert, A.; Ozawa, S.; Stack, M.; Murray, J.; Hutubessy, R. Estimating costs of care for meningitis infections in low- and middle-income countries. *Vaccine* **2015**, *33*, A240–A247. [CrossRef] [PubMed]
28. The World Bank. GDP per Capita, PPP (Current International $). Available online: https://data.worldbank.org/indicator/NY.GDP.PCAP.PP.CD (accessed on 11 January 2021).
29. World Health Organization. WHO-CHOICE Estimates of Cost for Inpatient and Outpatient Health Service Delivery Costs. Available online: https://www.who.int/teams/health-systems-governance-and-financing/economic-analysis/costing-and-technical-efficiency/quantities-and-unit-prices- (accessed on 22 January 2023).
30. United Nations. Department of Economic and Social Affairs, Population Division (2021). *World Population Prospects*. Available online: https://population.un.org/wpp/ (accessed on 7 January 2022).
31. The World Health Organization. Global Vaccine Market Report 2022. Available online: https://www.who.int/publications/i/item/9789240062726 (accessed on 23 January 2023).
32. Woods, B.; Revill, P.; Sculpher, M.; Claxton, K. Country-Level Cost-Effectiveness Thresholds: Initial Estimates and the Need for Further Research. *Value Health* **2016**, *19*, 929–935. [CrossRef] [PubMed]
33. Unicef. Vaccines Pricing Data. Available online: https://www.unicef.org/supply/vaccines-pricing-data (accessed on 25 February 2023).
34. The Pan American Health Organization. Revolving Fund Prices. Available online: https://www.paho.org/en/revolving-fund (accessed on 26 January 2023).
35. Sriudomporn, S.; Watts, E.; Yoon Sim, S.; Hutubessy, R.; Patenaude, B. Achieving immunization agenda 2030 coverage targets for 14 pathogens: Projected product and immunization delivery costs for 194 Countries, 2021–2030. *Vaccine X* **2023**, *13*, 100256. [CrossRef] [PubMed]
36. Canevari, J.; Von Mollendorf, C.; Nguyen, C.; Tsatsaronis, A.R.R.; Rusell, F. Impact of pneumococcal conjugate vaccine formulation and schedule against pneumonia in children under 9 years of age: A systematic Review and meta-analysis. In Proceedings of the 13th Meeting of the International Society of Pneumonia & Pneumococcal Diseases (ISPPD-13), Cape Town, South Africa, 17–20 March 2024.
37. Wannarong, T.; Ekpatanaparnich, P.; Boonyasiri, A.; Supapueng, O.; Vathanophas, V.; Tanphaichitr, A.; Ungkanont, K. Efficacy of Pneumococcal Vaccine on Otitis Media: A Systematic Review and Meta-Analysis. *Otolaryngol. Head Neck Surg.* **2023**, *169*, 765–779. [CrossRef] [PubMed]
38. World Health Organization. Global Health Observatory Data Repository. *Pneumococcal Conjugate (PCV3) Immunization Coverage Estimates by Country*. Available online: https://apps.who.int/gho/data/node.main.PCV3n?lang=en (accessed on 12 March 2023).
39. Mathers, C.D.; Lopez, A.D.; Murray, C.J.L. The Burden of Disease and Mortality by Condition: Data, Methods, and Results for 2001. In *Global Burden of Disease and Risk Factors*; Lopez, A.D., Mathers, C.D., Ezzati, M., Jamison, D.T., Murray, C.J.L., Eds.; Oxford University Press: Oxford, UK, 2006.
40. Ojal, J.; Griffiths, U.; Hammitt, L.L.; Adetifa, I.; Akech, D.; Tabu, C.; Scott, J.A.G.; Flasche, S. Sustaining pneumococcal vaccination after transitioning from Gavi support: A modelling and cost-effectiveness study in Kenya. *Lancet Glob. Health* **2019**, *7*, e644–e654. [CrossRef] [PubMed]

41. Edmond, K.; Clark, A.; Korczak, V.S.; Sanderson, C.; Griffiths, U.K.; Rudan, I. Global and regional risk of disabling sequelae from bacterial meningitis: A systematic review and meta-analysis. *Lancet Infect. Dis.* **2010**, *10*, 317–328. [CrossRef] [PubMed]
42. Lucas, M.J.; Brouwer, M.C.; van de Beek, D. Neurological sequelae of bacterial meningitis. *J. Infect.* **2016**, *73*, 18–27. [CrossRef]
43. Little, P.; Gould, C.; Williamson, I.; Moore, M.; Warner, G.; Dunleavey, J. Pragmatic randomised controlled trial of two prescribing strategies for childhood acute otitis media. *BMJ* **2001**, *322*, 336–342. [CrossRef]
44. Pfizer. Reports Fourth-Quarter and Full-Year Results. Available online: https://investors.pfizer.com/Investors/Financials/Annual-Reports/default.aspx (accessed on 13 December 2022).
45. US Securities and Exchange Commission. EDGAR Company Filings. Available online: https://www.sec.gov/edgar/searchedgar/companysearch (accessed on 2 March 2023).
46. Light, D.W.; Andrus, J.K.; Warburton, R.N. Estimated research and development costs of rotavirus vaccines. *Vaccine* **2009**, *27*, 6627–6633. [CrossRef]
47. Chit, A.; Parker, J.; Halperin, S.A.; Papadimitropoulos, M.; Krahn, M.; Grootendorst, P. Toward more specific and transparent research and development costs: The case of seasonal influenza vaccines. *Vaccine* **2014**, *32*, 3336–3340. [CrossRef] [PubMed]
48. World Health Organization. WHO Guide for Standardization of Economic Evaluations of Immunization Programmes. Available online: https://apps.who.int/iris/bitstream/handle/10665/329389/WHO-IVB-19.10-eng.pdf (accessed on 11 April 2023).
49. Jamison, D.T.; Summers, L.H.; Alleyne, G.; Arrow, K.J.; Berkley, S.; Binagwaho, A.; Bustreo, F.; Evans, D.; Feachem, R.G.; Frenk, J.; et al. Global health 2035: A world converging within a generation. *Lancet* **2013**, *382*, 1898–1955. [CrossRef] [PubMed]
50. Bertram, M.Y.; Lauer, J.A.; Stenberg, K.; Edejer, T.T.T. Methods for the Economic Evaluation of Health Care Interventions for Priority Setting in the Health System: An Update From WHO CHOICE. *Int. J. Health Policy Manag.* **2021**, *10*, 673–677. [CrossRef] [PubMed]
51. Care AGDoHaA. The Pharmaceutical Benefits Scheme. Available online: https://www.pbs.gov.au/pbs/news/2022/05/review-of-discount-rate-in-the-pbac-guidelines (accessed on 27 June 2024).
52. Brown, R.J.; Head, M.G. Sizing Up Pneumonia Research. *J. Contrib.* **2018**. [CrossRef]
53. Centers for Disease Control and Prevention. CDC Vaccine Price List. Available online: https://www.cdc.gov/vaccines/programs/vfc/awardees/vaccine-management/price-list/index.html (accessed on 11 August 2023).
54. Parmaksiz, K.; Pisani, E.; Bal, R.; Kok, M.O. A systematic review of pooled procurement of medicines and vaccines: Identifying elements of success. *Glob. Health* **2022**, *18*, 59. [CrossRef]
55. Temple, B.; Toan, N.T.; Uyen, D.Y.; Balloch, A.; Bright, K.; Cheung, Y.B.; Licciardi, P.; Nguyen, C.D.; Phuong, N.T.M.; Satzke, C.; et al. Evaluation of different infant vaccination schedules incorporating pneumococcal vaccination (The Vietnam Pneumococcal Project): Protocol of a randomised controlled trial. *BMJ Open* **2018**, *8*, e019795. [CrossRef]
56. U.S. National Library of Medicine: ClinicalTrials.gov. Trial of Pneumococcal Vaccine Schedules in Ho Chi Minh City, Vietnam (NCT01953510). Available online: https://clinicaltrials.gov/ct2/show/NCT01953510 (accessed on 11 November 2020).
57. Smith-Vaughan, H.; Temple, B.; Dai, V.T.T.; Hoan, P.T.; Thuy, H.N.L.; Phan, T.V.; Bright, K.; Toan, N.T.; Uyen, D.Y.; Nguyen, C.D. Effect of different schedules of ten-valent pneumococcal conjugate vaccine on pneumococcal carriage in Vietnamese infants: Results from a randomised controlled trial. *Lancet Reg. Health West. Pac.* **2022**, *32*, 100651. [CrossRef]
58. Temple, B.; Tran, H.P.; Dai, V.T.T.; Smith-Vaughan, H.; Licciardi, P.V.; Satzke, C.; Nguyen, T.V.; Mulholland, K. Efficacy against pneumococcal carriage and the immunogenicity of reduced-dose (0 + 1 and 1 + 1) PCV10 and PCV13 schedules in Ho Chi Minh City, Viet Nam: A parallel, single-blind, randomised controlled trial. *Lancet Infect. Dis.* **2023**, *23*, 933–944. [CrossRef]
59. Gavi. Pneumococcal AMC. Available online: https://www.gavi.org/investing-gavi/innovative-financing/pneumococcal-amc (accessed on 28 September 2023).
60. Gavi. Making Immunisation Sustainable: Gavi's Approach to Engaging with Middle-Income Countries. Available online: https://www.gavi.org/programmes-impact/types-support/sustainability (accessed on 19 December 2023).
61. Russell, F.M.; Bowen, A.; Cotton, M.; Mascareñas, A.; O'Ryan, M. World Society for Pediatric Infectious Diseases calls for action to ensure fair prices for vaccines. *Lancet Glob. Health* **2024**, *12*, e22–e24. [CrossRef]
62. Médecins Sans Frontières. The Right Shot: Bringing Down Barriers to af Fordable and Adapted Vaccines. Available online: https://msfaccess.org/right-shot-bringing-down-barriers-affordable-and-adapted-vaccines-2nd-ed-2015 (accessed on 6 May 2023).
63. ACIP Updates: Recommendations for Use of 20-Valent Pneumococcal Conjugate Vaccine in Children—United States, 2023. *MMWR Morb. Mortal. Wkly. Rep.* **2023**, *72*, 1072. [CrossRef]
64. Warren, S.; Barmpouni, M.; Kossyvaki, V.; Gourzoulidis, G.; Perdrizet, J. Estimating the Clinical and Economic Impact of Switching from the 13-Valent Pneumococcal Conjugate Vaccine (PCV13) to Higher-Valent Options in Greek Infants. *Vaccines* **2023**, *11*, 1369. [CrossRef] [PubMed]
65. James, S.L.; Abate, D.; Abate, K.H.; Abay, S.M.; Abbafati, C.; Abbasi, N.; Abbastabar, H.; Abd-Allah, F.; Abdela, J.; Abdelalim, A.; et al. Global, regional, and national incidence, prevalence, and years lived with disability for 354 diseases and injuries for 195 countries and territories, 1990–2017: A systematic analysis for the Global Burden of Disease Study 2017. *Lancet* **2018**, *392*, 1789–1858. [CrossRef]
66. Hayman, B.; Kumar Suri, R.; Downham, M. Sustainable vaccine manufacturing in low- and middle-Income countries. *Vaccine* **2022**, *40*, 7288–7304. [CrossRef]
67. PATH. Developing a More Affordable Pneumococcal Vaccine. Available online: https://www.path.org/our-impact/case-studies/developing-more-affordable-pneumococcal-vaccine/ (accessed on 18 January 2024).

68. World Intellectual Property Organization. Patentscope. WO/2011/151760; Streptococcus Pneumoniae Vaccine Formulations, Available online: https://patentscope.wipo.int/search/en/detail.jsf?docId=WO2011151760&recNum=1&maxRec=&office=&prevFilter=&sortOption=&queryString=&tab=PCT+Biblio (accessed on 23 August 2023).
69. Cernuschi, T.; Gilchrist, S.; Hajizada, A.; Malhame, M.; Mariat, S.; Widmyer, G. Price transparency is a step towards sustainable access in middle income countries. *BMJ* **2020**, *368*, l5375. [CrossRef]
70. Chan, J.; Lai, J.Y.R.; Nguyen, C.D.; Vilivong, K.; Dunne, E.M.; Dubot-Pérès, A.; Fox, K.; Hinds, J.; Moore, K.A.; Nation, M.L.; et al. Indirect effects of 13-valent pneumococcal conjugate vaccine on pneumococcal carriage in children hospitalised with acute respiratory infection despite heterogeneous vaccine coverage: An observational study in Lao People's Democratic Republic. *BMJ Glob. Health* **2021**, *6*, e005187. [CrossRef] [PubMed]
71. Hammitt, L.L.; Etyang, A.O.; Morpeth, S.C.; Ojal, J.; Mutuku, A.; Mturi, N.; Moisi, J.C.; Adetifa, I.M.; Karani, A.; Akech, D.O.; et al. Effect of ten-valent pneumococcal conjugate vaccine on invasive pneumococcal disease and nasopharyngeal carriage in Kenya: A longitudinal surveillance study. *Lancet* **2019**, *393*, 2146–2154. [CrossRef]
72. Bar-Zeev, N.; Swarthout, T.D.; Everett, D.B.; Alaerts, M.; Msefula, J.; Brown, C.; Bilima, S.; Mallewa, J.; King, C.; von Gottberg, A.; et al. Impact and effectiveness of 13-valent pneumococcal conjugate vaccine on population incidence of vaccine and non-vaccine serotype invasive pneumococcal disease in Blantyre, Malawi, 2006–18: Prospective observational time-series and case-control studies. *Lancet Glob. Health* **2021**, *9*, e989–e998. [CrossRef] [PubMed]
73. Faye, P.M.; Sonko, M.A.; Diop, A.; Thiongane, A.; Ba, I.D.; Spiller, M.; Ndiaye, O.; Dieye, B.; Mwenda, J.M.; Sow, A.I.; et al. Impact of 13-Valent Pneumococcal Conjugate Vaccine on Meningitis and Pneumonia Hospitalizations in Children aged <5 Years in Senegal, 2010–2016. *Clin. Infect. Dis.* **2019**, *69*, S66–S71. [CrossRef]
74. Advisory Committee on Immunization Practices. *Preventing Pneumococcal Disease among Infants and Young Children: Recommendations of the Advisory Committee on Immunization Practices (ACIP)*; Levine, O.S., Schwartz, B.A., Beneden, C.A.V., Whitney, C.G., Eds.; MMWR Recommendations and Reports; ACIP: Atlanta, GA, USA, 2000.
75. Zhao, Y.; Li, G.; Xia, S.; Ye, Q.; Yuan, L.; Li, H.; Li, J.; Chen, J.; Yang, S.; Jiang, Z.; et al. Immunogenicity and Safety of a Novel 13-Valent Pneumococcal Vaccine in Healthy Chinese Infants and Toddlers. *Front. Microbiol.* **2022**, *13*, 870973. [CrossRef]
76. Rodgers, G. The Future of Pneumococcal Conjugate Vaccines: The Need and Challenges for Higher Valency Vaccines. In Proceedings of the 13th Meeting of the International Society of Pneumonia & Pneumococcal Diseases (ISPPD-13), Cape Town, South Africa, 17–20 March 2024.
77. Said, M.A.; Johnson, H.L.; Nonyane, B.A.S.; Deloria-Knoll, M.; O'Brien, K.L.; AGEDD Adult Pneumococcal Burden Study Team. Estimating the Burden of Pneumococcal Pneumonia among Adults: A Systematic Review and Meta-Analysis of Diagnostic Techniques. *PLoS ONE* **2013**, *8*, e60273. [CrossRef] [PubMed]
78. Källander, K.; Hildenwall, H.; Waiswa, P.; Galiwango, E.; Peterson, S.; Pariyo, G. Delayed care seeking for fatal pneumonia in children aged under five years in Uganda: A case-series study. *Bull. World Health Organ.* **2008**, *86*, 332–338. [CrossRef] [PubMed]
79. US Bureau of Labor Statistics. Consumer Price Index. Available online: https://www.bls.gov/cpi/ (accessed on 21 March 2023).
80. DiMasi, J.A.; Grabowski, H.G.; Hansen, R.W. Innovation in the pharmaceutical industry: New estimates of R&D costs. *J. Health Econ.* **2016**, *47*, 20–33.
81. Head, M.G.; Fitchett, J.R.; Newell, M.-L.; Scott, J.A.G.; Harris, J.N.; Clarke, S.C.; Atun, R. Mapping pneumonia research: A systematic analysis of UK investments and published outputs 1997–2013. *eBioMedicine* **2015**, *2*, 1193–1199. [CrossRef]
82. Burdman, J.R. *Vaccine Design: The Subunit and Adjuvant Approach*; Springer: Berlin/Heidelberg, Germany, 2012.
83. Anderson, P.W.; Eby, R.J. Immunogenic Conjugates of Streptococcus Pneumonial Capsular Polymer and Toxin or in Toxiad. U.S. Patent US5360897A, 1 November 1994.
84. NIH. Research Portfolio Online Reporting Tools (RePORT). Available online: https://report.nih.gov/report-funding (accessed on 12 May 2023).
85. University of Rochester. Childhood Vaccine with Rochester Roots Recognized. Available online: https://www.rochester.edu/pr/Review/V70N1/gazette2.html (accessed on 13 May 2023).
86. Kumar, B.R.; Kumar, B.R. Acquisitions by Pfizer. In *Wealth Creation in the World's Largest Mergers and Acquisitions: Integrated Case Studies*; Springer: Cham, switzerland, 2019; pp. 85–99.
87. Wouters, O.J.; McKee, M.; Luyten, J. Estimated Research and Development Investment Needed to Bring a New Medicine to Market, 2009–2018. *JAMA* **2020**, *323*, 844–853. [CrossRef] [PubMed]
88. Harrington, S. *Cost of Capital for Pharmaceutical, Biotechnology, and Medical Device Firms*; The Oxford Handbook of the Economics of the Biopharmaceutical Industry; Oxford University Press: Oxford, UK, 2009.
89. Wong, C.H.; Siah, K.W.; Lo, A.W. Estimation of clinical trial success rates and related parameters. *Biostatistics* **2019**, *20*, 273–286. [CrossRef] [PubMed]
90. Clendinen, C.; Zhang, Y.; Warburton, R.N.; Light, D.W. Manufacturing costs of HPV vaccines for developing countries. *Vaccine* **2016**, *34*, 5984–5989. [CrossRef]
91. Munira, S.L.; Hendriks, J.T.; Atmosukarto, I.I.; Friede, M.H.; Carter, L.M.; Butler, J.R.G.; Clements, A.C. A cost analysis of producing vaccines in developing countries. *Vaccine* **2019**, *37*, 1245–1251. [CrossRef]

92. Mahoney, R.T.; Francis, D.P.; Frazatti-Gallina, N.M.; Precioso, A.R.; Raw, I.; Watler, P.; Whitehead, P.; Whitehead, S.S. Cost of production of live attenuated dengue vaccines: A case study of the Instituto Butantan, Sao Paulo, Brazil. *Vaccine* **2012**, *30*, 4892–4896. [CrossRef]
93. Kornfield, R.; Donohue, J.; Berndt, E.R.; Alexander, G.C. Promotion of Prescription Drugs to Consumers and Providers, 2001–2010. *PLoS ONE* **2013**, *8*, e55504. [CrossRef]

Disclaimer/Publisher's Note: The statements, opinions and data contained in all publications are solely those of the individual author(s) and contributor(s) and not of MDPI and/or the editor(s). MDPI and/or the editor(s) disclaim responsibility for any injury to people or property resulting from any ideas, methods, instructions or products referred to in the content.

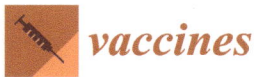

Review

Inequality in Childhood Immunization Coverage: A Scoping Review of Data Sources, Analyses, and Reporting Methods

Carrie Lyons, Devaki Nambiar, Nicole E. Johns, Adrien Allorant, Nicole Bergen and Ahmad Reza Hosseinpoor *

Department of Data and Analytics, World Health Organization, 20 Avenue Appia, 1211 Geneva, Switzerland; lyonsc@who.int (C.L.); nambiard@who.int (D.N.); johnsn@who.int (N.E.J.); allorranta@who.int (A.A.); bergenn@who.int (N.B.)
* Correspondence: hosseinpoora@who.int; Tel.: +41-22-791-3205

Abstract: Immunization through vaccines among children has contributed to improved childhood survival and health outcomes globally. However, vaccine coverage among children is unevenly distributed across settings and populations. The measurement of inequalities is essential for understanding gaps in vaccine coverage affecting certain sub-populations and monitoring progress towards achieving equity. Our study aimed to characterize the methods of reporting inequalities in childhood vaccine coverage, inclusive of the settings, data source types, analytical methods, and reporting modalities used to quantify and communicate inequality. We conducted a scoping review of publications in academic journals which included analyses of inequalities in vaccination among children. Literature searches were conducted in PubMed and Web of Science and included relevant articles published between 8 December 2013 and 7 December 2023. Overall, 242 publications were identified, including 204 assessing inequalities in a single country and 38 assessing inequalities across more than one country. We observed that analyses on inequalities in childhood vaccine coverage rely heavily on Demographic Health Survey (DHS) or Multiple Indicator Cluster Surveys (MICS) data (39.3%), and papers leveraging these data had increased in the last decade. Additionally, about half of the single-country studies were conducted in low- and middle-income countries. We found that few studies analyzed and reported inequalities using summary measures of health inequality and largely used the odds ratio resulting from logistic regression models for analyses. The most analyzed dimensions of inequality were economic status and maternal education, and the most common vaccine outcome indicator was full vaccination with the recommended vaccine schedule. However, the definition and construction of both dimensions of inequality and vaccine coverage measures varied across studies, and a variety of approaches were used to study inequalities in vaccine coverage across contexts. Overall, harmonizing methods for selecting and categorizing dimensions of inequalities as well as methods for analyzing and reporting inequalities can improve our ability to assess the magnitude and patterns of inequality in vaccine coverage and compare those inequalities across settings and time.

Keywords: health inequalities; infant and child health; immunization; vaccination; scoping review

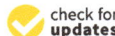

Citation: Lyons, C.; Nambiar, D.; Johns, N.E.; Allorant, A.; Bergen, N.; Hosseinpoor, A.R. Inequality in Childhood Immunization Coverage: A Scoping Review of Data Sources, Analyses, and Reporting Methods. *Vaccines* **2024**, *12*, 850. https://doi.org/10.3390/vaccines12080850

Academic Editor: Pedro Plans-Rubió

Received: 14 June 2024
Revised: 12 July 2024
Accepted: 20 July 2024
Published: 29 July 2024

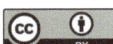

Copyright: © World Health Organization 2024. Licensee MDPI. This article is distributed under the terms of the Creative Commons Attribution IGO License. (https://creativecommons.org/licenses/by/3.0/igo/) which permits unrestricted use, distribution, and reproduction in any medium, provided the original work is properly cited. In any reproduction of this article there should not be any suggestion that WHO or this article endorse any specific organization or products. The use of the WHO logo is not permitted.

1. Introduction

Vaccine development and distribution for children has contributed to improved childhood survival and health outcomes globally [1–4]. Immunization through vaccines in childhood serves not only as a vital intervention for disease prevention for individuals but also as an effective community intervention for controlling infectious diseases among populations. Unfortunately, progress in childhood vaccination coverage in the last decade has stalled, with over 14 million children worldwide remaining completely unvaccinated and substantially higher levels of children not receiving all recommended vaccines [5–9].

In response, the Immunization Agenda 2030 (IA2030) was developed as a global strategy for vaccines and immunization coverage [10].

Vaccine coverage among children is unevenly distributed across settings and populations. Globally, 60% of those children who have not received any vaccines reside in 10 low- or middle-income countries (Nigeria, India, Pakistan, Indonesia, Ethiopia, the Philippines, the Democratic Republic of Congo, Brazil, Angola, and Vietnam). This is indicative of inequalities, or observable differences, in vaccine coverage between countries [8]. Variations in vaccine coverage have also been widely observed within countries. In low- and middle-income countries, inequalities in vaccination coverage have been associated with socioeconomic status, rural vs. urban residence, and maternal education [11]. Although high-income countries generally have higher overall vaccine coverage, inequalities in childhood vaccination based on socioeconomic status have also been observed [12,13]. Across settings, marginalized or devalued communities are consistently disproportionately unvaccinated and under-vaccinated [14]. Not only do inequalities experienced in early childhood result in adverse health outcomes for children, but these inequalities will also likely be perpetuated or amplified throughout the life course. Given the existing evidence on inequalities in vaccination coverage and the implications for health outcomes, IA2030 has incorporated goals for the reduction in global inequities in vaccine coverage [10]. Specifically, IA2023 aims to extend immunization services to under-immunized children and communities and improve immunization coverage nationally and sub-nationally in a sustainable manner.

The measurement of inequalities allows for the understanding of the magnitude, context, and trends in inequalities across settings and populations and is also essential for monitoring progress towards achieving equity [15–17]. However, the methods used to assess and report inequalities vary, given the diverse data available, the multiple disciplines conducting research on inequalities, and the wide range of potential audiences and applications for inequality evidence [18]. Social inequalities measure how a health indicator varies between subgroups, which are defined by different dimensions of inequality such as socio-economic status. Inequalities can be assessed quantitatively using disaggregated data or summary measures, which can capture either absolute or relative inequalities. The World Health Organization recommends reporting both absolute and relative measures for tracking health inequalities [19–23]. The literature about the use and application of health inequality summary measures highlights that the selection of measures may influence the interpretation of results about trends over time and the level of inequalities based on settings, populations, or health conditions [24–26]. A systematic review found that health inequalities overall are most commonly reported using only relative measures, although this has not been formally assessed specifically for childhood vaccine coverage inequalities [27]. The ability to improve childhood immunization relies on having an accurate and comprehensive understanding of inequalities affecting populations based on socioeconomic, demographic or geographic dimensions. Therefore, assessing the landscape of inequality analyses and reporting for childhood vaccination will provide insight into the quality of evidence and identify opportunities for improvement.

In response, the objectives of the paper are to characterize the methods of reporting inequalities in childhood vaccine coverage, inclusive of the settings, data source types, analysis methods, and reporting modalities used to quantify and communicate inequality.

2. Materials and Methods

2.1. Protocol Development

We conducted a scoping review of publications in academic journals which included analyses of inequalities in vaccine coverage among children. The search strategy was developed using Medical Subject Headings (MeSH) and key terms focused on three concepts related to inequality, immunization, and children/infants. The literature searches were conducted in PubMed and Web of Science. The protocol was developed in adherence with the JBI Manual for Evidence Synthesis, and we followed the Preferred Reporting Items for Systematic reviews and Meta-Analyses extension for Scoping Reviews (PRISMA-ScR) Checklist [28,29]. This protocol can be accessed in File S1.

2.2. Inclusion and Exclusion Criteria

Articles were included if published between 8 December 2013 and 7 December 2023. Studies were eligible for inclusion if the study population was children under 5 years of age; the outcome was vaccine coverage; inequalities in vaccine coverage were examined by one or more socioeconomic, demographic, or geographic dimension; and the study reported an objective of assessing inequalities. No language restrictions were applied; however, only English search terms were used within primarily English databases. The full inclusion and exclusion criteria are included in Table 1.

Table 1. Inclusion and exclusion criteria for articles obtained through the search for inequality analyses in childhood vaccine coverage.

Inclusion Criteria	Exclusion Criteria
Study population of children under the age of 5 years. Peer-reviewed research articles and research reports with the use of primary or secondary data published in academic journals. Studies examining an outcome of vaccination coverage or lack of coverage, including dropout and partial/incomplete vaccination. Reporting vaccination coverage by one or more socioeconomic, demographic, or geographic dimension(s) of inequality. Assessed within-country inequality.	Study population did not include results specific to children <5 years. The following document types: Short communications, comments, letters, editorials, biographies, reference materials, interviews, conference proceedings, news articles, pre-prints and systematic, scoping, and other reviews. Studies that exclusively used a qualitative methodology. Articles published more than 10 years before the search date. Only evaluates inequalities in vaccination coverage by medical factors, diagnoses, or comorbidities. Study includes multiple childhood health or related development outcomes, of which immunization is only one (e.g., includes immunization, nutrition, and education outcomes). Evaluates only between-country inequalities. Full text is not available.

2.3. Screening Process

The results from the literature search were reviewed using Covidence software (www.covidence.org, accessed on 18 March 2024) [30]. Title and abstract screening were conducted by one researcher (NJ), and the full text review was conducted by three reviewers (NJ, CL, AA). At the full text review stage, conflicts between reviewers were settled by a separate reviewer. Data extraction was carried out by four reviewers (NJ, CL, AA, DN). The flow chart of the review process is outlined in Figure 1.

2.4. Data Extraction and Synthesis

The data extraction tool was developed using the Covidence data extraction template. The template was designed to extract basic study characteristics, outcomes, dimensions of inequality, and results.

The summary measures of inequality used in this review are defined based on the World Health Organization Health Equity Assessment Toolkit [26]. Dimensions of inequality were reported using PROGRESS-Plus-defined categories of place; race, ethnicity, culture, and language; occupation; gender and sex; religion; education; socioeconomic status; social capital; and additional context-specific dimensions, such as subnational region [31]. Data on the specific vaccines for each article were extracted, as well as outcomes reporting full vaccination (either of a single vaccine or multiple vaccines); vaccination initiation (at least one dose); non-vaccination (with one vaccine or multiple vaccines) or zero-dose (as defined by the study); drop-out, partial vaccination, or incomplete vaccination; and age-appropriate vaccination receipt. Data sources for vaccine outcomes were identified and extracted.

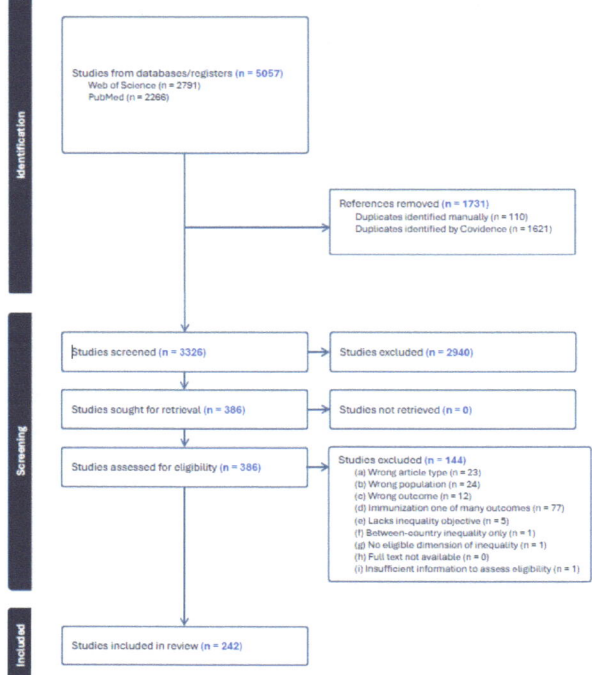

Figure 1. PRISMA flow diagram showing literature identification and screening.

Demographic and Health Surveys (DHS) and/or Multiple Indicator Cluster Surveys (MICS) are large multi-country household surveys that provide publicly available data. The DHS Program is funded primarily through the United States Agency for International Development (USAID) and is designed to collect key population, health, and nutrition information for the entire population of a country. MICS are implemented through support by UNICEF and designed specifically to assess the health of women and children. Additional data sources were administrative surveys and other surveys including households or schools.

We described the number of publications over time and the distribution of studies using different data sources on vaccine coverage indicators over time. We further explored the landscape of publications selected in our review using Multiple Correspondence Analysis (MCA), which is a data visualization technique used to identify and illustrate underlying patterns in categorical data [32]. Each axis represents a dimension along which the data variability is maximized. Typically, the first two axes capture the most significant patterns of variation among the variables. MCA was performed using the FactoMineR package version 2.11 in R version 4.4.1.

3. Results

A total of 5057 potential studies were identified through the literature search, and 1731 duplicates were removed before screening. Titles and abstracts for 3326 studies were screened. Of these, 386 met the inclusion criteria for full-text evaluation. Finally, 242 studies underwent extraction. The full list of articles included is in Table S1.

Overall, we observed an increase in the number of publications on inequalities in childhood vaccine coverage over the period of this review (Figure 2). There was a peak of 42 publications in 2022, noting that the literature search for years 2013 and 2023 did not include the entire calendar year. Differential increases in publications on inequalities in childhood vaccination by the data source of the vaccine indicators were observed over the review period. The number of publications using administrative or health surveillance data was relatively constant over the period, as were the publications based on other sources such as non-routine, study-specific, or small-scale surveys. However, publications utilizing DHS/MICS have increased in absolute numbers, as well as the overall proportion of manuscripts published since 2019. Across the entire period of the review, a total of 95 (39.3%) papers had utilized DHS/MICS data.

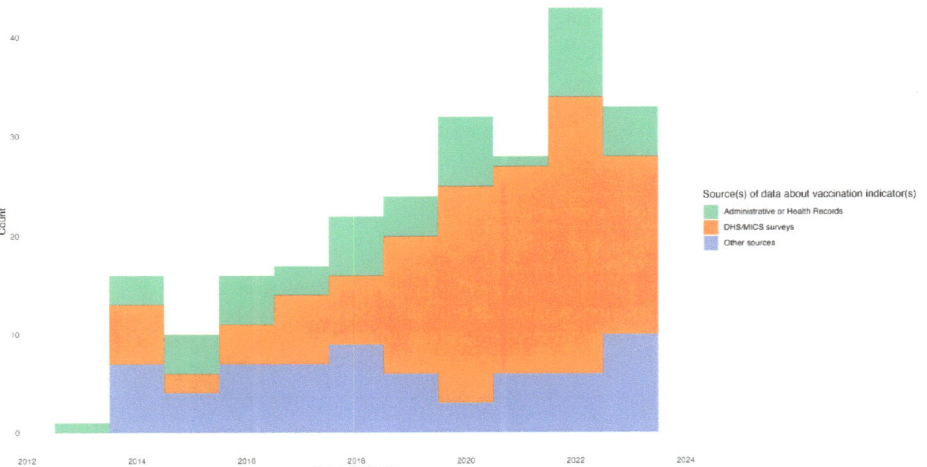

Figure 2. Publications of studies of inequalities in childhood vaccine coverage between 2013 and 2023 by data source for vaccine indicators (N = 242).

We described clusters of studies based on different categorical attributes in the MCA presented in Figure S1. Broadly, we observed a cluster of studies from low-income and lower-middle-income countries utilizing data from DHS/MICS. These studies primarily focus on full vaccination and zero-dose scenarios. In contrast, we observed another cluster of studies from high-income countries that use cohort data derived from administrative records.

Across all studies identified in this review (see Table 2), 15.7% (N = 38) of those included were multi-country studies, ranging from comparative studies of two countries within [33] or across regions [33,34] to a study that included 95 low- and middle-income countries [35] (Table 2). Most studies were cross-sectional in design (82.3% of all studies), followed by cohort (N = 39; 16.1%), as well as one study which was a randomized controlled trial. Of the studies with cohort study design, 87.2% of these used routine or administrative data sources (34 out of 39 studies). Most studies utilized DHS or MICS (53.3% of all studies) as well as survey data (25.6% of all studies) for the vaccine outcome. The study population was reported as the general population for 72.7% (N = 176) of all studies, while approximately one in five studies (22.3%) were focused on specific geographic regions. We also found that 223 out of 242 studies (92.1%) measured individual vaccine coverage as the outcome, while 15 studies (6.2%) computed vaccine coverage in small area units.

Table 2. Characteristics of studies on inequalities in childhood vaccination conducted between 2013 and 2023 (N = 242).

Country	N	%
Single-country	204	84.3%
Multi-country	38	15.7%
Study design		
Randomized control trial	1	0.4%
Cohort study	39	16.1%
Cross-sectional study	199	82.3%
Other	3	1%
Sources of data for vaccine indicator		
DHS or MICS	129	53.3%
Other surveys (household, school, etc.)	62	25.6%
Administrative	51	21.1%
Other	4	1.7%
Vaccine indicator classification		
Full vaccination of multiple vaccines	141	58.3%
Full vaccination of a specific vaccine	89	36.8%
Vaccination initiation (at least one dose of a multi-dose vaccine series)	27	11.2%
Non-vaccination (with one or multiple vaccines)/zero dose	45	19.0%
Drop-out, partial vaccination, or incomplete vaccination	36	14.9%
Age-appropriate vaccination receipt	16	6.6%
Other	8	3.3%

A range of indicators were used to characterize childhood vaccination. Over two-thirds of the studies (N = 163/242; 67.4%) used a single indicator, while the remaining used multiple indicators to report on vaccination. Overall, we found that the most commonly reported vaccine indicator was full coverage of multiple vaccines (58.3%), such as the coverage of WHO-recommended basic vaccine doses or the coverage of all countries' Essential Programme on Immunization-recommended vaccine doses. The second most common indicator, reported in 36.8% of studies, was full vaccination of a specific vaccine series, including pentavalent or DTP vaccines (57 studies), measles or MMR vaccines (50 studies), and polio vaccines (42 studies). Drop-out was reported as an outcome in just under 15% of studies. Notably, zero-dose or non-vaccination was reported in about a fifth of studies, appearing more prominently in studies published after 2022 [36,37]. The most common type of vaccine (78.5%, 190/242) analyzed among studies was the pentavalent (Diphtheria, Pertussis, Tetanus, Hepatitis B, and Hib) vaccine or DPT (Diphtheria, Pertussis, and Tetanus) vaccine.

We did not see great variation in the summary measures used to characterize inequality (see Table 3). The most common analysis was a regression-based measure: odds ratios resulting from multivariate or multivariable logistic regression (N = 150; 62% of studies). A third of studies (36.8% N = 89) employed simple summary measures of health inequality: over a quarter (25.6%; N = 62) of studies reported the ratio, while over one in ten (11.2%; N = 27) reported the difference. Relative Concentration Index measures were reported in 19.8% of studies (N = 48). Overall, 19.0% (N = 46) studies reported absolute summary measures; 50.0% (N = 212) reported relative summary measures; and about 8.3% (N = 20) reported both absolute and relative summary measures. For studies that reported more than one summary measure, all were included in Table 2.

Table 3. Summary measures or effect estimates of inequality used in studies on inequalities in childhood vaccination conducted between 2013 and 2023.

Type of Summary Measures or Regession Method	N	%
Regression-based odds ratios	150	62.0%
Ratio	62	25.6%
Relative concentration index	48	19.8%
Difference	27	11.2%
Slope Index of Inequality	13	5.4%
Population Attributable Risk	6	2.5%
Relative Index of Inequality	4	1.7%
Population Attributable Fraction	5	2.1%
Index of Disparity	1	0.4%
Theil Index	1	0.4%

3.1. Single-Country Studies

A total of 204 publications reported on inequalities in childhood vaccination in a single-country context (see Figure 3). Across these studies, 46 countries were represented. India had the largest number of papers, with a total of 34 publications in this period, followed by Ethiopia (N = 16), United Kingdom (N = 14), United States (N = 14), China (N = 12), and Nigeria (N = 12). Countries including Canada, Bangladesh, Ghana, and Nepal were featured in 5–10 publications in this period. We also found that 19 other countries had a single study published on this topic in the period studied.

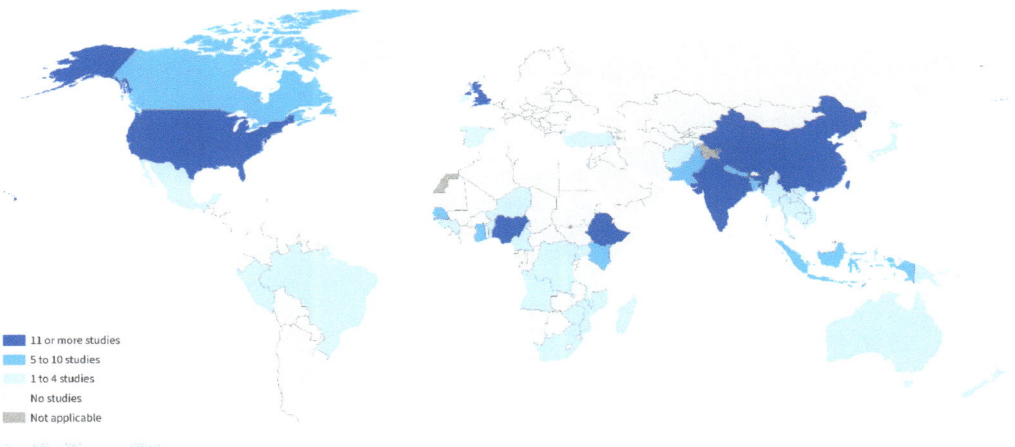

Figure 3. Global map of countries where studies on inequalities in childhood vaccination have been conducted between 2013 and 2023.

In single-country studies, the most commonly reported dimension of inequality overall was socioeconomic status (71.9% of studies; see Table 4). The measures used to define socioeconomic status varied based on whether the variable was measured at the individual, household, regional, or country level. Of these studies, the most commonly reported measure for socioeconomic status was the wealth index, which was treated as a quantile, as a tertile, and as continuous. Other proxies for socioeconomic status were personal income, type of household, deprivation index, poverty level, and GDP per capita at the subnational level.

Table 4. Dimensions of inequality assessed and reported in single-country studies on inequalities in childhood vaccination conducted between 2013 and 2023 (N = 204).

	Overall (N = 204)		2023 World Bank Group Country Income Category							
			Low Income (N = 30)		Lower-Middle Income (N = 102)		Upper Middle Income (N = 26)		High Income (N = 46)	
PROGRESS-Plus characteristic	N	%	N	%	N	%	N	%	N	%
Place of residence (rural/urban)	118	58.1%	21	70.0%	71	69.6%	18	69.2%	8	17.4%
Race, ethnicity, culture, language	89	43.8%	6	20.0%	48	47.1%	8	30.8%	27	58.7%
Occupation (maternal)	53	25.6%	11	36.7%	30	29.4%	10	38.5%	2	4.3%
Gender and sex (Child's sex)	133	65.0%	18	60.0%	79	77.4%	21	80.8%	15	32.6%
Religion	60	29.6%	8	26.7%	48	47.1%	1	3.8%	3	6.5%
Education (maternal)	138	67.5%	25	83.3%	84	82.42%	18	69.2%	11	23.9%
Socioeconomic status	146	71.9%	25	83.3%	76	75.2%	21	80.8%	24	52.2%
Subnational region	99	48.8%	16	53.3%	58	57.4%	10	38.5%	15	32.6%
+ Vulnerability index	21	10.3%	0	0.0%	4	4.0%	1	3.8%	16	34.8%

The next more commonly reported dimension of inequality overall was maternal education (67.5% of studies), followed by child's sex (65.0%). This pattern was seen in countries across World Bank classification categories, although among high-income countries, there was a greater relative quantity of studies looking at race, ethnicity, culture, or language (58.7% of studies). Further, vulnerability indices were much more commonly applied in high-income country contexts. Religion as a dimension of inequality was much more commonly used in low- (N = 8) and lower-middle-income (N = 48) countries compared to in upper-middle-income (N = 1) and high-income (N = 3) countries. Lastly, we found that about a quarter of the single-country papers (N = 50) looked at multiple dimensions of inequality, and 28 used multiple disaggregation of inequality dimensions.

We also found an increasing use of vaccination indicators that may serve as proxies of inequity and disadvantage: zero-dose or non-vaccination was measured in 34 (or 16.7% of single-country) studies. Among these studies, the most commonly reported dimension of inequality was maternal education (76.5% of single-country studies reporting non-vaccination or zero-dose), followed closely by socioeconomic inequality (67.6% of single-country studies reporting non-vaccination or zero-dose), place of residence (64.7% of single-country studies reporting on this indicator), as well as gender and sex (58.5% of single-country studies reporting on this indicator). No studies examining zero-dose or non-vaccination utilized a vulnerability index. The findings broadly matched the patterns seen in full vaccine coverage studies, meaning that higher education and socio-economic statuses were associated with a lower zero-dose prevalence. Further, minoritized racial and ethnic groups, as well as religious groups, reported a higher zero-dose prevalence. However, for certain dimensions of inequality, like gender and sex as well as place of residence, a number of studies reported no association or associations that became insignificant in the multivariate analysis. The full results of the evidence for single-country studies are included in Table S2.

3.2. Multi-Country Studies

Of the 38 multi-country studies identified in our review, the most commonly reported dimension of inequality was socioeconomic status, defined as the wealth index, household wealth, or household disposable income. Of the multi-country studies, 20 had data on full coverage of multiple vaccines. Among multi-country studies, 94.7% (N = 36) used DHS/MICS data. Four studies (10.5%) used multiple disaggregation, and over a quarter of the studies (N = 10) looked at inequality trends over time. Finally, subnational inequalities in vaccination were reported in a number of multi-country studies [38–40]. The full results of evidence for single-country studies are included in Table S3.

4. Discussion

Our scoping review aimed to characterize the methods of reporting inequalities in childhood vaccine coverage, inclusive of the settings, data source types, analysis methods, and reporting modalities used to quantify and communicate inequality. We observed that analyses on inequalities in childhood vaccination rely heavily on DHS or MICS data and that papers leveraging these data had increased in the last decade. We found that few studies analyzed and reported inequalities using summary measures and instead largely used multivariate or multivariable logistic regression models for analyses. The most commonly analyzed dimensions of inequality were economic status and maternal education, and the most common vaccine outcome indicator was full vaccination of multiple vaccines. However, the definition and construction of both dimensions of inequality and outcome measures varied across studies.

Summary measures allow inequalities to be described by a single number and can be useful in describing, monitoring, and comparing inequality across settings and over time [26]. However, a low proportion of studies identified in this review used summary measures of inequalities. Overwhelmingly, the studies used multivariate or multivariate logistic regression models. While these models provide valuable insights by simultaneously examining the influence of multiple factors on the outcome of interest, they do not strictly qualify as summary measures of inequality. Estimates from logistic regression provide an estimate of the direct effect of a dimension of inequality, while summary measures of inequality provide a measure of the total effect of a dimension of inequality. By accounting for various potential confounders, these models offer a more nuanced understanding of the association between socioeconomic status and vaccine coverage. However, their reliance on specific sets of covariates, which are tailored to the author's conceptual framework and the available data, complicates the comparability of effect estimates between studies. This variability in model specifications can lead to inconsistencies in findings and hinder efforts to synthesize evidence across diverse research endeavors. Additionally, the construction of models may come with limitations, especially when not accounting for the study design and sampling approaches. For example, several studies identified in our review leveraged DHS or MICS data and included the place of residence but not regions in the regression models. DHS and MICS use both the place of residence and regions as strata for survey sampling and therefore oversample certain regions as needed [41,42]. Thus, if vaccine coverage is greater in certain regions than others, then this omission of both place of residence and regions as potential confounders would likely introduce a bias into the estimate. Multivariate and multivariable logistic regression models serve an important purpose; however, there is a need for more studies reporting summary measures to inform the monitoring and tracking of inequalities across countries and over time.

Among the studies identified in this review, approximately one in five reported absolute summary measures, while half reported relative summary measures and about one-tenth reported both absolute and relative summary measures [19–23]. The selection of reporting absolute vs. relative summary measures may influence the interpretation, conclusions, and implications of the study results [24–26]. For example, one study used multiple inequality summary measures, which all led to fairly consistent findings for the presence of inequalities but inconsistent findings for trends of inequality over time [43]. Although eight percent of studies reported both absolute and relative summary measures, there is an opportunity for more studies to leverage both types of measures to provide more meaningful and informative results and reduce reporting bias. Simple measures of inequality, such as the difference and ratio, were used in a large proportion of analyses identified in this review and allow for comparisons of vaccination outcomes in two population subgroups. However, the selection of only two subgroups may not reflect the level of inequalities across diverse subgroups in the population. Conversely, complex measures allow for comparison with more than two population subgroups and were used in about one-third of the studies identified in this review. Most of the complex summary measures reported in this review leveraged disproportionality measures such as the relative concentration index, which is a measure of inequality that shows the gradient across population subgroups and indicates the extent to which inequality is concentrated among certain subgroups.

Impact summary measures are used to estimate the potential benefits of addressing inequalities in childhood vaccination coverage. Overall, only 2% of studies (N = 4) identified in this review used impact measures—specifically, the population attributable fraction—to show the potential improvement that could be achieved if all population subgroups had the same level of vaccine coverage as a reference subgroup. Several other studies were focused on assessing the potential for inequality reduction. For example, one study used an equity outcome in program evaluation [44] and another study aimed at evaluating changes in inequalities as a result of a policy [45]. Although measuring the state of inequalities and monitoring inequalities are essential, there is a need for more studies to look forward towards how to reduce inequalities and improve childhood vaccination coverage.

This review highlighted that the most commonly analyzed dimensions of inequality were economic status and maternal education. However, the distribution of the use of these varied based on country-level income, as a higher proportion of studies in low- and middle-income settings utilized these dimensions than in high-income settings. Conversely, race and ethnicity were explored in a high proportion of studies in high-income settings compared to those in lower- and middle-income settings. The selection of dimensions of inequalities may reflect the differences in the drivers and conceptual pathways in inequalities in high-income settings compared to those in lower- and middle-income settings. Importantly, the definitions and categorizations of the dimensions differed, with over ten different ways in which economic status was defined and the measure was constructed. Studies may have leveraged data-driven or conceptual approaches for categorizing dimensions of inequalities; however, using conceptual approaches for categorization may allow for uniform measures across different settings and datasets.

Across studies identified in this scoping review, vaccine outcome indicators varied in how they were constructed. For example, the most commonly reported vaccine indicator was full vaccination of multiple vaccines. However, not all of these studies utilized the same set of vaccines in their definition of full vaccination coverage. Almost half of the studies in this review used non-vaccination as a vaccine outcome, and this was defined as non-vaccination with one specific vaccine, non-vaccination of multiple vaccines, or as 'zero dose' (children who have not received any routine vaccinations). The choice and construction of vaccine outcomes may influence the inequality observed, the interpretation of the results, and the utility of the findings. For example, analyzing full coverage in vaccination may provide insight into inequalities in subgroups who are not achieving the recommended vaccination coverage and provide insight into how programs may fill gaps in reaching goals for full coverage. Conversely, assessing inequalities in non-vaccination or zero coverage provides insights into the sub-populations that may be most marginalized and not obtaining any vaccine coverage, highlighting subgroups with a severe need for interventions.

Our scoping review highlights the patterns in data sources used for assessing inequalities among children. Across studies, DHS or MICS were the most commonly used data source for vaccine indicators. Importantly, the utilization of DHS or MICS appears to have increased over the last decade and is contributing to a larger proportion of the literature on inequalities in childhood vaccinations. Notably, almost all the multi-country studies utilized DHS or MICS data, highlighting the reliance on these data for regional and global analyses of inequalities. Therefore, the quality of this body of literature is heavily tied to the quality of these data. Both DHS and MICS are household surveys and are designed to be nationally representative samples. Given that DHS and MICS use consistent indicators across countries, and the recruitment methods are standardized, cross-country comparisons are feasible. Both DHS and MICS have publicly available datasets and are therefore accessible to researchers who wish to analyze and report on disaggregated data. However, there are some limitations of using these data, such as the lack of control over the selection and measurement of the dimensions of inequalities available. Additionally, there is generally a large lag in the release of data and reports from when the data are collected.

Lastly, DHS/MICS may have limited data on marginalized populations of interest for inequality studies.

Our scoping review highlights that there are challenges in comparing results of inequalities in childhood vaccination across settings and over time. These challenges arise from the differences in the data used for analyses, indicator definitions for vaccinations as well and dimensions of inequalities, and summary measures. Although the goal of our review was not to summarize the evidence of studies, we explored the evidence in Table S2 for the purpose of understanding the patterns and potential implications of the methods used. Given the differences in the data, indicators, methods, and summary measures used, we expect to observe inconsistencies in the results across settings. For example, studies assessing residence using rural vs. urban settings as the dimension of inequality varied in terms of inequalities favoring either urban or rural. One may conclude that these findings highlight that rural–urban inequalities are likely very context- and setting-dependent and that this variation likely depends on the funding and programmatic priorities and efforts towards vaccination in either setting. However, the variation in results may alternatively be a product of the methods used for assessment, including definitions of vaccine coverage or of urbanicity, rather than actual inequalities. Despite challenges and limitations, some consistencies in the results were observed across studies. For example, maternal education and economic status are widely used dimensions of inequality for assessing vaccination among children, with more than half of the studies identified in this review analyzing at least one of these dimensions. Across studies, the results were largely consistent with inequalities favoring higher education and a higher economic status. This may highlight the persistent and universal role that education and economic statuses may serve in inequalities in childhood vaccines, regardless of the country, setting, or methods used. However, harmonizing methods used in assessing inequalities will improve our ability to accurately compare across countries, across populations, and over time.

There are several limitations that should be considered for this scoping review. The results from this search strategy are subject to how the manuscripts were indexed into each database. Therefore, relevant manuscripts may not have been detected in the search. For our search strategy, only predominately English-language databases were searched, and therefore, relevant articles in non-English databases may not have been identified in the search. Our search was limited to articles published in academic journals, and therefore, literature such as project reports, normative agency reports, or other studies may not have been identified in our search strategy.

5. Conclusions

Measuring and monitoring inequalities in childhood immunization is essential to achieving health equity. Currently, the evidence on inequalities in childhood vaccination in academic journals relies on the use of various approaches including data, analytical methods, and measures of results, which makes comparisons across settings and time difficult. The harmonization of approaches may allow for improved monitoring through academic studies.

Supplementary Materials: The following supporting information can be downloaded at: https://www.mdpi.com/article/10.3390/vaccines12080850/s1, File S1: Search Protocol; Table S1. Full list of articles identified in the scoping review on inequality in childhood immunization coverage; Figure S1: Multiple Correspondence Analysis of Article Characteristics on Child Vaccine Coverage Inequalities; Table S2. Summary of findings of single-country studies on inequalities in child vaccine coverage conducted between 2013 and 2023; Table S3. Summary of findings of multi-country studies on inequalities in child vaccine coverage conducted between 2013 and 2023 [46–157].

Author Contributions: The conceptualization was led by A.R.H., N.E.J., and N.B. The methodology was led by A.R.H., N.E.J., N.B., D.N., C.L., and A.A. The analysis was led by D.N. and supported by C.L. and A.A. The writing was led by C.L. and supported by D.N. and N.E.J. All authors contributed to the review and finalization of the manuscript (A.R.H., N.E.J., N.B., D.N., C.L., and A.A). All authors have read and agreed to the published version of the manuscript. NEJ is affiliated with University of California San Diego, San Diego, USA at the time of publication of the article.

Funding: This research was funded by Gavi, the Vaccine Alliance. The funders had no role in the design of the study; in the collection, analyses, or interpretation of the data; in the writing of the manuscript; or in the decision to publish the results.

Institutional Review Board Statement: Not applicable.

Informed Consent Statement: Not applicable.

Data Availability Statement: Not applicable.

Conflicts of Interest: The authors declare that they have no conflicts of interest. The authors are staff of the World health Organization. The authors alone are responsible for the views expressed in this publication, and they do not necessarily represent the views, decisions, or policies of the World Health Organization.

References

1. McGovern, M.E.; Canning, D. Vaccination and all-cause child mortality from 1985 to 2011: Global evidence from the Demographic and Health Surveys. *Am. J. Epidemiol.* **2015**, *182*, 791–798. [CrossRef] [PubMed]
2. Patel, M.K.; Goodson, J.L.; Alexander, J.P., Jr.; Kretsinger, K.; Sodha, S.V.; Steulet, C.; Gacic-Dobo, M.; Rota, P.A.; McFarland, J.; Menning, L.; et al. Progress Toward Regional Measles Elimination—Worldwide, 2000–2019. *MMWR Morb. Mortal. Wkly. Rep.* **2020**, *69*, 1700–1705. [CrossRef] [PubMed]
3. Li, X.; Mukandavire, C.; Cucunubá, Z.M.; Echeverria Londono, S.; Abbas, K.; Clapham, H.E.; Jit, M.; Johnson, H.L.; Papadopoulos, T.; Vynnycky, E.; et al. Estimating the health impact of vaccination against ten pathogens in 98 low-income and middle-income countries from 2000 to 2030: A modelling study. *Lancet* **2021**, *397*, 398–408. [CrossRef] [PubMed]
4. Chang, A.Y.; Riumallo-Herl, C.; Perales, N.A.; Clark, S.; Clark, A.; Constenla, D.; Garske, T.; Jackson, M.L.; Jean, K.; Jit, M.; et al. The Equity Impact Vaccines May Have On Averting Deaths And Medical Impoverishment In Developing Countries. *Health Aff. (Proj. Hope)* **2018**, *37*, 316–324. [CrossRef] [PubMed]
5. Measuring routine childhood vaccination coverage in 204 countries and territories, 1980–2019: A systematic analysis for the Global Burden of Disease Study 2020, Release 1. *Lancet* **2021**, *398*, 503–521. [CrossRef] [PubMed]
6. Verrier, F.; de Lauzanne, A.; Diouf, J.N.; Zo, A.Z.; Ramblière, L.; Herindrainy, P.; Sarr, F.D.; Sok, T.; Vray, M.; Collard, J.M.; et al. Vaccination Coverage and Risk Factors Associated With Incomplete Vaccination Among Children in Cambodia, Madagascar, and Senegal. *Open Forum Infect. Dis.* **2023**, *10*, ofad136. [CrossRef] [PubMed]
7. Yendewa, G.A.; James, P.B.; Mohareb, A.; Barrie, U.; Massaquoi, S.P.E.; Yendewa, S.A.; Ghazzawi, M.; Bockarie, T.; Cummings, P.E.; Diallo, I.S.; et al. Determinants of incomplete childhood hepatitis B vaccination in Sierra Leone, Liberia, and Guinea: Analysis of national surveys (2018–2020). *Epidemiol. Infect.* **2023**, *151*, e193. [CrossRef] [PubMed]
8. Peck, M.; Gacic-Dobo, M.; Diallo, M.S.; Nedelec, Y.; Sodha, S.V.; Wallace, A.S. Global Routine Vaccination Coverage, 2018. *MMWR Morb. Mortal. Wkly. Rep.* **2019**, *68*, 937–942. [CrossRef] [PubMed]
9. Cata-Preta, B.O.; Santos, T.M.; Mengistu, T.; Hogan, D.R.; Barros, A.J.D.; Victora, C.G. Zero-dose children and the immunisation cascade: Understanding immunisation pathways in low and middle-income countries. *Vaccine* **2021**, *39*, 4564–4570. [CrossRef]
10. World Health Organization. *Immunization Agena 2030: A Global Strategy to Leave No One Behind*; World Health Organization: Geneva, Switzerland, 2020.
11. Ali, H.A.; Hartner, A.M.; Echeverria-Londono, S.; Roth, J.; Li, X.; Abbas, K.; Portnoy, A.; Vynnycky, E.; Woodruff, K.; Ferguson, N.M.; et al. Vaccine equity in low and middle income countries: A systematic review and meta-analysis. *Int. J. Equity Health* **2022**, *21*, 82. [CrossRef]
12. Bocquier, A.; Ward, J.; Raude, J.; Peretti-Watel, P.; Verger, P. Socioeconomic differences in childhood vaccination in developed countries: A systematic review of quantitative studies. *Expert Rev. Vaccines* **2017**, *16*, 1107–1118. [CrossRef]
13. Bergen, N.; Cata-Preta, B.O.; Schlotheuber, A.; Santos, T.M.; Danovaro-Holliday, M.C.; Mengistu, T.; Sodha, S.V.; Hogan, D.R.; Barros, A.J.D.; Hosseinpoor, A.R. Economic-Related Inequalities in Zero-Dose Children: A Study of Non-Receipt of Diphtheria-Tetanus-Pertussis Immunization Using Household Health Survey Data from 89 Low- and Middle-Income Countries. *Vaccines* **2022**, *10*, 633. [CrossRef]
14. Lai, X.; Zhang, H.; Pouwels, K.B.; Patenaude, B.; Jit, M.; Fang, H. Estimating global and regional between-country inequality in routine childhood vaccine coverage in 195 countries and territories from 2019 to 2021: A longitudinal study. *EClinicalMedicine* **2023**, *60*, 102042. [CrossRef]
15. Hosseinpoor, A.R.; Bergen, N. Health Inequality Monitoring: A Practical Application of Population Health Monitoring. In *Population Health Monitoring: Climbing the Information Pyramid*; Verschuuren, M., van Oers, H., Eds.; Springer International Publishing: Cham, Switzerland, 2019; pp. 151–173.
16. Hosseinpoor, A.R.; Bergen, N.; Schlotheuber, A.; Grove, J. Measuring health inequalities in the context of sustainable development goals. *Bull. World Health Organ.* **2018**, *96*, 654–659. [CrossRef] [PubMed]

17. Health Inequality Monitoring. *Harnessing Data to Advance Health Equity (In Development)*; World Health Organization: Geneva, Switzerland, 2023.
18. O'Donnell, O.; Van Doorslaer, E.; Wagstaff, A.; Lindelow, M. *Analyzing Health Equity Using Household Survey Data: A Guide to Techniques and Their Implementation*; World Bank Group: Washington, DC, USA, 2018.
19. Kelly, M.P.M.A.; Bonnefoy, J.; Butt, J.; Bergmann, V. *The Social Determinants of Health: Developing an Evidence Base for Action*; World Health Organization Commission on Social Determinants of Health: Geneva, Switzerland, 2007.
20. *Handbook on Health Inequality Monitoring: With a Special Focus on Low- and Middle-Income Countries*; The World Health Organization: Geneva, Switzerland, 2013.
21. *Inequality Monitoring in Immunization: A Step-by-Step Manual*; The World Health Organization: Geneva, Switzerland, 2019.
22. Kjellsson, G.; Gerdtham, U.G.; Petrie, D. Lies, Damned Lies, and Health Inequality Measurements: Understanding the Value Judgments. *Epidemiology* 2015, 26, 673–680. [CrossRef]
23. Asada, Y. On the choice of absolute or relative inequality measures. *Milbank Q.* 2010, 88, 616–622; discussion 623–627. [CrossRef] [PubMed]
24. Houweling, T.A.; Kunst, A.E.; Huisman, M.; Mackenbach, J.P. Using relative and absolute measures for monitoring health inequalities: Experiences from cross-national analyses on maternal and child health. *Int. J. Equity Health* 2007, 6, 15. [CrossRef] [PubMed]
25. Moser, K.; Frost, C.; Leon, D.A. Comparing health inequalities across time and place--rate ratios and rate differences lead to different conclusions: Analysis of cross-sectional data from 22 countries 1991–2001. *Int. J. Epidemiol.* 2007, 36, 1285–1291. [CrossRef]
26. Schlotheuber, A.; Hosseinpoor, A.R. Summary Measures of Health Inequality: A Review of Existing Measures and Their Application. *Int. J. Environ. Res. Public Health* 2022, 19, 3697. [CrossRef]
27. King, N.B.; Harper, S.; Young, M.E. Use of relative and absolute effect measures in reporting health inequalities: Structured review. *BMJ (Clin. Res. Ed)* 2012, 345, e5774. [CrossRef] [PubMed]
28. Aromataris, E.; Munn, Z. (Eds.) Chapter 11. Scoping reviews. In *JBI Manual for Evidence Synthesis*; JBI: Miami, FL, USA, 2017; Available online: https://jbi-global-wiki.refined.site/space/MANUAL/4687342/Chapter+11:+Scoping+reviews (accessed on 18 March 2024).
29. Tricco, A.C.; Lillie, E.; Zarin, W.; O'Brien, K.K.; Colquhoun, H.; Levac, D.; Moher, D.; Peters, M.D.J.; Horsley, T.; Weeks, L.; et al. PRISMA Extension for Scoping Reviews (PRISMA-ScR): Checklist and Explanation. *Ann. Intern. Med.* 2018, 169, 467–473. [CrossRef] [PubMed]
30. *Covidence Systematic Review Software*; Veritas Health Innovation: Melbourne, Australia, 2020.
31. O'Neill, J.; Tabish, H.; Welch, V.; Petticrew, M.; Pottie, K.; Clarke, M.; Evans, T.; Pardo Pardo, J.; Waters, E.; White, H.; et al. Applying an equity lens to interventions: Using progress ensures consideration of socially stratifying factors to illuminate inequities in health. *J. Clin. Epidemiol.* 2014, 67, 56–64. [CrossRef] [PubMed]
32. Le Roux, B.; Rouanet, H. *Multiple Correspondence Analysis*; Series: Quantitative Applications in the Social Sciences; SAGE: Thousand Oaks, CA, USA, 2010; Volume 163.
33. Alaba, O.A.; Hongoro, C.; Thulare, A.; Lukwa, A.T. Leaving No Child Behind: Decomposing Socioeconomic Inequalities in Child Health for India and South Africa. *Int. J. Environ. Res. Public Health* 2021, 18, 7114. [CrossRef]
34. Siddiqui, N.T.; Owais, A.; Agha, A.; Karim, M.S.; Zaidi, A.K. Ethnic disparities in routine immunization coverage: A reason for persistent poliovirus circulation in Karachi, Pakistan? *Asia Pac. J. Public Health* 2014, 26, 67–76. [CrossRef] [PubMed]
35. Wendt, A.; Hellwig, F.; Saad, G.E.; Faye, C.; Mokomane, Z.; Boerma, T.; Barros, A.J.D.; Victora, C. Are children in female-headed households at a disadvantage? An analysis of immunization coverage and stunting prevalence: In 95 low- and middle-income countries. *SSM Popul. Health* 2021, 15, 100888. [CrossRef] [PubMed]
36. Sissoko, D.; Trottier, H.; Malvy, D.; Johri, M. The Influence of Compositional and Contextual Factors on Non-Receipt of Basic Vaccines among Children of 12–23-Month Old in India: A Multilevel Analysis. *PLoS ONE* 2014, 9, e106528. [CrossRef]
37. Prusty, R.K.; Kumar, A. Socioeconomic dynamics of gender disparity in childhood immunization in India, 1992–2006. *PLoS ONE* 2014, 9, e104598. [CrossRef]
38. Dimitrova, A.; Carrasco-Escobar, G.; Richardson, R.; Benmarhnia, T. Essential childhood immunization in 43 low- and middle-income countries: Analysis of spatial trends and socioeconomic inequalities in vaccine coverage. *PLoS Med.* 2023, 20, e1004166. [CrossRef]
39. Fullman, N.; Correa, G.C.; Ikilezi, G.; Phillips, D.E.; Reynolds, H.W. Assessing Potential Exemplars in Reducing Zero-Dose Children: A Novel Approach for Identifying Positive Outliers in Decreasing National Levels and Geographic Inequalities in Unvaccinated Children. *Vaccines* 2023, 11, 647. [CrossRef]
40. Gao, Y.; Kc, A.; Chen, C.; Huang, Y.; Wang, Y.; Zou, S.; Zhou, H. Inequality in measles vaccination coverage in the "big six" countries of the WHO South-East Asia region. *Hum Vaccin Immunother* 2020, 16, 1485–1497. [CrossRef] [PubMed]
41. DHS Methodology. Available online: https://dhsprogram.com/Methodology/Survey-Types/DHS-Methodology.cfm (accessed on 1 February 2024).
42. MICS7 TOOLS. Available online: https://mics.unicef.org/tools#survey-design (accessed on 1 February 2024).

43. Zegeye, B.; El-Khatib, Z.; Oladimeji, O.; Ahinkorah, B.O.; Ameyaw, E.K.; Seidu, A.A.; Budu, E.; Yaya, S. Demographic and health surveys showed widening trends in polio immunisation inequalities in Guinea. *Acta Paediatr.* **2021**, *110*, 3334–3342. [CrossRef] [PubMed]
44. Katz, A.; Enns, J.E.; Chateau, D.; Lix, L.; Jutte, D.; Edwards, J.; Brownell, M.; Metge, C.; Nickel, N.; Taylor, C.; et al. Does a pay-for-performance program for primary care physicians alleviate health inequity in childhood vaccination rates? *Int. J. Equity Health* **2015**, *14*, 114. [CrossRef] [PubMed]
45. Sowe, A.; Namatovu, F.; Cham, B.; Gustafsson, P.E. Does a pay-for-performance health service model improve overall and rural-urban inequity in vaccination rates? A difference-in-differences analysis from the Gambia. *Vaccine X* **2022**, *12*, 100206. [CrossRef]
46. Shenton, L.M.; Wagner, A.L.; Carlson, B.F.; Mubarak, M.Y.; Boulton, M.L. Vaccination status of children aged 1–4 years in Afghanistan and associated factors, 2015. *Vaccine* **2018**, *36*, 5141–5149. [CrossRef]
47. Boulton, M.L.; Carlson, B.F.; Power, L.E.; Wagner, A.L. Socioeconomic factors associated with full childhood vaccination in Bangladesh, 2014. *Int. J. Infect. Dis.* **2018**, *69*, 35–40. [CrossRef]
48. Budu, E.; Ahinkorah, B.O.; Guets, W.; Ameyaw, E.K.; Essuman, M.A.; Yaya, S. Socioeconomic and residence-based related inequality in childhood vaccination in Sub-Saharan Africa: Evidence from Benin. *Health Sci. Rep.* **2023**, *6*, e1198. [CrossRef]
49. Zhang, H.; Lai, X.; Mak, J.; Sriudomporn, S.; Fang, H.; Patenaude, B. Coverage and Equity of Childhood Vaccines in China. *JAMA Netw. Open* **2022**, *5*, e2246005. [CrossRef] [PubMed]
50. Dheresa, M.; Dessie, Y.; Negash, B.; Balis, B.; Getachew, T.; Ayana, G.M.; Merga, B.T.; Regassa, L.D. Child Vaccination Coverage, Trends and Predictors in Eastern Ethiopia: Implication for Sustainable Development Goals. *J. Multidiscip. Healthc.* **2021**, *14*, 2657–2667. [CrossRef]
51. Tola, H.H.; Gamtesa, D.F. High Inequality and Slow Services Improvement in Newborn and Child Health Interventions in Ethiopia. *Pediatr. Health Med. Ther.* **2020**, *11*, 513–523. [CrossRef]
52. Asmare, G.; Madalicho, M.; Sorsa, A. Disparities in full immunization coverage among urban and rural children aged 12–23 months in southwest Ethiopia: A comparative cross-sectional study. *Hum. Vaccin. Immunother.* **2022**, *18*, 2101316. [CrossRef] [PubMed]
53. Debie, A.; Lakew, A.M.; Tamirat, K.S.; Amare, G.; Tesema, G.A. Complete vaccination service utilization inequalities among children aged 12–23 months in Ethiopia: A multivariate decomposition analyses. *Int. J. Equity Health* **2020**, *19*, 65. [CrossRef] [PubMed]
54. Yibeltal, K.; Tsegaye, S.; Zelealem, H.; Worku, W.; Demissie, M.; Worku, A.; Berhane, Y. Trends, projection and inequalities in full immunization coverage in Ethiopia: In the period 2000–2019. *BMC Pediatr.* **2022**, *22*, 193. [CrossRef] [PubMed]
55. Budu, E.; Opoku Ahinkorah, B.; Okyere, J.; Seidu, A.A.; Ofori Duah, H. Inequalities in the prevalence of full immunization coverage among one-year-olds in Ghana, 1993–2014. *Vaccine* **2022**, *40*, 3614–3620. [CrossRef] [PubMed]
56. Sharma, S.; Maheshwari, S.; Jaiswal, A.K.; Mehra, S. Income-based inequality in full immunization coverage of children aged 12–23 months in Eastern India: A decomposition analysis. *Clin. Epidemiol. Glob. Health* **2021**, *11*, 100738. [CrossRef]
57. Goli, S.; James, K.S.; Pallikadavath, S.; Mishra, U.S.; Irudaya Rajan, S.; Prasad, R.D.; Salve, P.S. Perplexing condition of child full immunisation in economically better off Gujarat in India: An assessment of associated factors. *Vaccine* **2020**, *38*, 5831–5841. [CrossRef] [PubMed]
58. Bettampadi, D.; Carlson, B.F.; Mathew, J.L. Impact of Multiple Risk Factors on Vaccination Inequities: Analysis in Indian Infants Over 2 Decades. *Am. J. Prev. Med.* **2021**, *60* (Suppl. S1), S34–S43. [CrossRef] [PubMed]
59. Bettampadi, D.; Lepkowski, J.M.; Sen, A.; Power, L.E.; Boulton, M.L. Vaccination Inequality in India, 2002–2013. *Am. J. Prev. Med.* **2021**, *60* (Suppl. S1), S65–S76. [CrossRef] [PubMed]
60. Francis, M.R.; Nohynek, H.; Larson, H.; Balraj, V.; Mohan, V.R.; Kang, G.; Nuorti, J.P. Factors associated with routine childhood vaccine uptake and reasons for non-vaccination in India: 1998–2008. *Vaccine* **2018**, *36*, 6559–6566. [CrossRef]
61. Holroyd, T.A.; Wahl, B.; Gupta, M.; Sauer, M.; Blunt, M.; Gerste, A.K.; Erchick, D.J.; Santosham, M.; Limaye, R.J. Characterizing mothers and children at risk of being under-immunized in India: A latent class analysis approach. *Int. J. Infect. Dis.* **2020**, *100*, 59–66. [CrossRef]
62. Khan, N.; Saggurti, N. Socioeconomic inequality trends in childhood vaccination coverage in India: Findings from multiple rounds of National Family Health Survey. *Vaccine* **2020**, *38*, 4088–4103. [CrossRef] [PubMed]
63. Herliana, P.; Douiri, A. Determinants of immunisation coverage of children aged 12–59 months in Indonesia: A cross-sectional study. *BMJ Open* **2017**, *7*, e015790. [CrossRef]
64. Win, Z.M.; Traill, T.; Kyaw, Z.L.; Hnin, K.T.; Chit, P.T.; La, T.; Deshpande, A.S.; Ogbuoji, O.; Mao, W. Equity assessment of childhood immunisation at national and subnational levels in Myanmar: A benefit incidence analysis. *BMJ Glob. Health* **2022**, *7*, e007800. [CrossRef] [PubMed]
65. Kc, A.; Nelin, V.; Raaijmakers, H.; Kim, H.J.; Singh, C.; Målqvist, M. Increased immunization coverage addresses the equity gap in Nepal. *Bull. World Health Organ.* **2017**, *95*, 261–269. [CrossRef] [PubMed]
66. Chidiebere, O.D.I.; Uchenna, E.; Kenechi, O.S. Maternal sociodemographic factors that influence full child immunisation uptake in Nigeria. *S. Afr. J. Child. Health* **2014**, *8*, 138–142. [CrossRef]

67. Ogundele, O.A.; Ogundele, T.; Fehintola, F.O.; Fagbemi, A.T.; Beloved, O.O.; Osunmakinwa, O.O. Determinants of incomplete vaccination among children 12–23 months in Nigeria: An analysis of a national sample. *Tzu Chi Med. J.* **2022**, *34*, 448–455. [CrossRef] [PubMed]
68. Seck, I.; Diop, B.; Leyé, M.M.; Mboup, B.M.; Ndiaye, A.; Seck, P.A.; Doucoure, A.; Ba, T.A.; Diongue, M.; Faye, A.; et al. Social determinants of routine immunization coverage of children aged 72 to 23 months in the Kaolack region of Senegal. *Sante Publique* **2016**, *28*, 807–815. [CrossRef] [PubMed]
69. Jammeh, A.; Muhoozi, M.; Kulane, A.; Kajungu, D. Comparing full immunisation status of children (0–23 months) between slums of Kampala City and the rural setting of Iganga District in Uganda: A cross-sectional study. *BMC Health Serv. Res.* **2023**, *23*, 856. [CrossRef] [PubMed]
70. Ataguba, J.E.; Ojo, K.O.; Ichoku, H.E. Explaining socio-economic inequalities in immunization coverage in Nigeria. *Health Policy Plan.* **2016**, *31*, 1212–1224. [CrossRef]
71. Asif, A.M.; Akbar, M.; Tahir, M.R.; Arshad, I.A. Role of Maternal Education and Vaccination Coverage: Evidence From Pakistan Demographic and Health Survey. *Asia Pac. J. Public Health* **2019**, *31*, 679–688. [CrossRef]
72. Al-Kassab-Córdova, A.; Silva-Perez, C.; Maguiña, J.L. Spatial distribution, determinants and trends of full vaccination coverage in children aged 12–59 months in Peru: A subanalysis of the Peruvian Demographic and Health Survey. *BMJ Open* **2022**, *12*, e050211. [CrossRef] [PubMed]
73. Debnath, A.; Bhattacharjee, N. Wealth-Based Inequality In Child Immunization In India: A Decomposition Approach. *J. Biosoc. Sci.* **2018**, *50*, 312–325. [CrossRef]
74. Mishra, P.S.; Choudhary, P.K.; Anand, A. Migration and child health: Understanding the coverage of child immunization among migrants across different socio-economic groups in India. *Child. Youth Serv. Rev.* **2020**, *119*, 105684. [CrossRef]
75. Hu, Y.; Wang, Y.; Chen, Y.; Li, Q. Determinants of inequality in the up-to-date fully immunization coverage among children aged 24–35 months: Evidence from Zhejiang province, East China. *Hum. Vaccin. Immunother.* **2017**, *13*, 1902–1907. [CrossRef] [PubMed]
76. Lu, X.; Fu, C.; Wang, Q.; Hee, J.; Takesue, R.; Tang, K. Women's Empowerment and Children's Complete Vaccination in the Democratic Republic of the Congo: A Cross-Sectional Analysis. *Vaccines* **2021**, *9*, 1117. [CrossRef]
77. Tesfa, G.A.; Yehualashet, D.E.; Getnet, A.; Bimer, K.B.; Seboka, B.T. Spatial distribution of complete basic childhood vaccination and associated factors among children aged 12–23 months in Ethiopia. A spatial and multilevel analysis. *PLoS ONE* **2023**, *18*, e0279399. [CrossRef] [PubMed]
78. Asuman, D.; Ackah, C.G.; Enemark, U. Inequalities in child immunization coverage in Ghana: Evidence from a decomposition analysis. *Health Econ. Rev.* **2018**, *8*, 9. [CrossRef]
79. Moran, E.B.; Wagner, A.L.; Asiedu-Bekoe, F.; Abdul-Karim, A.; Schroeder, L.F.; Boulton, M.L. Socioeconomic characteristics associated with the introduction of new vaccines and full childhood vaccination in Ghana, 2014. *Vaccine* **2020**, *38*, 2937–2942. [CrossRef]
80. Singh, C.M.; Mishra, A.; Agarwal, N.; Ayub, A.; Mishra, S.; Lohani, P. Gender discrimination and other factors affecting Full Immunization Coverage (FIC) in 59 low performing blocks of Bihar. *Indian J. Community Health* **2020**, *32*, 101–107. [CrossRef]
81. Saikia, N.; Kumar, K.; Bora, J.K.; Mondal, S.; Phad, S.; Agarwal, S. What Determines the District-Level Disparities in Immunization Coverage in India: Findings from Five Rounds of the National Family Health Survey. *Vaccines* **2023**, *11*, 851. [CrossRef]
82. Kumar, C.; Singh, P.K.; Singh, L.; Rai, R.K. Socioeconomic disparities in coverage of full immunisation among children of adolescent mothers in India, 1990–2006: A repeated cross-sectional analysis. *BMJ Open* **2016**, *6*, e009768. [CrossRef]
83. Chu, H.; Rammohan, A. Childhood immunization and age-appropriate vaccinations in Indonesia. *BMC Public Health* **2022**, *22*, 2023. [CrossRef] [PubMed]
84. Setiawan, M.S.; Wijayanto, A.W. Determinants of immunization status of children under two years old in Sumatera, Indonesia: A multilevel analysis of the 2020 Indonesia National Socio-Economic Survey. *Vaccine* **2022**, *40*, 1821–1828. [CrossRef]
85. Joseph, N.K.; Macharia, P.M.; Ouma, P.O.; Mumo, J.; Jalang'o, R.; Wagacha, P.W.; Achieng, V.O.; Ndung'u, E.; Okoth, P.; Muñiz, M.; et al. Spatial access inequities and childhood immunisation uptake in Kenya. *BMC Public Health* **2020**, *20*, 1407. [CrossRef]
86. Sowe, A.; Johansson, K. Disentangling the rural-urban immunization coverage disparity in The Gambia: A Fairlie decomposition. *Vaccine* **2019**, *37*, 3088–3096. [CrossRef] [PubMed]
87. Shrivastwa, N.; Gillespie, B.W.; Kolenic, G.E.; Lepkowski, J.M.; Boulton, M.L. Predictors of vaccination in India for children aged 12–36 months. *Vaccine* **2015**, *33*, D99–D105. [CrossRef]
88. Gram, L.; Soremekun, S.; ten Asbroek, A.; Manu, A.; O'Leary, M.; Hill, Z.; Danso, S.; Amenga-Etego, S.; Owusu-Agyei, S.; Kirkwood, B.R. Socio-economic determinants and inequities in coverage and timeliness of early childhood immunisation in rural Ghana. *Trop. Med. Int. Health* **2014**, *19*, 802–811. [CrossRef]
89. Wahl, B.; Gupta, M.; Erchick, D.J.; Patenaude, B.N.; Holroyd, T.A.; Sauer, M.; Blunt, M.; Santosham, M.; Limaye, R.J. Change in full immunization inequalities in Indian children 12–23 months: An analysis of household survey data. *BMC Public Health* **2021**, *21*, 841. [CrossRef] [PubMed]
90. Utazi, C.E.; Pannell, O.; Aheto, J.M.K.; Wigley, A.; Tejedor-Garavito, N.; Wunderlich, J.; Hagedorn, B.; Hogan, D.; Tatem, A.J. Assessing the characteristics of un- and under-vaccinated children in low- and middle-income countries: A multi-level cross-sectional study. *PLOS Glob. Public Health* **2022**, *2*, e0000244. [CrossRef]
91. Allan, S.; Adetifa, I.M.O.; Abbas, K. Inequities in childhood immunisation coverage associated with socioeconomic, geographic, maternal, child, and place of birth characteristics in Kenya. *BMC Infect. Dis.* **2021**, *21*, 553. [CrossRef]

92. Devkota, S.; Butler, C. Caste-ethnic disparity in vaccine use among 0- to 5-year-old children in Nepal: A decomposition analysis. *Int. J. Public Health* **2016**, *61*, 693–699. [CrossRef] [PubMed]
93. Ali, A.; Zar, A.; Wadood, A. Factors associated with incomplete child immunization in Pakistan: Findings from Demographic and Health Survey 2017–18. *Public Health* **2022**, *204*, 43–48. [CrossRef] [PubMed]
94. Marek, L.; Hobbs, M.; McCarthy, J.; Wiki, J.; Tomintz, M.; Campbell, M.; Kingham, S. Investigating spatial variation and change (2006–2017) in childhood immunisation coverage in New Zealand. *Soc. Sci. Med.* **2020**, *264*, 113292. [CrossRef] [PubMed]
95. Oliveira, M.F.; Martinez, E.Z.; Rocha, J.S. Factors associated with vaccination coverage in children < 5 years in Angola. *Rev. Saude Publica* **2014**, *48*, 906–915. [PubMed]
96. Zhao, Y.; Mak, J.; de Broucker, G.; Patenaude, B. Multivariate Assessment of Vaccine Equity in Cambodia: A Longitudinal VERSE Tool Case Study Using Demographic and Health Survey 2004, 2010, and 2014. *Vaccines* **2023**, *11*, 795. [CrossRef] [PubMed]
97. Yakum, M.N.; Atanga, F.D.; Ajong, A.B.; Eba Ze, L.E.; Shah, Z. Factors associated with full vaccination and zero vaccine dose in children aged 12–59 months in 6 health districts of Cameroon. *BMC Public Health* **2023**, *23*, 1693. [CrossRef]
98. Nda'chi Deffo, R.; Fomba Kamga, B. Do the dynamics of vaccine programs improve the full immunization of children under the age of five in Cameroon? *BMC Health Serv. Res.* **2020**, *20*, 953. [CrossRef] [PubMed]
99. Geweniger, A.; Abbas, K.M. Childhood vaccination coverage and equity impact in Ethiopia by socioeconomic, geographic, maternal, and child characteristics. *Vaccine* **2020**, *38*, 3627–3638. [CrossRef] [PubMed]
100. Patenaude, B.; Odihi, D.; Sriudomporn, S.; Mak, J.; Watts, E.; de Broucker, G. A standardized approach for measuring multivariate equity in vaccination coverage, cost-of-illness, and health outcomes: Evidence from the Vaccine Economics Research for Sustainability & Equity (VERSE) project. *Soc. Sci. Med.* **2022**, *302*, 114979.
101. Siramaneerat, I.; Agushybana, F. Inequalities in immunization coverage in Indonesia: A multilevel analysis. *Rural Remote Health* **2021**, *21*, 6348. [CrossRef]
102. Masters, N.B.; Wagner, A.L.; Carlson, B.F.; Muuo, S.W.; Mutua, M.K.; Boulton, M.L. Childhood vaccination in Kenya: Socioeconomic determinants and disparities among the Somali ethnic community. *Int. J. Public Health* **2019**, *64*, 313–322. [CrossRef]
103. Ntenda, P.A.M.; Chuang, K.Y.; Tiruneh, F.N.; Chuang, Y.C. Analysis of the effects of individual and community level factors on childhood immunization in Malawi. *Vaccine* **2017**, *35*, 1907–1917. [CrossRef]
104. Nozaki, I.; Hachiya, M.; Kitamura, T. Factors influencing basic vaccination coverage in Myanmar: Secondary analysis of 2015 Myanmar demographic and health survey data. *BMC Public Health* **2019**, *19*, 242. [CrossRef] [PubMed]
105. Song, I.H.; Palley, E.; Atteraya, M.S. Inequalities in complete childhood immunisation in Nepal: Results from a population-based cross-sectional study. *BMJ Open* **2020**, *10*, e037646. [CrossRef]
106. Patel, P.N.; Hada, M.; Carlson, B.F.; Boulton, M.L. Immunization status of children in Nepal and associated factors, 2016. *Vaccine* **2021**, *39*, 5831–5838. [CrossRef]
107. Acharya, K.; Paudel, Y.R.; Dharel, D. The trend of full vaccination coverage in infants and inequalities by wealth quintile and maternal education: Analysis from four recent demographic and health surveys in Nepal. *BMC Public Health* **2019**, *19*, 1673. [CrossRef]
108. Mak, J.; Odihi, D.; Wonodi, C.; Ali, D.; de Broucker, G.; Sriudomporn, S.; Patenaude, B. Multivariate assessment of vaccine equity in Nigeria: A VERSE tool case study using demographic and health survey 2018. *Vaccine X* **2023**, *14*, 100281. [CrossRef] [PubMed]
109. Uthman, O.A.; Adedokun, S.T.; Olukade, T.; Watson, S.; Adetokunboh, O.; Adeniran, A.; Oyetoyan, S.A.; Gidado, S.; Lawoko, S.; Wiysonge, C.S. Children who have received no routine polio vaccines in Nigeria: Who are they and where do they live? *Hum. Vaccin. Immunother.* **2017**, *13*, 2111–2122. [CrossRef]
110. Al-Kassab-Córdova, A.; Silva-Perez, C.; Mendez-Guerra, C.; Sangster-Carrasco, L.; Arroyave, I.; Cabieses, B.; Mezones-Holguin, E. Inequalities in infant vaccination coverage during the COVID-19 pandemic: A population-based study in Peru. *Vaccine* **2023**, *41*, 564–572. [CrossRef] [PubMed]
111. Sarker, A.R.; Akram, R.; Ali, N.; Chowdhury, Z.I.; Sultana, M. Coverage and Determinants of Full Immunization: Vaccination Coverage among Senegalese Children. *Medicina* **2019**, *55*, 480. [CrossRef]
112. Vo, H.L.; Huynh, L.T.; Anh, H.N.S.; Do, D.A.; Doan, T.N.; Nguyen, T.H.; Nguyen Van, H. Trends in Socioeconomic Inequalities in Full Vaccination Coverage among Vietnamese Children aged 12–23 Months, 2000–2014: Evidence for Mitigating Disparities in Vaccination. *Vaccines* **2019**, *7*, 188. [CrossRef] [PubMed]
113. Kriss, J.L.; Goodson, J.; Machekanyanga, Z.; Shibeshi, M.E.; Daniel, F.; Masresha, B.; Kaiser, R. Vaccine receipt and vaccine card availability among children of the apostolic faith: Analysis from the 2010–2011 Zimbabwe demographic and health survey. *Pan Afr. Med. J.* **2016**, *24*, 47. [CrossRef] [PubMed]
114. Hu, Y.; Liang, H.; Wang, Y.; Chen, Y. Inequities in Childhood Vaccination Coverage in Zhejiang, Province: Evidence from a Decomposition Analysis on Two-Round Surveys. *Int. J. Environ. Res. Public Health* **2018**, *15*, 2000. [CrossRef] [PubMed]
115. Rahman, A.; Reza, A.A.S.; Bhuiyan, B.A.; Alam, N.; Dasgupta, S.K.; Mostari, S.; Anwar, I. Equity and determinants of routine child immunisation programme among tribal and non-tribal populations in rural Tangail subdistrict, Bangladesh: A cohort study. *BMJ Open* **2018**, *8*, e022634. [CrossRef] [PubMed]
116. Roy, D.; Debnath, A.; Sarma, M.; Das, K. A Decomposition Analysis to Understand the Wealth-Based Inequalities in Child Vaccination in Rural Southern Assam: A Cross-Sectional Study. *Indian J. Community Med.* **2023**, *48*, 112–125. [CrossRef] [PubMed]
117. Oyefara, J.L. Mothers' Characteristics and Immunization Status of Under-Five Children in Ojo Local Government Area, Lagos State, Nigeria. *SAGE Open* **2014**, *4*, 2158244014545474. [CrossRef]

118. Bryden, G.M.; Browne, M.; Rockloff, M.; Unsworth, C. The privilege paradox: Geographic areas with highest socio-economic advantage have the lowest rates of vaccination. *Vaccine* **2019**, *37*, 4525–4532. [CrossRef] [PubMed]
119. Hu, Y.; Wang, Y.; Chen, Y.; Liang, H. Analyzing the Urban-Rural Vaccination Coverage Disparity through a Fair Decomposition in Zhejiang Province, China. *Int. J. Environ. Res. Public Health* **2019**, *16*, 4575. [CrossRef] [PubMed]
120. Adebowale, A.; Obembe, T.; Bamgboye, E. Relationship between household wealth and childhood immunization in core-North Nigeria. *Afr. Health Sci.* **2019**, *19*, 1582–1593. [CrossRef]
121. Hu, Y.; Chen, Y.; Wang, Y.; Liang, H.; Lv, H. The trends of socioeconomic inequities in full vaccination coverage among children aged 12–23 months from 2000 to 2017: Evidence for mitigating disparities in vaccination service in Zhejiang province. *Hum. Vaccin. Immunother.* **2021**, *17*, 810–817. [CrossRef]
122. Doherty, E.; Walsh, B.; O'Neill, C. Decomposing socioeconomic inequality in child vaccination: Results from Ireland. *Vaccine* **2014**, *32*, 3438–3444. [CrossRef] [PubMed]
123. Xeuatvongsa, A.; Hachiya, M.; Miyano, S.; Mizoue, T.; Kitamura, T. Determination of factors affecting the vaccination status of children aged 12–35 months in Lao People's Democratic Republic. *Heliyon* **2017**, *3*, e00265. [CrossRef] [PubMed]
124. Adedokun, S.T.; Uthman, O.A.; Adekanmbi, V.T.; Wiysonge, C.S. Incomplete childhood immunization in Nigeria: A multilevel analysis of individual and contextual factors. *BMC Public Health* **2017**, *17*, 236. [CrossRef] [PubMed]
125. Adokiya, M.N.; Baguune, B.; Ndago, J.A. Evaluation of immunization coverage and its associated factors among children 12–23 months of age in Techiman Municipality, Ghana, 2016. *Arch Public Health* **2017**, *75*, 28. [CrossRef] [PubMed]
126. Ahuja, R.; Rajpurohit, A.C. Gender inequalities in immunization of children in a rural population of Barabanki, Uttar Pradesh. *Indian J. Community Health* **2014**, *26*, 370–373.
127. Pal, R. Decomposing Inequality of Opportunity in Immunization by Circumstances: Evidence from India. *Eur. J. Dev. Res.* **2016**, *28*, 431–446. [CrossRef]
128. Shrivastwa, N.; Wagner, A.L.; Boulton, M.L. Analysis of State-Specific Differences in Childhood Vaccination Coverage in Rural India. *Vaccines* **2019**, *7*, 24. [CrossRef] [PubMed]
129. Devasenapathy, N.; Ghosh Jerath, S.; Sharma, S.; Allen, E.; Shankar, A.H.; Zodpey, S. Determinants of childhood immunisation coverage in urban poor settlements of Delhi, India: A cross-sectional study. *BMJ Open* **2016**, *6*, e013015. [CrossRef]
130. Joe, W. Intersectional inequalities in immunization in India, 1992–1993 to 2005–06: A progress assessment. *Health Policy Plan* **2015**, *30*, 407–422. [CrossRef]
131. Obanewa, O.A.; Newell, M.L. The role of place of residency in childhood immunisation coverage in Nigeria: Analysis of data from three DHS rounds 2003–2013. *BMC Public Health* **2020**, *20*, 123. [CrossRef]
132. Shanawaz, M.; Sundar, J.S. An Evaluation of Primary Immunization Coverage Among Icds Children Under Urban Field Practice Area of Osmania Medical College, Hyderabad. *J. Evol. Med. Dent. Sci. -Jemds* **2014**, *3*, 1012–1019.
133. Srivastava, S.; Fledderjohann, J.; Upadhyay, A.K. Explaining socioeconomic inequalities in immunisation coverage in India: New insights from the fourth National Family Health Survey (2015–16). *BMC Pediatr.* **2020**, *20*, 295. [CrossRef] [PubMed]
134. Asresie, M.B.; Fekadu, G.A.; Dagnew, G.W. Urban-rural disparities in immunization coverage among children aged 12–23 months in Ethiopia: Multivariate decomposition analysis. *BMC Health Serv. Res.* **2023**, *23*, 969. [CrossRef] [PubMed]
135. Kattan, J.A.; Kudish, K.S.; Cadwell, B.L.; Soto, K.; Hadler, J.L. Effect of vaccination coordinators on socioeconomic disparities in immunization among children after the 2006 Connecticut birth cohort. *Am J Public Health* **2014**, *104*, e74–e81. [CrossRef] [PubMed]
136. Michels, S.Y.; Niccolai, L.M.; Hadler, J.L.; Freeman, R.E.; Albers, A.N.; Glanz, J.M.; Daley, M.F.; Newcomer, S.R. Failure to Complete Multidose Vaccine Series in Early Childhood. *Pediatrics* **2023**, *152*, e2022059844. [CrossRef] [PubMed]
137. Santorelli, G.; West, J.; Mason, D.; Cartwright, C.; Inamdar, L.; Tomes, C.; Wright, J. Factors associated with the uptake of the UK routine childhood immunization schedule in a bi-ethnic population. *Eur. J. Public Health* **2020**, *30*, 697–702. [CrossRef] [PubMed]
138. Wondimu, A.; van der Schans, J.; van Hulst, M.; Postma, M.J. Inequalities in Rotavirus Vaccine Uptake in Ethiopia: A Decomposition Analysis. *Int. J. Environ. Res. Public Health* **2020**, *17*, 2696. [CrossRef] [PubMed]
139. Khan, J.; Shil, A.; Prakash, R. Exploring the spatial heterogeneity in different doses of vaccination coverage in India. *PLoS ONE* **2018**, *13*, e0207209. [CrossRef] [PubMed]
140. Atteraya, M.S.; Song, I.H.; Ebrahim, N.B.; Gnawali, S.; Kim, E.; Dhakal, T. Inequalities in Childhood Immunisation in South Asia. *Int. J. Environ. Res. Public Health* **2023**, *20*, 1755. [CrossRef]
141. Fenta, S.M.; Biresaw, H.B.; Fentaw, K.D.; Gebremichael, S.G. Determinants of full childhood immunization among children aged 12–23 months in sub-Saharan Africa: A multilevel analysis using Demographic and Health Survey Data. *Trop. Med. Health* **2021**, *49*, 29. [CrossRef]
142. Hajizadeh, M. Decomposing socioeconomic inequality in child vaccination in the Gambia, the Kyrgyz Republic and Namibia. *Vaccine* **2019**, *37*, 6609–6616. [CrossRef] [PubMed]
143. Cata-Preta, B.O.; Santos, T.M.; Wendt, A.; Hogan, D.R.; Mengistu, T.; Barros, A.J.D.; Victora, C.G. Ethnic disparities in immunisation: Analyses of zero-dose prevalence in 64 countries. *BMJ Glob. Health* **2022**, *7*, e008833. [CrossRef] [PubMed]
144. Ameyaw, E.K.; Kareem, Y.O.; Ahinkorah, B.O.; Seidu, A.A.; Yaya, S. Decomposing the rural-urban gap in factors associated with childhood immunisation in sub-Saharan Africa: Evidence from surveys in 23 countries. *BMJ Glob. Health* **2021**, *6*, e003773. [CrossRef] [PubMed]
145. Arat, A.; Norredam, M.; Baum, U.; Jónsson, S.H.; Gunlaugsson, G.; Wallby, T.; Hjern, A. Organisation of preventive child health services: Key to socio-economic equity in vaccine uptake? *Scand. J. Public Health* **2020**, *48*, 491–494. [CrossRef] [PubMed]

146. Singh, P.K.; Parsuraman, S. Sibling composition and child immunization in India and Pakistan, 1990–2007. *World J. Pediatr.* **2014**, *10*, 145–150. [CrossRef] [PubMed]
147. Singh, A. Gender based within-household inequality in immunization status of children: Some evidence from South Asian countries. *Econ. Bull.* **2015**, *35*, 911–923.
148. Arsenault, C.; Harper, S.; Nandi, A.; Mendoza Rodríguez, J.M.; Hansen, P.M.; Johri, M. Monitoring equity in vaccination coverage: A systematic analysis of demographic and health surveys from 45 Gavi-supported countries. *Vaccine* **2017**, *35*, 951–959. [CrossRef] [PubMed]
149. Restrepo-Méndez, M.C.; Barros, A.J.; Wong, K.L.; Johnson, H.L.; Pariyo, G.; França, G.V.; Wehrmeister, F.C.; Victora, C.G. Inequalities in full immunization coverage: Trends in low- and middle-income countries. *Bull. World Health Organ.* **2016**, *94*, 794B–805B. [CrossRef] [PubMed]
150. Santos, T.M.; Cata-Preta, B.O.; Wendt, A.; Arroyave, L.; Hogan, D.R.; Mengistu, T.; Barros, A.J.D.; Victora, C.G. Religious affiliation as a driver of immunization coverage: Analyses of zero-dose vaccine prevalence in 66 low- and middle-income countries. *Front. Public Health* **2022**, *10*, 977512. [CrossRef]
151. Acharya, K.; Dharel, D.; Subedi, R.K.; Bhattarai, A.; Paudel, Y.R. Inequalities in full vaccination coverage based on maternal education and wealth quintiles among children aged 12–23 months: Further analysis of national cross-sectional surveys of six South Asian countries. *BMJ Open* **2022**, *12*, e046971. [CrossRef]
152. Bobo, F.T.; Asante, A.; Woldie, M.; Dawson, A.; Hayen, A. Child vaccination in sub-Saharan Africa: Increasing coverage addresses inequalities. *Vaccine* **2022**, *40*, 141–150. [CrossRef] [PubMed]
153. Donfouet, H.P.P.; Agesa, G.; Mutua, M.K. Trends of inequalities in childhood immunization coverage among children aged 12–23 months in Kenya, Ghana, and Côte d'Ivoire. *BMC Public Health* **2019**, *19*, 988. [CrossRef] [PubMed]
154. Soura, A.B.; Mberu, B.; Elungata, P.; Lankoande, B.; Millogo, R.; Beguy, D.; Compaore, Y. Understanding inequities in child vaccination rates among the urban poor: Evidence from Nairobi and Ouagadougou health and demographic surveillance systems. *J. Urban. Health* **2015**, *92*, 39–54. [CrossRef] [PubMed]
155. Wariri, O.; Edem, B.; Nkereuwem, E.; Nkereuwem, O.O.; Umeh, G.; Clark, E.; Idoko, O.T.; Nomhwange, T.; Kampmann, B. Tracking coverage, dropout and multidimensional equity gaps in immunisation systems in West Africa, 2000–2017. *BMJ Glob Health* **2019**, *4*, e001713. [CrossRef] [PubMed]
156. Wendt, A.; Santos, T.M.; Cata-Preta, B.O.; Arroyave, L.; Hogan, D.R.; Mengistu, T.; Barros, A.J.D.; Victora, C.G. Exposure of Zero-Dose Children to Multiple Deprivation: Analyses of Data from 80 Low- and Middle-Income Countries. *Vaccines* **2022**, *10*, 1568. [CrossRef]
157. Tur-Sinai, A.; Gur-Arie, R.; Davidovitch, N.; Kopel, E.; Glazer, Y.; Anis, E.; Grotto, I. Vaccination uptake and income inequalities within a mass vaccination campaign. *Isr. J. Health Policy Res.* **2019**, *8*, 63. [CrossRef]

Disclaimer/Publisher's Note: The statements, opinions and data contained in all publications are solely those of the individual author(s) and contributor(s) and not of MDPI and/or the editor(s). MDPI and/or the editor(s) disclaim responsibility for any injury to people or property resulting from any ideas, methods, instructions or products referred to in the content.

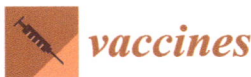

Article

The Impact of the Coronavirus Pandemic on Vaccination Coverage in Latin America and the Caribbean

Ignacio E. Castro-Aguirre [1], Dan Alvarez [1], Marcela Contreras [1], Silas P. Trumbo [2], Oscar J. Mujica [3], Daniel Salas Peraza [1] and Martha Velandia-González [1,*]

[1] Comprehensive Family Immunization Unit, Pan American Health Organization, Washington, DC 20037, USA; castroign@paho.org (I.E.C.-A.); alvarezdan@paho.org (D.A.)
[2] Department of Medicine, University of Central Florida College of Medicine, Orlando, FL 32827, USA
[3] Department of Evidence and Intelligence for Action in Health, Pan American Health Organization, Washington, DC 20037, USA; mujicaos@paho.org
* Correspondence: velandiam@paho.org; Tel.: +1-(202)-974-3000

Abstract: Background: Routine vaccination coverage in Latin America and the Caribbean declined prior to and during the coronavirus pandemic. We assessed the pandemic's impact on national coverage levels and analyzed whether financial and inequality indicators, immunization policies, and pandemic policies were associated with changes in national and regional coverage levels. Methodology: We compared first- and third-dose coverage of diphtheria–pertussis–tetanus-containing vaccine (DTPcv) with predicted coverages using time series forecast modeling for 39 LAC countries and territories. Data were from the PAHO/WHO/UNICEF Joint Reporting Form. A secondary analysis of factors hypothesized to affect coverages during the pandemic was also performed. Results: In total, 31 of 39 countries and territories (79%) had greater-than-predicted declines in DTPcv1 and DTPcv3 coverage during the pandemic, with 9 and 12 of these, respectively, falling outside the 95% confidence interval. Within-country income inequality (i.e., Gini coefficient) was associated with significant declines in DTPcv1 coverage, and cross-country income inequality was associated with declines in DTPcv1 and DTPcv3 coverages. Observed absolute and relative inequality gaps in DTPcv1 and DTPcv3 coverage between extreme country quintiles of income inequality (i.e., Q1 vs. Q5) were accentuated in 2021, as compared with the 2019 observed and 2021 predicted values. We also observed a trend between school closures and greater-than-predicted declines in DTPcv3 coverage that approached statistical significance ($p = 0.06$). Conclusion: The pandemic exposed vaccination inequities in LAC and significantly impacted coverage levels in many countries. New strategies are needed to reattain high coverage levels.

Keywords: coronavirus pandemic; immunization coverage levels; diphtheria–tetanus–pertussis-containing vaccine; vaccination of newborns; zero-dose children; health disparities

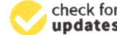

Citation: Castro-Aguirre, I.E.; Alvarez, D.; Contreras, M.; Trumbo, S.P.; Mujica, O.J.; Salas Peraza, D.; Velandia-González, M. The Impact of the Coronavirus Pandemic on Vaccination Coverage in Latin America and the Caribbean. *Vaccines* **2024**, *12*, 458. https://doi.org/10.3390/vaccines12050458

Academic Editor: Pedro Plans-Rubió

Received: 29 January 2024
Revised: 14 March 2024
Accepted: 27 March 2024
Published: 25 April 2024

Copyright: © 2024 by the authors. Licensee MDPI, Basel, Switzerland. This article is an open access article distributed under the terms and conditions of the Creative Commons Attribution (CC BY) license (https://creativecommons.org/licenses/by/4.0/).

1. Introduction

Following the establishment of national immunization programs in the 1970s, countries in Latin America and the Caribbean (LAC) have made marked improvements in the control of vaccine-preventable diseases (VPDs) [1,2]. Over the last decade, however, third-dose coverage of diphtheria–pertussis–tetanus-containing vaccine (DTPcv3) has declined from 93% in 2010 to 84% in 2019, with rising numbers of children with incomplete schedules and those who have not received any doses ("zero-dose" children) (Figure 1) [1,3]. Decreases in DTPcv1 and DTPcv3 coverages have also been observed in other routine vaccines; in an analysis of coverage trends from 2015 to 2019, Plans-Rubió found that 10 out of 13 vaccines in the Americas decreased during this period [4]. Coverage declines have been pronounced among children living in poverty and other vulnerable situations, as well as those in hard-to-reach areas [5,6].

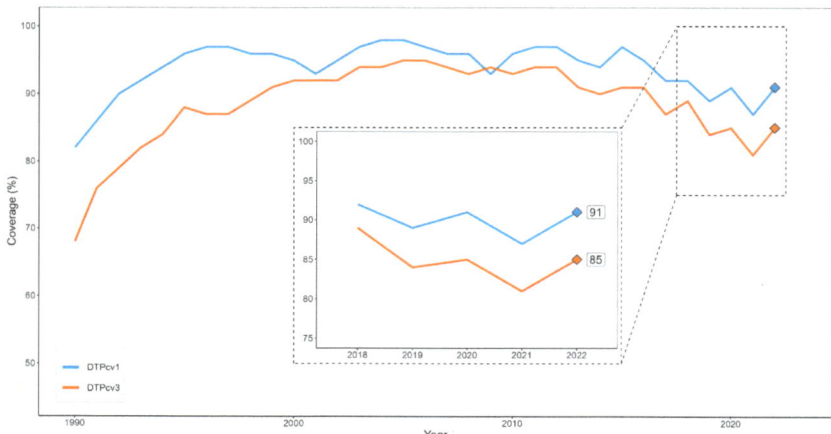

Figure 1. DTPcv1 and DTPcv3 coverage levels in Latin America and the Caribbean, 1990–2022.

Causes of low vaccination coverage vary among countries but include health system factors (e.g., a lack of access to vaccination services), communication factors (e.g., vaccine hesitancy), and sociopolitical factors (e.g., poverty and political instability) [6]. The COVID-19 pandemic has exacerbated many of these problems. Containment measures; the suspension of school vaccination strategies and mass vaccination campaigns; the interruption of routine immunization services; the population's reluctance to go to health centers due to fear of contracting the virus; and the diversion of resources for the coronavirus pandemic have resulted in the delayed administration of routine vaccines [7–11]. Additionally, the pandemic has politicized vaccination, worsening mistrust in health systems [12], coronavirus vaccines [13,14], and immunization services more generally [15]. As a result, coverages for DTP1cv1 and DTPcv3 in 2021 reached levels not seen in LAC since the early 1990s.

Against this backdrop, the Pan American Health Organization and World Health Organization (PAHO/WHO) have continued efforts to control and eliminate VPDs. Immunization Agenda 2030 (IA2030) and PAHO's strategic document "Reinvigorating Immunization as a Public Good for Universal Health" provide concrete steps to aid countries in reaching all people, especially vulnerable populations and zero-dose children [1,16]. To support these goals, there is a need for an updated analysis of national coverage trends in LAC before and after the pandemic and the factors that may explain changes in coverage.

In this article, we estimate the effect of the COVID-19 pandemic on vaccination coverage for countries and territories in LAC. We then analyze whether national financial indicators, vaccine policies, and pandemic policies are associated with changes in coverage levels and cross-country distributive inequality. We conclude by discussing the causes of declining coverage rates and propose strategies to reverse these declines.

2. Methodology

PAHO/WHO and UNICEF publish annual vaccination coverages based on country reports collected through the Joint Reporting Form (JRF) [3]. We performed an analysis of these data in LAC from 1990 to 2022 [3]. Of the 49 countries and territories in LAC, 39 were included in the analysis, accounting for 99% of the region's population [3].

We chose first-dose coverage of diphtheria–tetanus–pertussis-containing vaccine in children aged <12 months (DTPcv1) as an indicator of access to health services and third-dose coverage (DTPcv3) as an indicator of immunization program follow-up and performance. Consistent with IA2030, "zero-dose" children—i.e., those not receiving any dose of DTPcv before age <12 months—were considered to have limited access to health services [16].

As an initial analysis, we compared absolute coverage changes in DTPcv1 and DTPcv3 between 2019 and 2021. To distinguish between pre-pandemic trends in vaccination coverage and the impact of the pandemic on DTPcv1 and DTPcv3 coverages, we then used time series forecast modeling to compare predicted coverages (i.e., those expected if a pandemic had not occurred) with country-reported coverage levels in 2021. DTPcv1 and DTPcv3 coverages from 1990 to 2019 were used in the forecast model. Although concerns about COVID-19 began in late 2019, countries did not implement significant pandemic measures until 2020. As such, we defined all years before 2020 as pre-pandemic. Predicted coverages were estimated through Holt's linear trend model, which aims to describe the behavior of a trending time series [17].

We performed a secondary analysis of factors hypothesized to affect coverages during the pandemic, comparing observed to predicted coverage changes for DTPcv1 and DTPcv3 in 2021. Supplemental Table S1 outlines the data source, categories, methodology, and statistical test used for each variable [3,18–22]. Furthermore, we conducted an exploratory analysis of vaccination coverage inequalities across countries ranked by their mean income per capita (deflated and purchase-power-adjusted), calculating standard summary measures of health inequality, including Kuznets-like inequality gaps and the slope index of inequality (SII) through a log-linear weighted regression model, as described elsewhere [22,23].

We analyzed data with Microsoft Excel and the R statistical software (version 4.3.2) [24]. Time series modeling was performed using the fpp2 package (version 2.5) [17]. During one phase of the article's development, generative AI was used for general editing and to draft a preliminary version of the discussion section (which was then significantly modified); however, the technology was not subsequently utilized, and the content presented is the creation and responsibility of the authors.

3. Results

From 2019 to 2021, 30 of 39 countries and territories had absolute declines in DTPcv1 coverage, with 13 declining <5 percentage points (%pt), 12 declining 5–10 %pt, and five declining >10 %pt (Supplemental Table S2). Four countries and territories reported increased DTPcv1 coverage during the pandemic, most notably Anguilla (79% in 2019 vs. 88% in 2021). During the same period, 32 of 39 countries experienced decreases in DTPcv3 coverage, with 13 declining <5 %pt, 12 declining 5–10 %pt, and 7 declining >10 %pt. Haiti reported the greatest increase in DTPcv3 coverage (66% in 2019 vs. 73% in 2021) during the pandemic.

For 2021, time series forecast modeling showed that 31 countries and territories experienced greater-than-predicted declines in DTPcv1 coverage, with 9 falling outside the 95% confidence interval (CI) (Figure 2). For DTPcv3 coverage, 31 countries and territories experienced greater-than-predicted declines; 12 of these were outside the CI. Coverage in Belize for DPTcv1, for example, decreased by 20 %pt with respect to the prediction's mean, falling outside the CI and suggesting that the decline may be due to the pandemic.

Figure 2 compares observed to predicted changes in coverage for DTPcv1 and DTPcv3 and, thus, a country or territory's access to vaccines (DTPcv1) and to follow-up immunization services (DTPcv3). In 27 of 39 countries and territories, access and follow-up to immunization services both worsened. But some countries did not follow this pattern. For example, in Mexico, follow-up worsened by 2 %pt more than predicted, but access improved by 1% more than predicted. Conversely, in Brazil, follow-up improved by 3 %pt more than predicted, but access worsened by 2 %pt.

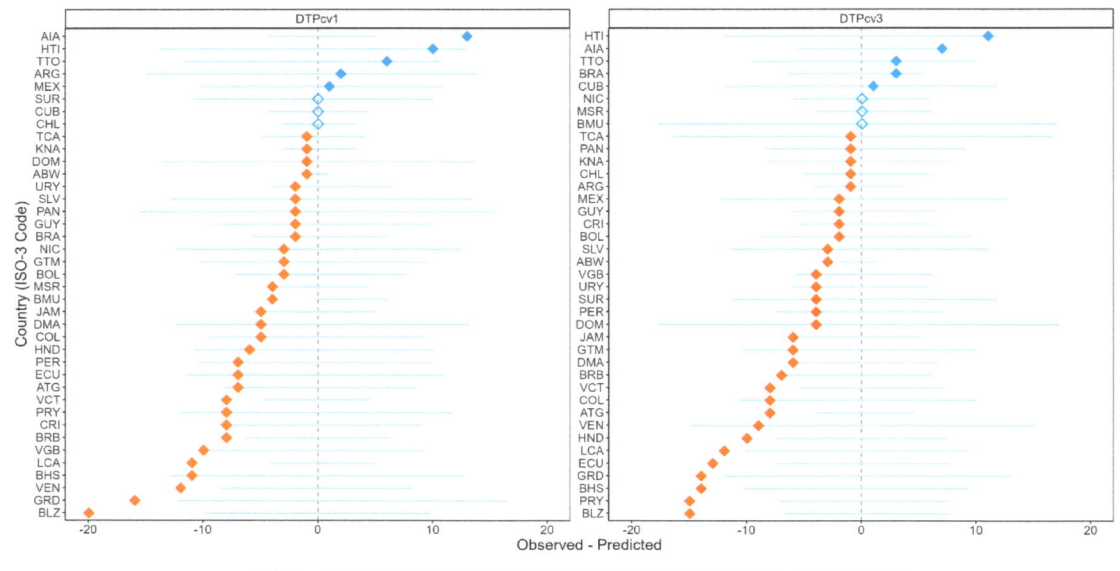

Figure 2. Observed versus predicted changes in DTPcv1 and DTPcv3 coverage in 2021 in Latin America and the Caribbean, 39 countries and territories with available data.

A secondary analysis of explanatory variables showed that vaccine administration in schools and national pandemic policies regarding public transportation and stay-at-home orders were not associated with statistically significant changes in DTPcv1 or DTPCv3 coverages at the regional level (Table 1). We observed a trend between school closures and greater-than-predicted declines in DTPcv3 coverage that did not reach statistical significance ($p = 0.06$). Of the three financial indicators evaluated, only the Gini index of income inequality was statistically significant at the regional level. Countries with greater income inequality had greater DTPcv1 coverage declines than countries with less income inequality (-5 %pt vs. -1.5 %pt, $p = 0.04$).

An exploratory analysis of DTPcv1 and DTPcv3 coverage inequalities showed the effect of income inequality *between* countries on their magnitude and trends at the regional level (Table 2). When ranking countries from poorest to richest by their mean GDP per capita, those in the poorest quintile fared consistently worse than those in the richest quintile; indeed, in 2021, the observed absolute and relative inequality gaps in DTPcv1 and DTPcv3 coverage between these extreme quintiles were larger than predicted.

Moreover, there were clear regional inequality gradients in DTPcv1 and DTPcv3 coverage that were evident across the social hierarchy ("social hierarchy" refers to the cross-country gradient formed when countries are ranked by GDP per capita from poorest to richest) as defined by country GDP per capita (Table 2). The pro-poor inequality pattern in DTPcv1 coverage, initially observed in 2019 (and predicted by 2021), was inverted in 2021; the SII increased from -2.10 %pt DTPcv1 in 2019 to 5.08 %pt in 2021. The pro-rich inequality pattern in DTPcv3 coverage became more evident between 2019 and 2021, with the SII rising from 4.92 %pt in 2019 to 9.68 %pt in 2021 (Figure 3).

Table 1. Factors associated with changes in observed versus predicted DTPcv1 and DTPcv3 coverages during the coronavirus pandemic, 2019–2022.

Variable	DTPcv1 Median (IQR)	p-Value	DTPcv3 Median (IQR)	p-Value
Vaccine administration in school				
Yes	−4.00 (−8.00; −1.00)	0.98	−3.00 (−8.00; −1.00)	0.55
No	−3.00 (−6.00; −1.50)		−4.00 (−7.50; −1.50)	
School-closing policies				
None/recommended	−2.50 (−3.75; −1.25)	0.37	−1.50 (−3.75; 0.00)	0.06
Required	−3.00 (−7.25; −0.75)		−4.00 (−8.25; −1.75)	
Stay-at-home policies				
None/recommended	−3.00 (−5.00; −2.00)	0.60	−3.00 (−6.00; −2.00)	0.82
Required	−3.00 (−7.00; 0.00)		−4.00 (−8.00; −1.00)	
Closing of public transportation				
None	−3.00 (−5.00; −1.00)	0.95	−2.00 (−4.00; −1.00)	0.40
Recommended/required	−3.00 (−7.00; −1.00)		−4.00 (−8.00; −1.00)	
WB income group				
High	−2.00 (−7.25; −1.00)	0.57	−2.00 (−4.75; −1.00)	0.41
Middle	−4.00 (−7.25; −1.75)		−4.00 (−8.50; −2.00)	
GDP per capita				
High	−1.85 (−4.00; −1.00)	0.18	−2.08 (−4.00; 0.00)	0.14
Middle	−4.85 (−8.00; −1.00)		−5.15 (−8.00; −2.00)	
Low	−5.08 (−7.00; −3.00)		−5.46 (−10.00; −2.00)	
GINI index				
Less unequal	−1.50 (−2.75; 0.75)	0.04 *	−2.50 (−4.00; −1.25)	0.54
More unequal	−5.00 (−7.00; −3.00)		−6.00 (−10.00; −1.00)	
SDIx 2021				
High	−2.00 (−7.00; 0.00)	0.42	−1.00 (−7.00; −1.00)	0.65
Middle	−6.00 (−8.00; −1.00)		−4.00 (−8.25; −2.00)	
Low	−4.00 (−6.25; −2.75)		−6.00 (−10.50; −1.50)	

IQR: interquartile range; WB: World Bank; GDP: gross domestic product; SDIx: PAHO Sustainable Development Index; * p-Value < 0.05.

Table 2. DTPcv1 and DTPcv3 vaccine coverage by country quintiles of income per capita, regional average, and Kuznets-like inequality gap metrics. Latin America and the Caribbean, 2019 and 2021.

| Vaccine | Timepoint, Scenario | Vaccine Coverage (%) | | | | | Setting Average | Q1 v Q5 Inequality Gap | |
		Q1	Q2	Q3	Q4	Q5		Absolute Gap	Relative Gap
DTPcv1	2019 observed	86.9	91.9	82.5	87.3	91.5	86.0	−4.6	0.95
	2021 predicted	86.2	85.8	82.6	92.4	89.8	84.7	−3.6	0.96
	2021 observed	82.4	80.9	80.6	93.1	91.9	82.5	−9.5	0.90
DTPcv3	2019 observed	76.7	87.1	75.3	84.0	92.4	79.8	−15.7	0.83
	2021 predicted	75.5	82.9	75.7	86.8	90.9	77.8	−15.4	0.83
	2021 observed	72.8	73.6	75.1	85.1	90.3	75.9	−17.5	0.81

Notes: Q1 = poorest; Q3 = median; Q5 = richest.

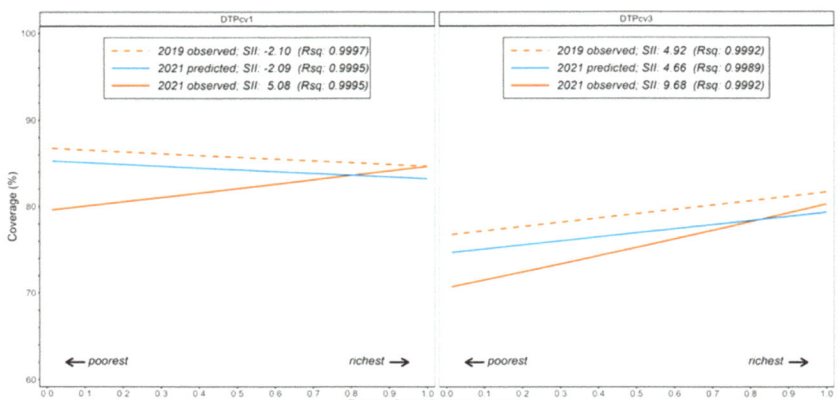

Figure 3. Income-related cross-country inequality gradients in DTPcv1 and DTPcv3 coverage, Latin America and the Caribbean, 2019 and 2021.

4. Discussion

We found that routine vaccination coverage in most LAC countries and territories declined during the COVID-19 pandemic. While only 9 and 12 LAC countries and territories, respectively, experienced statistically significant greater-than-predicted declines in DTPcv1 and DTPcv3 coverage, there was a clear trend toward lower-than-predicted coverages. For both DTPcv1 and DTPcv3, 79% of countries had larger-than-expected declines in coverage based on the pattern observed over the last 30 years.

Large studies have shown that the coronavirus pandemic negatively impacted routine vaccination rates in countries around the world [25–28]. Consistent with previous research, the decrease in coverage in LAC countries and territories likely stems from service disruptions, a lack of vaccine availability, the population's fear of visiting health centers, and the diversion of resources to pandemic-related activities [25–30]. This being acknowledged, the fact that eight LAC countries and territories had no decreases in DPTcv3 coverage suggests that some countries may have been able to quickly recover from service disruptions in early 2020 due to their strong immunization programs [25], relatively mild income inequality, or other factors. Further research, potentially in the form of country case studies, could explore what factors were associated with immunization program resilience during the pandemic.

We found income inequality to be associated with declines in DTPcv1 coverage during the pandemic. Previous research has shown that lower-middle-income countries (LMICs) experienced greater declines than high-income countries (HICs) during the pandemic [25]. Similarly, we observed a significant slope index of inequality in DTPcv1 and DTPcv3 coverages across the cross-country gradient defined by GDP per capita (i.e., a measure of *between-country* income inequality), a pro-rich slope that was steeper in 2021. Furthermore, we found that *within-country* income inequality, as measured by the Gini index, predicted greater-than-expected coverage declines, aligning with other reports highlighting how the pandemic revealed and deepened existing health inequities [31–33]. Our research also revealed a possible association between school closures and greater-than-predicted declines in DTPcv3 coverage, although statistical significance was not reached ($p = 0.06$).

Previous research has shown that DTPcv1 and DTPCv3 coverages in the Americas declined by 3.0% and 2.7%, respectively, from 2015 to 2019 [4]. We found that coverage levels rebounded to pre-pandemic levels in 2022 but remained well below 2015 levels. The improvement suggests that LAC countries can reverse the decline. Still, the overall trend remains concerning, and new challenges have emerged in the wake of the COVID-19 pandemic. For example, the politicization of the pandemic has created misinformation on vaccines [13], and the pandemic may have decreased the public's confidence in immunization programs [25]. Amid this complexity, the pandemic may serve as a "wake-up call" for the region to re-prioritize immunization and re-evaluate the strategies needed to ensure high and homogenous coverages.

Recommendations based on our findings, a review of the literature, and expert opinion include addressing vaccine hesitancy, targeting socioeconomic factors driving undervaccination, and focusing on reducing the number of zero-dose children while avoiding unintended negative impacts on follow-up schedules [1,34,35]. Vaccine hesitancy in LAC is multifactorial, likely to vary among and within countries, and is arguably the largest factor affecting coverages [6]. Using the Strategic Advisory Group of Experts (SAGE) working group's framework for vaccine hesitancy, Guzman-Holst found that hesitancy in the region centered on individual/group influences (e.g., safety misconceptions), contextual influences (e.g., low socioeconomic status), and vaccine and vaccination-specific issues (e.g., negative experiences at health centers) [6,36]. Countries should identify specific causes of vaccine hesitancy at the local level, develop strategies to combat misinformation, and educate healthcare workers who themselves may be hesitant toward vaccines [1,14].

Countries must also develop contingency plans to reach children who missed vaccines and to minimize disruptions during future public health emergencies [13]. Strategies, such as campaigns and periodic outreach activities, must be in place to maintain routine immunization in schools and integrate immunization with all essential health services across primary healthcare. This is particularly important in areas with significant income inequality, since lockdowns may disproportionately affect the most vulnerable and economically disadvantaged children [31].

Finally, the decrease in coverage due to the pandemic may lead to an increase in the prevalence of VPDs. This may be especially true for diseases with high transmissibility rates, such as measles, where a decrease in coverage can result in increased prevalence in the short term [37]. The pandemic highlights an opportunity for countries to reaffirm their commitment to immunization and make the investments needed to increase coverage. Early results suggest that countries may already be making such an investment. In April 2023, Caribbean countries and territories signed the Declaration of Nassau to strengthen national immunization programs [38]. In Brazil, the president championed a national movement in favor of vaccination [39], and the senate held sessions to discuss vaccination as a public good [40]. Meanwhile, Argentina held a very successful Vaccination Week, resulting in more than 1.1 million vaccines being administered and culminating with a community event called "El Festival de las Vacunas" [41]. Such post-pandemic activities and commitments are vital to raising coverage levels.

The principal strengths of this study include the use of time series modeling to differentiate pre-existing coverage trends from changes in coverage that might be attributed to the pandemic and a robust secondary analysis of the role of within- and between-country inequality in vaccination outcomes. However, this study has several notable limitations. Data submitted by countries to the JRF are administrative and subject to occasional issues in quality and recording (e.g., outdated census data) [42,43]. Although the PAHO/WHO and UNICEF strive to address these concerns by triangulating administrative data with coverage surveys, resulting coverage adjustments may be inaccurate. Additionally, our model assumed a linear trend in coverage patterns, but some countries and territories may have seasonal patterns, thereby limiting our model's accuracy. It is also worth noting that the pandemic may have caused fluctuations in monthly vaccination coverages not detected in our model. Lastly, LAC includes many countries and territories with small populations; in these cases, minor changes in coverages may not be statistically significant but still meaningfully impact patients. We have accordingly argued that it is important to consider both trends and statistical significance when evaluating coverage changes following the pandemic.

Our secondary analysis was constrained by limited data on factors that may have affected vaccination coverage during the pandemic. We attempted to incorporate factors like "trust in science" and "trust in the government" that were included in other studies on changes in vaccination coverage during the pandemic [18,44]. Unfortunately, only a small proportion of countries in LAC had available data for these factors. A valuable area of future research would be the creation of a multivariable model to explain changes in coverage levels that incorporates the factors in our secondary analysis, as well as others related to confidence in the health system, government, and immunization programs [45].

5. Conclusions

The COVID-19 pandemic exposed vaccination inequities in LAC and significantly impacted coverage levels in specific countries and territories. Although coverage levels continued to decrease during the pandemic, they have rebounded to pre-pandemic levels. This signals an opportunity for continued improvement and suggests that the pandemic may have prompted a renewed investment in immunization in the Americas. Strategies to reattain and maintain high coverage include conducting outreach activities for marginalized groups, targeting socioeconomic factors driving vaccination inequities, employing a multifaceted approach to confront vaccine hesitancy, reaffirming national commitment to vaccination, and developing plans to minimize disruptions in future public health emergencies [1,13,34,35].

Supplementary Materials: The following supporting information can be downloaded at: https://www.mdpi.com/article/10.3390/vaccines12050458/s1. Supplemental Table S1 (Data sources and methodology for factors hypothesized to be associated with changes in DTPcv1 and DTPcv3 coverage rates during the coronavirus pandemic, 2019–2021) and Supplemental Table S2 ("Data dictionary" and "Observed versus predicted changes in DTPcv1 and DTPcv3 coverage and associated variables, Latin America and the Caribbean, 2019 and 2021").

Author Contributions: I.E.C.-A., D.A., M.C. and M.V.-G. developed and implemented a preliminary version of this study. I.E.C.-A., D.A. and S.P.T. revised the study design. I.E.C.-A., D.A., S.P.T. and O.J.M. performed the secondary analysis with feedback from M.C. and M.V.-G. S.P.T. drafted the manuscript with multiple revisions and significant input from I.E.C.-A., D.A., M.C., M.V.-G., D.S.P. and O.J.M. All authors have read and agreed to the published version of the manuscript.

Funding: This research received no external funding. However, Silas Trumbo received a consultancy fee for his participation.

Institutional Review Board Statement: Not applicable.

Informed Consent Statement: Not applicable.

Data Availability Statement: Data are contained within the article and also presented in Supplemental Table S2.

Acknowledgments: We wish to acknowledge the efforts of healthcare workers in the Americas who tirelessly provided health services to the population during the pandemic. We also thank officials in each country's ministry of health, as well as the PAHO immunization focal points, for their efforts in providing high-quality immunization data for this analysis. Lastly, we appreciate the peer reviewers who provided helpful feedback on our manuscript; their contributions resulted in a stronger article. Generative AI (Chat GPT4 and Notion) was used to edit and draft parts of this article, as explained above. The ideas presented are original to the authors or else cited accordingly. The authors take full responsibility for the information presented.

Conflicts of Interest: The authors are staff members of the Pan American Health Organization. The author alone is responsible for the views expressed in this publication, and they do not necessarily represent the decisions or policies of the Pan American Health Organization.

References

1. Pan American Health Organization. Reinvigorating Immunization as a Public Good for Universal Health. 2021. Available online: https://www.paho.org/en/documents/ce16814-reinvigorating-immunization-public-good-universal-health (accessed on 7 January 2024).
2. Chan, I.L.; Mowson, R.; Alonso, J.P.; Roberti, J.; Contreras, M.; Velandia-González, M. Promoting immunization equity in Latin America and the Caribbean: Case studies, lessons learned, and their implication for COVID-19 vaccine equity. *Vaccine* **2022**, *40*, 1977–1986. [CrossRef] [PubMed]

3. Pan American Health Organization. Immunization Dashboard. 2024. Available online: https://immunizationdata.who.int (accessed on 7 January 2024).
4. Plans-Rubió, P. Vaccination coverage for routine vaccines and herd immunity levels against measles and pertussis in the world in 2019. *Vaccines* **2021**, *9*, 256. [CrossRef] [PubMed]
5. Matta-Chuquisapon, J.; Gianella, C.; Carrasco-Escobar, G. Missed opportunities for vaccination in Peru 2010–2020, A study of socioeconomic inequalities. *Lancet Reg. Health—Am.* **2022**, *14*, 100321. [CrossRef] [PubMed]
6. Guzman-Holst, A.; DeAntonio, R.; Prado-Cohrs, D.; Juliao, P. Barriers to vaccination in Latin America: A systematic literature review. *Vaccine* **2020**, *38*, 470–481. [CrossRef] [PubMed]
7. Cardoso Pinto, A.M.; Ranasinghe, L.; Dodd, P.J.; Budhathoki, S.S.; Seddon, J.A.; Whittaker, E. Disruptions to routine childhood vaccinations in low- and middle-income countries during the COVID-19 pandemic: A systematic review. *Front. Pediatr.* **2022**, *10*, 979769. [CrossRef] [PubMed]
8. Matos, C.C.S.A.; Barbieri, C.L.A.; Couto, M.T. COVID-19 and its impact on immunization programs: Reflections from Brazil. *Rev. Saude Publica* **2020**, *54*, 114. [CrossRef] [PubMed]
9. Sato, A.P.S. Pandemic and vaccine coverage: Challenges of returning to schools. *Rev. Saude Publica* **2020**, *54*, 115. [CrossRef] [PubMed]
10. World Health Organization. Routine Immunization Services during the Coronavirus (COVID-19) Pandemic. 2020. Available online: https://apps.who.int/iris/bitstream/handle/10665/331925/Routine-immunization-services-COVID-19-eng.pdf?sequence=1&isAllowed=y (accessed on 26 December 2023).
11. La Organización Panamericana de la Salud. Cuarta Ronda de la Encuesta Nacional Sobre la Continuidad de los Servicios Esenciales de Salud Durante la Pandemia de COVID-19. Resumen de Resultados y Conclusiones para la Región de las Américas. Noviembre 2022–Enero 2023. 2023. Available online: https://iris.paho.org/bitstream/handle/10665.2/57793/OPSHSSPH230003_spa.pdf?sequence=7&isAllowed=y (accessed on 26 December 2023).
12. Edelman. Edelman Trust Barometer 2022. Special Report: Trust and Health. 2022. Available online: https://www.edelman.com/sites/g/files/aatuss191/files/2022-08/2022%20Trust%20Barometer%20Special%20Report%20Trust%20and%20Health%20with%20Talk%20Track.pdf (accessed on 14 March 2024).
13. Halpern, B.; Ranzani, O.T. Lessons From the COVID-19 Pandemic in Latin America: Vulnerability Leading to More Vulnerability. *Am. J. Public Health* **2022**, *112*, S579–S580. [CrossRef] [PubMed]
14. Puertas, E.B.; Velandia-Gonzalez, M.; Vulanovic, L.; Bayley, L.; Broome, K.; Ortiz, C.; Rise, N.; Antelo, M.V.; Rhoda, D.A. Concerns, attitudes, and intended practices of Caribbean healthcare workers concerning COVID-19 vaccination: A cross-sectional study. *Lancet Reg. Health—Am.* **2022**, *9*, 100193. [CrossRef]
15. Siani, A.; Tranter, A. Is vaccine confidence an unexpected victim of the COVID-19 pandemic? *Vaccine* **2022**, *40*, 7262–7269. [CrossRef]
16. World Health Organization. Immunization Agenda 2030. A Global Strategy to Leave No One Behind. 2021, pp. 1–24. Available online: https://cdn.who.int/media/docs/default-source/immunization/strategy/ia2030/ia2030-draft-4-wha_b8850379-1fce-4847-bfd1-5d2c9d9e32f8.pdf?sfvrsn=5389656e_69&download=true (accessed on 26 December 2023).
17. Hyndman, R.J.; Athanasopoulos, G. Forecasting: Principles and Practice. 2018. Available online: https://otexts.com/fpp2/ (accessed on 10 February 2023).
18. Hale, T.; Angrist, N.; Goldszmidt, R.; Kira, B.; Petherick, A.; Phillips, T.; Webster, S.; Cameron-Blake, E.; Hallas, L.; Majumdar, S.; et al. A global panel database of pandemic policies (Oxford COVID-19 Government Response Tracker). *Nat. Hum. Behav.* **2021**, *5*, 529–538. [CrossRef] [PubMed]
19. The World Bank. The World by Income and Region. 2022. Available online: https://datatopics.worldbank.org/world-development-indicators/the-world-by-income-and-region.html (accessed on 15 January 2024).
20. Global Health Data Exchange. Gross Domestic Product per Capita 1960–2050. 2021. Available online: https://ghdx.healthdata.org/record/ihme-data/global-gdp-per-capita-1960-2050-fgh-2021 (accessed on 28 July 2023).
21. The World Bank. Gini Index. 2023. Available online: https://data.worldbank.org/indicator/SI.POV.GINI (accessed on 26 December 2023).
22. Mújica, Ó.J.; Moreno, C.M. De la retórica a la acción: Medir desigualdades en salud para "no dejar a nadie atrás" [From words to action: Measuring health inequalities to "leave no one behind"Da retórica à ação: Mensurar as desigualdades em saúde para não deixar ninguém atrás]. *Rev. Panam. Salud Publica* **2019**, *43*, e12. [CrossRef] [PubMed]
23. World Health Organization. *Inequality Monitoring in Immunization: A Step-by-Step Manual*; World Health Organization: Geneva, Switzerland, 2019.
24. The R Foundation. The R Project for Statistical Computing. 2023. Available online: https://www.r-project.org (accessed on 10 February 2023).
25. Yunusa, A.; Cabral, C.; Anderson, E. The impact of the COVID-19 pandemic on the uptake of routine maternal and infant vaccines globally: A systematic review. *PLoS Glob. Public Health* **2022**, *2*, e0000628. [CrossRef] [PubMed]
26. Causey, K.; Fullman, N.; Sorensen, R.J.D.; Galles, N.C.; Zheng, P.; Aravkin, A.; Danovaro-Holliday, M.C.; Martinez-Piedra, R.; Sodha, S.V.; Velandia-González, M.P.; et al. Estimating global and regional disruptions to routine childhood vaccine coverage during the COVID-19 pandemic in 2020, a modelling study. *Lancet* **2021**, *398*, 522–534. [CrossRef] [PubMed]

27. Lassi, Z.S.; Naseem, R.; Salam, R.A.; Siddiqui, F.; Das, J.K. The impact of the COVID-19 pandemic on immunization campaigns and programs: A systematic review. *Int. J. Environ. Res. Public Health* **2021**, *18*, 988. [CrossRef] [PubMed]
28. Dalton, M.; Sanderson, B.; Robinson, L.J.; Homer, C.S.; Pomat, W.; Danchin, M.; Vaccher, S. Impact of COVID-19 on routine childhood immunisations in low- and middle-income countries: A scoping review. *PLoS Glob. Public Health* **2023**, *3*, e0002268. [CrossRef] [PubMed]
29. Essoh, T.A.; Adeyanju, G.C.; Adamu, A.A.; Ahawo, A.K.; Aka, D.; Tall, H.; Aplogan, A.; Wiysonge, C.S. Early Impact of SARS-CoV-2 Pandemic on Immunization Services in Nigeria. *Vaccines* **2022**, *10*, 1107. [CrossRef] [PubMed]
30. Firman, N.; Marszalek, M.; Gutierrez, A.; Homer, K.; Williams, C.; Harper, G.; Dostal, I.; Ahmed, Z.; Robson, J.; Dezateux, C. Impact of the COVID-19 pandemic on timeliness and equity of measles, mumps and rubella vaccinations in North East London: A longitudinal study using electronic health records. *BMJ Open* **2022**, *12*, e066288. [CrossRef]
31. Bambra, C.; Riordan, R.; Ford, J.; Matthews, F. The COVID-19 pandemic and health inequalities. *J. Epidemiol. Community Health* **2020**, *74*, 964–968. [CrossRef]
32. Spencer, N.; Markham, W.; Johnson, S.; Arpin, E.; Nathawad, R.; Gunnlaugsson, G.; Homaira, N.; Rubio, M.L.M.; Trujillo, C.J. The Impact of COVID-19 Pandemic on Inequity in Routine Childhood Vaccination Coverage: A Systematic Review. *Vaccines* **2022**, *10*, 1013. [CrossRef]
33. Ahmed Ali, H.; Hartner, A.M.; Echeverria-Londono, S.; Roth, J.; Li, X.; Abbas, K.; Portnoy, A.; Vynnycky, E.; Woodruff, K.; Ferguson, N.M.; et al. Correction: Vaccine equity in low and middle income countries: A systematic review and meta-analysis. *Int. J. Equity Health* **2022**, *21*, 92. [CrossRef] [PubMed]
34. Wigley, A.; Lorin, J.; Hogan, D.; Utazi, C.E.; Hagedorn, B.; Dansereau, E.; Tatem, A.J.; Tejedor-Garavito, N. Estimates of the number and distribution of zero-dose and under-immunised children across remote-rural, urban, and conflict-affected settings in low and middle-income countries. *PLoS Glob. Public Health* **2022**, *2*, e0001126. [CrossRef] [PubMed]
35. Harrison, E.A.; Wu, J.W. Vaccine confidence in the time of COVID-19. *Eur. J. Epidemiol.* **2020**, *35*, 325–330. [CrossRef] [PubMed]
36. MacDonald, N.E.; SAGE Working Group on Vaccine Hesitancy. Vaccine hesitancy: Definition, scope and determinants. *Vaccine* **2015**, *33*, 4161–4164. [CrossRef] [PubMed]
37. Pan American Health Organization/World Health Organization. Epidemiological Alert Epidemiological situation in the Region of the Americas—29 January 2024. 2024. Available online: https://www.paho.org/en/documents/epidemiological-alert-measles-region-americas-29-january-2024 (accessed on 14 March 2024).
38. Countries of the Caribbean Agree to Strengthen National Immunization Programs through Declaration of Nassau. 2023. Available online: https://www.paho.org/en/news/27-4-2023-countries-caribbean-agree-strengthen-national-immunization-programs-through (accessed on 15 August 2023).
39. Organização Pan-Americana da Saúde. Brasil Lança Movimento Nacional para Ampliar Vacinação. 2023. Available online: https://www.paho.org/pt/noticias/28-2-2023-brasil-lanca-movimento-nacional-para-ampliar-vacinacao (accessed on 4 September 2023).
40. Organização Pan-Americana da Saúde. No Senado do Brasil, Diretor da OPAS Destaca Importância de Intersetorialidade, Compromisso Político e Participação Social para Manter Alta a Cobertura de Vacinação. 2023. Available online: https://www.paho.org/pt/noticias/4-7-2023-no-senado-do-brasil-diretor-da-opas-destaca-importancia-intersetorialidade (accessed on 4 September 2023).
41. La Organización Panamericana de la Salud. Al Ritmo de Muchachos, Argentina Tuvo su Festival de Vacunas, Música y Color. 2023. Available online: https://www.paho.org/es/noticias/27-4-2023-al-ritmo-muchachos-argentina-tuvo-su-festival-vacunas-musica-color (accessed on 4 September 2023).
42. World Health Organization. Report of the SAGE Working Group on Quality and Use of Immunization and Surveillance Data 2019. Available online: https://terrance.who.int/mediacentre/data/sage/SAGE_Docs_Ppt_Oct2019/8_session_immunization_data/Oct2019_session8_SAGE-Data_WGreport.pdf (accessed on 10 August 2023).
43. Velandia-González, M.; Vilajeliu, A.; Contreras, M.; Trumbo, S.P.; Pacis, C.; Ropero, A.M.; Ruiz-Matus, C. Monitoring progress of maternal and neonatal immunization in Latin America and the Caribbean. *Vaccine* **2021**, *39*, B55–B63. [CrossRef] [PubMed]
44. COVID-19 National Preparedness Collaborators. Pandemic preparedness and COVID-19, an exploratory analysis of infection and fatality rates, and contextual factors associated with preparedness in 177 countries, from 1 Jan 2020, to 30 Sept 2021. *Lancet* **2022**, *399*, 1489–1512. [CrossRef]
45. Llau, A.F.; Williams, M.L.; Tejada, C.E. National vaccine coverage trends and funding in Latin America and the Caribbean. *Vaccine* **2021**, *39*, 317–323. [CrossRef]

Disclaimer/Publisher's Note: The statements, opinions and data contained in all publications are solely those of the individual author(s) and contributor(s) and not of MDPI and/or the editor(s). MDPI and/or the editor(s) disclaim responsibility for any injury to people or property resulting from any ideas, methods, instructions or products referred to in the content.

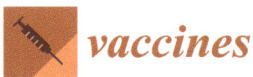 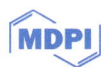

Article

Analyzing Subnational Immunization Coverage to Catch Up and Reach the Unreached in Seven High-Priority Countries in the Eastern Mediterranean Region, 2019–2021

Kamal Fahmy [1,*], Quamrul Hasan [1], Md Sharifuzzaman [1] and Yvan Hutin [2]

1. Universal Health Coverage (UHC)/Department of Communicable Disease Prevention and Control (DCD), Immunization, Vaccine Preventable Diseases and Polio Transition (IVP), World Health Organization Regional Office for the Eastern Mediterranean, Cairo 34222, Egypt; hasanq@who.int (Q.H.); sharifuzzamanm@who.int (M.S.)
2. Universal Health Coverage (UHC)/Department of Communicable Disease Prevention and Control (DCD), World Health Organization Regional Office for the Eastern Mediterranean, Cairo 11371, Egypt; hutiny@who.int
* Correspondence: fahmyk@who.int; Tel.: +20-120-123-6330

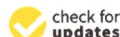

Citation: Fahmy, K.; Hasan, Q.; Sharifuzzaman, M.; Hutin, Y. Analyzing Subnational Immunization Coverage to Catch Up and Reach the Unreached in Seven High-Priority Countries in the Eastern Mediterranean Region, 2019–2021. *Vaccines* **2024**, *12*, 285. https://doi.org/10.3390/vaccines12030285

Academic Editor: Pedro Plans-Rubió

Received: 29 December 2023
Revised: 27 January 2024
Accepted: 30 January 2024
Published: 8 March 2024

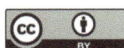

Copyright: © 2024 by the authors. Licensee MDPI, Basel, Switzerland. This article is an open access article distributed under the terms and conditions of the Creative Commons Attribution (CC BY) license (https://creativecommons.org/licenses/by/4.0/).

Abstract: Yearly national immunization coverage reporting does not measure performance at the subnational level throughout the year and conceals inequalities within countries. We analyzed subnational immunization coverage from seven high-priority countries in our region. We analyzed subnational, monthly immunization data from seven high-priority countries. Five were Gavi eligible (i.e., Afghanistan, Pakistan, Somalia, Syria, and Yemen); these are countries that according to their low income are eligible for support from the Global Alliance on Vaccine and Immunization, while Iraq and Jordan were included because of a recent decrease in immunization coverage and contribution to the regional number of under and unimmunized children. DTP3 coverage, which is considered as the main indicator for the routine immunization coverage as the essential component of the immunization program performance, varied monthly in 2019–2021 before reaching pre-pandemic coverage in the last two months of 2021. Somalia and Yemen had a net gain in DTP3 coverage at the end of 2021, as improvement in 2021 exceeded the regression in 2020. In Pakistan and Iraq, DTP3 improvement in 2021 equaled the 2020 regression. In Afghanistan, Syria and Jordan, the regression in DTP3 coverage continued in 2020 and 2021. The number of districts with at least 6000 zero-dose children improved moderately in Afghanistan and substantially in Somalia throughout the follow-up period. In Pakistan, the geographical distribution differed between 2020 and 2021.Of the three countries with the highest number of zero-dose children, DTP1 coverage reached 109% in Q4 of 2020 after a sharp drop to 69% in Q2 of 2020. However, in Pakistan, the number of zero-dose children decreased to 1/10 of its burden in Q4 of 2021. In Afghanistan, the number of zero-dose children more than a doubled. Among the even countries, adaptation of immunization service to the pandemic varied, depending on the agility of the health system and the performance of the components of the expanded program on immunization. We recommended monitoring administrative monthly immunization coverage data at the subnational level to detect low-performing districts, plan catchup, identify bottlenecks towards reaching unvaccinated children and customize strategies to improve the coverage in districts with zero-dose children throughout the year and monitor progress.

Keywords: subnational immunization coverage; under-immunized children; immunization inequality; zero-dose children; COVID pandemic

1. Introduction

In 2011, the World Health Organization (WHO) has set a global plan to improve immunization coverage and reduce vaccine-preventable diseases. This Global Vaccine Action Plan [GVAP] proposed to strengthen immunization systems worldwide and achieve equitable access to vaccines for all populations. The plan set dual targets of 90% national coverage and 80% coverage for all districts within countries by 2020, using the third dose of Diphtheria, Pertussis and Tetanus [DPT] coverage as a marker [1]. The plan also emphasized the integration of immunization goals with the Sustainable Development Goals [SDGs] to ensure that vaccines contribute to overall health and development outcomes. In 2020, immunization partners adapted the global strategy for immunization as per the Immunization Agenda [IA] 2030 that focuses on leaving no one behind. IA2030 envisions a world where everyone, everywhere, at every age, fully benefits from vaccines to improve health and well-being [2]. Key strategies to address some challenges in implementing the IA2030 are (1) increasing the financing of health systems, (2) addressing vaccine hesitancy, (3) building a strong partnership and making decisions based on data. Data at the subnational level drive the decision to address immunization service delivery gaps at the district level. All countries commit to report on their immunization coverage, among other indicators, at the end of every year. The joint reporting form (JRF) is the basis of the globally approved immunization coverage through the WHO–UNICEF Estimates of National Immunization Coverage based on administrative reported coverage and available surveys (WUNEIC) [3]. However, yearly reporting on immunization coverage lacks the ability to measure performance at the subnational level throughout the year. Further, national coverage data often conceal inequalities in coverage and access within the country [4]. During the COVID-19 pandemic, it could not be used to measure continuity of immunization service delivery and subsequent recovery. In contrast, analyzing immunization coverage at the district level allows for targeted interventions to improve immunization rates and prioritize intervention to reduce disparities [5,6]. Subnational immunization coverage analysis gained a global interest to identify low-performing districts. In some countries, data are available at the subdistrict level which allows for better consideration of any reduction in immunization coverage throughout the year.

The WHO Eastern Mediterranean Region (EMR) is one of the six World Health Organization regions with the lowest immunization coverage, with significant disparities between and within its 22 countries. Several countries of the region face numerous economic, social, and political challenges that affect the delivery of immunization services. Factors such as armed conflicts, population displacement, poverty, weak health systems, and cultural beliefs contribute to disparities in immunization coverage and hinder efforts to reach vulnerable populations. In 2012, the Eastern Mediterranean Regional Office (EMRO) developed as a regional framework aligned with the GVAP: the Eastern Mediterranean Vaccine Action Plan (EMVAP). EMVAP took into consideration regional specificities, specific needs of Member States and the challenges that these countries faced [7]. EMVAP had put a specific focus on all countries reaching the DTP3 coverage at 90% at the national level and at least 80% at the district (subnational) level. In 2023, the EMR was developing the regional framework in coherence with the IA 2030. Challenges in vaccination coverage in the EMR are considerable. Prior to the pandemic, in the Eastern Mediterranean region, the mean percentages of routine vaccination coverage increased from 2015 to 2019 for five (38.5%) vaccines and decreased for eight (61.5%) vaccines. Vaccination coverage increases from 2015 to 2019 ranged from 0.2% for the DTP1 vaccine and MCV2 to 11.9% for the first dose of inactivated poliovirus vaccine. Vaccination coverage reductions from 2015 to 2019 ranged from −0.2% for five vaccines (DTP3 vaccine, the first dose of hepatitis B vaccine, the third dose of hepatitis B vaccine, the third dose of poliovirus vaccine, and the first dose of rubella-containing vaccine) to −5% for the last dose of rotavirus vaccine. While in 2022, the coverage for DTP3 and MCV1 were 84% and *83%, respectively [8]. In 2019, in EMR, 1.8 million children did not get their first dose of DTP [zero-dose children]. EMRO identified seven high-priority countries in the region. Five of these are Gavi eligible countries (i.e., Afghanistan, Pakistan, Somalia, Syria, and Yemen). Iraq and Jordan are included as well in the review process because of the decrease in their immunization coverage and contribution to the regional under and unimmunized children. Further, three of the seven priority countries (Pakistan, Afghanistan, and Somalia) report two-thirds of zero-dose children in the region. In addition, overall, 2.9 million children in all EMR countries in 2022 did not receive their third dose of DTP3.

Analyzing immunization coverage at the subnational level allows better tracking of unimmunized children [9]. Regular monitoring of monthly immunization coverage at the subnational level allows countries to take timely decisions sooner rather than later. The EMRO started to support countries in analyzing their immunization coverage at the lowest possible subnational level. In 2018, the EMRO decided at the regional level to start collecting monthly immunization coverage data at the subnational level from high-priority countries. The objective was to obtain a greater understanding of disparities in the coverage and access within each country and to identify areas where immunization services were not reaching the population effectively. In the meantime, in 2020, the EPI in the region had to face the COVID-19 pandemic and organize the recovery of immunization services. Countries reported differences in immunization performance, as reflected by different antigens coverage, with a primarily focus on DTP3 and MCV2 coverage. The pandemic impacted one or more of the components of the expanded program on immunization (e.g., governance, work force, finance, vaccine and cold chain, immunization service delivery, surveillance, and demand generation). Taking advantage of our new system, we reviewed the monthly subnational immunization coverage in 2019–2021 in our seven priority countries. The objective was to document backslide and recovery in immunization coverage during and after the COVID-19 pandemic period. The expected outcome of this work was to contribute to regional efforts of countries' support to identify low-performing districts early to develop strategies to improve performance before final reporting at the end of the year.

2. Methods

2.1. Data Collection

Immunization data managers at the subnational and national level of the countries' EPI program collected immunization data on a monthly basis for all antigens. On a quarterly basis, immunization officers in respective countries' WHO country offices shared with the immunization unit in the EMRO the monthly immunization data of all antigens based on countries' immunization administrative coverage at the district level.

2.2. Data Analysis

The EMRO prepared and shared an automated spreadsheet with all WHO country offices to ensure standardization of reporting among all countries. The WHO-generated sheet had an automatic calculation of immunization coverage based on administered doses of every antigen with a subsequent color-coded level of coverage and equipped with some antigen (DTP1-DTP3 and MCV1-MCV2) dropout calculations and districts classification based on their coverage performance. The dropout rate is calculated as the proportion of drop in immunization coverage between the first and third dose of DTP or the first and second dose of MCV. WHO staff in countries filled in this spreadsheet, with an automatic calculation of immunization coverage, on a monthly basis at district and national levels. Each trimester, countries' offices sent an updated spreadsheet. The EMRO merged data from individual countries at the end of each year, including an update of data of all quarters when applicable. As per the regular information sharing within the WHO, the EMRO shared the data regularly with the global central data repository in a database with access restricted to inside the organization. The EMRO team received data, reviewed it, and cleaned it before the analysis including an analysis for data quality issues.

The EMRO then analyzed the district-level performance as per all antigens' coverage. Every quarter, the EMRO compared immunization coverage with the previous quarter and with the same quarter of the previous year. Zero-dose children, who are the children who never received their first dose of DTP, were analyzed separately.

At the end of every year, we analyzed the monthly coverage based on the most updated data received in the last quarter of every year. For 2019–2021, in the seven countries, we described the monthly DTP3 coverage and described the proportion of districts with at least 80% DTP3 coverage every quarter. Within every year, we compared quarters in terms of coverage. Across the years, we compared the same quarters in terms of coverage.

To estimate the coverage net gain between 2019 and 2021, we broke down the comparison by biennium. First, we calculated the difference in coverage in 2019–2020. Second, we calculated the difference in 2020–2021. Third, we plotted the net difference of the total period.

We mapped the distribution of zero-dose children at district level in the three countries with the highest number of zero-dose children for 2019–2021. Throughout the review period, for the three highest-priority countries with the highest burden of zero-dose children, we plotted by quarter the total number of zero-dose children according to DTP1 coverage.

2.3. Feedback

The EMRO provided feedback to the WHO country office in the form of a detailed analytic report on a quarterly basis that included sections on immunization data quality and immunization coverage analysis of all antigens. The report included conclusions of the findings and suggested recommendations for the countries' immunization program. The EMRO then suggested that the WHO country office share the report with the immunization program counterpart for their consideration and corrective action whenever needed. The detailed analysis of the immunization coverage reflected the most important components of countries' immunization program performance.

3. Results

3.1. Variations in Coverage throughout the Year

In 2020, the first year of the pandemic, the monthly DTP3 coverage dropped between March and June (Figure 1). Continuous monthly variation in DTP3 coverage occurred in the review period before the increase in the initial coverage in the last two months of 2021. The proportion of districts that exceeded 80% DTP3 coverage always improved in the last quarter every year (Figure 2). In 2021, the proportion of districts exceeding 80% DTP3 coverage was higher than in 2020. However, it did not reach the pre-pandemic performance level of 2019.

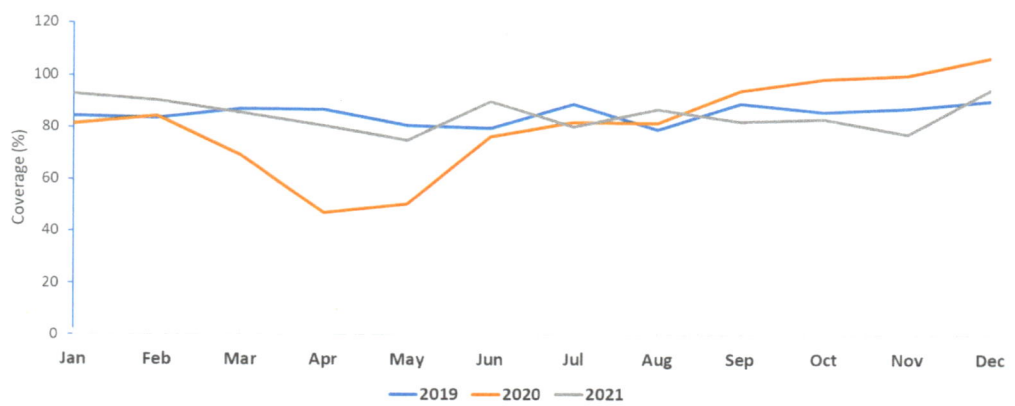

Figure 1. DTP3 monthly coverage in high-priority countries in the Eastern Mediterranean Region, 2019–2021. Afghanistan, Iraq, Jordan, Pakistan, Somalia, Syria, and Yemen.

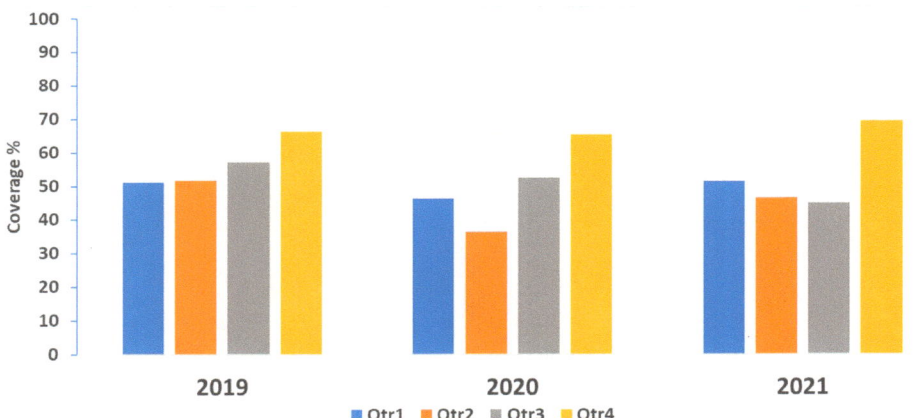

Figure 2. Proportion of districts with at least 80% DTP3 coverage by quarter in high-priority countries, in the Eastern Mediterranean Region, 2019–2021.

3.2. Recovery of Coverage following the Effect of the Pandemic

When we compared 2019 with 2020 and 2020 with 2021 according the DTP3 coverage net gain and net loss, three types of DTP3 coverage pattern emerged (Figure 3). First, some countries improved overall. Somalia and Yemen had a net gain of DTP3 coverage at the end of the review period because the improvement in 2021 exceeded the regression in 2020. Second, some countries recuperated just as much as they lost. DTP3 improvement in 2021 was equal to the 2020 regression in Pakistan and Iraq. Third, some countries did not recover enough. In Afghanistan, Syria and Jordan, the regression in DTP3 coverage continued in 2020 and 2021.

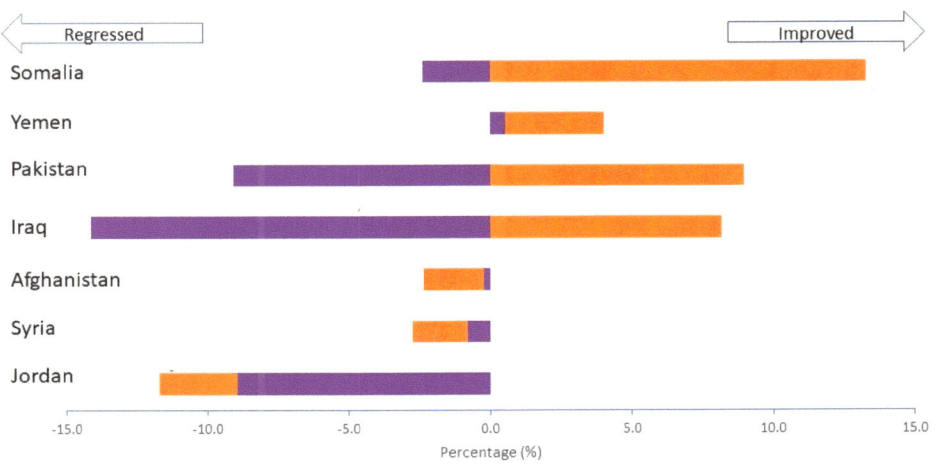

Figure 3. Difference in DTP3 coverage based on subnational coverage in high-priority countries in the Eastern Mediterranean Region, 2019–2021.

3.3. Distribution of Zero_Dose Children

The distribution of zero-dose children in the three countries with the highest burden in the region evolved over time (Figure 4). The number of districts with at least

6000 zero-dose children improved moderately in Afghanistan and substantially in Somalia throughout the follow-up period. In Pakistan, the geographical distribution differed between 2020 and 2021.

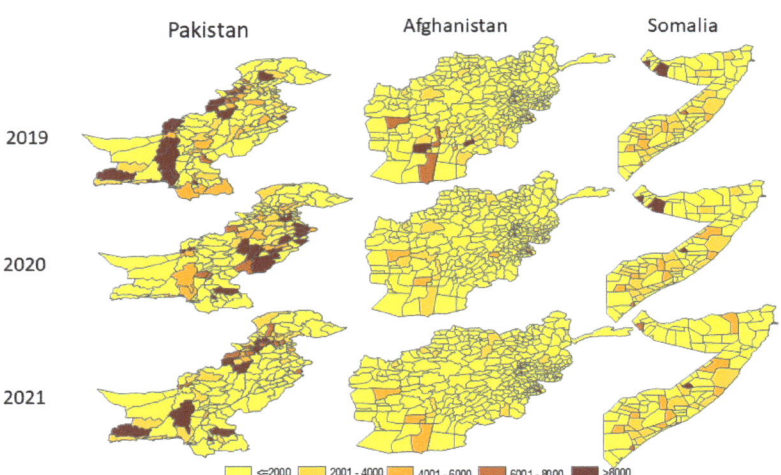

Figure 4. Subnational distribution of zero-dose children in the three highest burden zero-dose countries in the Eastern Mediterranean Region, 2019–2021.

3.4. DTP1 Coverage

DTP1 coverage of the three countries with highest number of zero-dose children reached 109% in Q4 of 2020 after a sharp drop to 69% in Q2 of 2020. However, the number of zero-dose children in Pakistan decreased to 1/10 of its burden in 2021 at Q4. In Afghanistan, the number of zero-dose children more than doubled throughout 2021 (Figure 5).

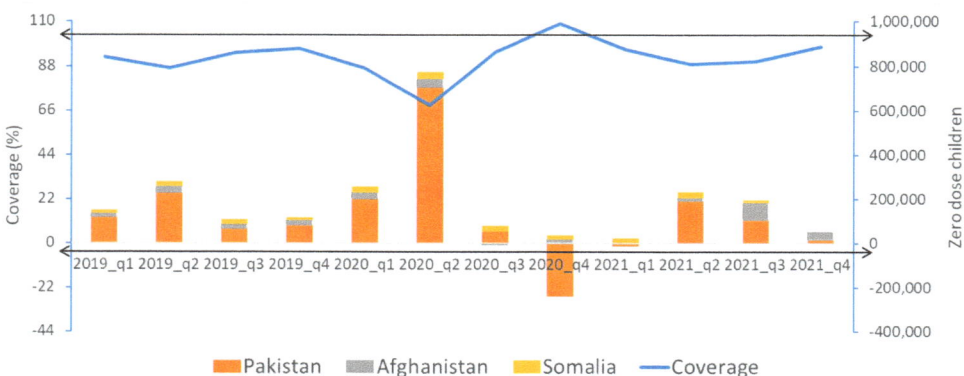

Figure 5. DTP1 coverage vs. zero-dose^2 children in three high-priority countries in the Eastern Mediterranean Region, 2019–2021. ^{2}Zero_dose children: DTP1-unvaccinated children. Source: monthly subnational immunization coverage data.

4. Discussion

There was a sharp drop in DTP3 coverage from March to June in 2020, the first year of the pandemic when countries started to sift attention to the pandemic control measures, and most of the immunization staff were concentrating on working on this initial phase of the outbreak response. Afterwards, it started to recuperate by the end of the year. The pre-pandemic level of DTP3 coverage continued to improve throughout the review period. Another study analyzing the disruption and recovery of immunization services in 170 countries depicted a similar trend [10]. More generally, in 2019–2021, the low proportion of districts achieving at least 80% DTP3 coverage at the beginning of the year started to improve in the second half of the year, with the best performances during the last quarter of every year. Countries identified missed children throughout the first three-quarters to guide the catching up of under-immunized children during the fourth quarter of every year. Some high-priority countries in the region reported coverage exceeding 100%. Experience from other countries suggests that this is mainly due to the inability to estimate the correct denominator at the district level. Other reasons could include the catchup of a backlog of unimmunized children in one month or quarter of the year [11,12]. In 2021, the performance of districts followed the same improving trend in terms of the proportion of districts reaching 80% DTP3 coverage by the end of the year. However, in the high-priority countries, coverage did not reach the pre-pandemic level of 2019. This delay varied in magnitude between countries involved in the analysis. Countries' programs to improve immunization coverage also competed with the introduction of COVID-19 vaccination and were taking place under stretched conditions of the ministries of health generally and the immunization programs specifically, sometimes aggravated by humanitarian situations in some countries, which increasingly needed more effort to cope with those situations [13].

Immunization service delivery adapted to the pandemic differently from country to country. These differences depended on the agility of the health system and the performance of one or more of the different components of expanded programs on immunization (i.e., governance, work force, finance, vaccine and cold chain, immunization service delivery, surveillance, and demand generation). The EMRO initiative to analyze monthly subnational immunization coverage on a quarterly basis provided support to the stretched country system. It facilitated the identification of unimmunized and under-immunized children before the end of the year to prevent a larger backsliding of immunization coverage. Backsliding of immunization, due to the pandemic, has been depicted in almost all countries in the world regardless of their income. Low- and middle-income countries have been most affected in terms of vaccination coverage of most of the antigens [14]. The World Health Organization [15] provided guidance on aspects of immunization recovery and catchup of missed children. This called for strengthening routine service delivery, conducting antigen specific or multiantigen campaigns and undertaking Periodic Intensification of Routine Immunization (PIRI). Somalia and Yemen responded early to the reduction in DTP3 coverage in 2020. The 2021 coverage reflected this response. In Pakistan and Iraq, the regression in DTP3 coverage in 2020 was compensated in 2021. Instant corrective measures were taken to address the backslide in immunization in high-priority districts based on their identification in the subnational coverage analysis. Afghanistan, Syria, and Jordan continued to regress throughout the period until the last quarter of 2021. This was mainly attributed to the delayed response of immunization service recovery in the lowest-performing districts.

Almost all EMR high-priority countries depend on outreach and mobile approaches that support fixed centers to deliver immunization services. The cancellation of outreach services following the COVID-19 lockdown meant that many children missed vaccination which resulted in backsliding of the immunization coverage and magnification of the number of zero-dose children [16]. Gavi in its support for low- and middle-income countries, among which included countries in this analysis, emphasized reaching zero-dose children at the subnational level (i.e., the last administrative level where data could be generated and reported). However, reaching zero-dose communities within districts becomes a long term goal, when identifying the target of zero-dose children in those communities becomes available [17]. Our analysis has confirmed that immunization coverage at the national level masks the heterogeneity of the coverage at the district level on a monthly basis in the reported countries. Hard-to-reach areas are the most affected areas with poor immunization coverage and host the biggest number of zero-dose children in all countries [18].

The constant decrease in the number of zero-dose children in the same districts throughout the years has led to an overall decrease in the number of zero-dose children in countries. This improvement is mainly related to the timely implementation of catch-up multi-antigen campaigns or an enhanced immunization outreached approach at the subnational level. These campaign and enhanced outreached strategies succeeded in catching up with underimmunization so more children have been reached with all missing antigens within a reduced timeline. Changes in geographical location in zero-dose children in Pakistan is related to different responses by districts and to substantial mobile populations between districts and provinces. Similar findings were also depicted in other similar-income countries [16,19]. In other settings [20], missed children are constantly located in the same districts and provinces due to a continuous lack of resources allocated and available to the expanded program in immunization. In Pakistan, the same number of districts had the same number of zero-dose children in 2019–2020, but the location changed. Yet, overall districts with zero-dose children have much decreased throughout the last quarter of 2021 due to a decrease in the overall number of zero-dose districts nationwide. In Afghanistan, the situation was very different. The number of zero-dose children increased in 2021, despite the decrease in zero-dose children in a number of districts compared to the great increase in zero-dose children in a different number of districts. This is mainly related to the worsening of the immunization performance and increased number of zero-dose children in several other districts. In the Laghman province of Afghanistan, Abid et al. reported [21] a period of improvement in immunization performance in most of the 400 districts through 2020 and 2021 during the pandemic period. An earlier study [22] did not suggest that the conflict situation in Afghanistan significantly affected DTP3 immunization coverage in most Afghanistan districts. However, the conflicts referred to were shorter than the pandemic. Finally, Somalia improved throughout the last two years of the review period, which resulted in recuperation of unimmunized and under-immunized children vaccination because of their early response since the first year of the pandemic. Focusing on reaching zero-dose children is the ultimate objective for reaching the sustainable development goals [23].

Our review suffered from several limitations. First, countries lacked accurate estimations of their monthly immunization target. This led to coverage exceeding 100% for several antigens in some districts, with a subsequent impact on the overall estimate of national immunization coverage. This has led to reflecting a negative number of zero-dose children in Q4 2020. The WHO [24] formulated guidelines for the estimation of denominators to accurately calculate the immunization coverage. The different methods to calculate denominators can be customized to the country context. Second, inaccurate and delayed reporting of monthly immunization data along with the existence of mobile, migrant and internal displaced populations (IDPs) may reflect unrealistic recovery of immunization coverage in some districts. Because of the inaccurate estimation of the target population, frequent mapping of mobile populations to include them in the denominator of the districts' catchment area will improve the estimation of immunization-targeted children. Third, cross-district vaccination and geographical redistribution of some districts may have impeded the real estimation of the subnational burden of zero-dose children, especially in countries with no cross notification of immunization coverage on a monthly basis. This hindered effective planning of catchup immunization campaigns. Electronic immunization registries with instant registration of immunization, which could be monitored centrally, and GPS-based home-based records could help in identifying missed children in a timely manner.

5. Conclusions

Based on this review, we can draw several conclusions. First, DTP3 coverage decreased in 2020, in the first year of the COVID pandemic, and recovered in the fourth quarter of every year. Second, countries differed in their recovery in 2019–2021, with a positive net improvement in DTP 3 coverage, a compensation, or a sustained reduction. Third, the geographical distribution of districts with a high number of zero-dose children is dynamic from year to year. While some hotspots are being addressed, new ones emerge. Based on these conclusions, we recommended the following actions. First, we need to monitor administrative monthly immunization coverage data of all antigens with evaluation of the dropout rates at the subnational level to detect low-performing districts and plan for catchup. Second, we need to identify bottlenecks towards reaching unvaccinated children at the subnational level based on the number of unimmunized and under-immunized children with a high focus on the zero-dose children. Third, we need to customize strategies continuously to improve the coverage of the districts with a high number of zero-dose children throughout the four quarters every year and monitor the progress of other better-performing districts. In countries with highly populated districts, there is a need to address subdistrict level data so zero-dose children can be located at the community level. This analysis was proposed by the EMRO as a model approach. Ultimately, the management of this approach should be transferred to countries so that the national immunization programs own the process and start to have a close monitoring of the immunization coverage on a monthly basis for up-to-date consideration should districts show a decline in the immunization coverage.

Author Contributions: K.F. contributed in conceptulizing the article, adopting the methods, writing the manuscript, original draft preparation and finalzation of the article, M.S. contributed to data analysis, Y.H. contributed in structuring the manscript, adjusting the analyisi and edit the text, Q.H. supported the analytics, supervising and review in the article. All authors have read and agreed to the published version of the manuscript.

Funding: The research has received no external funding except publication fees paid by WHO.

Data Availability Statement: Data is available at WHO country office of contributing countries and at Eastern Mediterranean Regional office of WHO.

Acknowledgments: We appreciate our colleagues Firas AL-Khafaji, Mohamed Farid, Mehraban Sayedzai, Sohail Nasim, Muaadh Thabet, Ala'a Al Shaikh and Aschalew Teka Bekele from WHO country offices in Iraq, Somalia, Afghanistan, Pakistan, Syria, Jordan and Yemen, respectively, and EPI counterparts of the ministry of health of participating countries in EMR for sharing the subnational immunization coverage data for the review period and considering the feedback analytic report for taking action.

Conflicts of Interest: The authors declare no conflict of interest.

References

1. World Health Organization. *Global Vaccine Action Plan 2011–2020*; World Health Organization: Geneva, Switzerland, 2012. Available online: https://www.who.int/teams/immunization-vaccines-and-biologicals/strategies/global-vaccine-action-plan (accessed on 10 November 2023).
2. World Health Organization. *Immunization Agenda 2030: A Global Strategy to Leave No One Behind*; World Health Organization: Geneva, Switzerland, 2020.
3. WHO/UNICEF Joint Reporting Process. Available online: https://www.who.int/teams/immunization-vaccines-and-biologicals/immunization-analysis-and-insights/global-monitoring/who-unicef-joint-reporting-process (accessed on 17 September 2023).
4. Hosseinpoor, A.R.; Bergen, N.; Schlotheuber, A.; Gacic-Dobo, M.; Hansen, P.M.; Senouci, K.; Boerma, T.; Barros, A.J.D. State of inequality in diphtheria-tetanus-pertussis immunisation coverage in low-income and middle-income countries: A multicountry study of household health surveys. *Lancet Glob. Health.* **2016**, *4*, e617–e626. [CrossRef] [PubMed]
5. Reaching Every District (RED). Available online: https://www.who.int/teams/immunization-vaccines-and-biologicals/essential-programme-on-immunization/implementation/reaching-every-district-(red) (accessed on 17 September 2023).
6. Vandelaer, J.; Bilous, J.; Nshimirimana, D. Reaching Every District (RED) approach: A way to improve immunization performance. Bull World Health Organ. 2008. Available online: https://www.ncbi.nlm.nih.gov/pmc/articles/PMC2647411/ (accessed on 17 September 2023).

7. World Health Organization. *Regional Office for the Eastern Mediterranean. Eastern Mediterranean Vaccine Action Plan 2016–2020: A Framework for Implementation of the Global Vaccine Action Plan*; World Health Organization, Regional Office for the Eastern Mediterranean: Geneva, Switzerland, 2019; 28p. Available online: https://apps.who.int/iris/handle/10665/311578 (accessed on 10 November 2023).
8. Plans-Rubió, P. Vaccination Coverage for Routine Vaccines and Herd Immunity Levels against Measles and Pertussis in the World in 2019. *Vaccines* **2021**, *9*, 256. [CrossRef] [PubMed]
9. Subnational Immunization Coverage Data. Available online: https://www.who.int/teams/immunization-vaccines-and-biologicals/immunization-analysis-and-insights/global-monitoring/immunization-coverage/subnational-immunization-coverage-data (accessed on 15 December 2023).
10. Shet, A.; Carr, K.; Danovaro-Holliday, M.C.; Sodha, S.V.; Prosperi, C.; Wunderlich, J.; Wonodi, C.; Reynolds, H.W.; Mirza, I.; Gacic-Dobo, M.; et al. Impact of the SARS-CoV-2 pandemic on routine immunization services: Evidence of disruption and recovery from 170 countries and territory. *Lancet* **2021**, *10*, E186–E194. [CrossRef]
11. Rau, C.; Lüdecke, D.; Dumolard, L.B.; Grevendonk, J.; Wiernik, B.M.; Kobbe, R.; Gacic-Dobo, M.; Danovaro-Holliday, M.C. Data quality of reported child immunization coverage in 194 countries between 2000 and 2019. *PLoS Glob. Public Health* **2022**, *2*, e000140. [CrossRef] [PubMed]
12. Brown, D.W.; Burton, A.H.; Feeney, G.; Gacic-Dobo, M. Avoiding the Will O' the Wisp: Challenges in Measuring High Levels of Immunization Coverage with Precision. *World J. Vaccines* **2014**, *4*, 97–99. [CrossRef]
13. Grundy, J.; Biggs, B.A. The impact of conflict on immunization coverage in 16 countries. *Int. J. Health Policy Manag.* **2019**, *8*, 211–221. [CrossRef] [PubMed]
14. World Health Organization. COVID-19 Pandemic Leads to Major Backsliding on Childhood Vaccinations, New WHO, UNICEF Data Shows. Available online: https://www.who.int/news/item/15-07-2021-covid-19-pandemic-leads-to-major-backsliding-on-childhood-vaccinations-new-who-unicef-data-shows (accessed on 7 July 2023).
15. World Health Organization. *Essential Programme on Immunization*; World Health Organization: Geneva, Switzerland. Available online: https://www.who.int/teams/immunization-vaccines-and-biologicals/essential-programme-on-immunization/implementation/immunization-campaigns (accessed on 7 July 2023).
16. Cata-Preta, B.; Santos, T.M.; Mengistu, T.; Hogan, D.R.; Barros, A.J.D.; Victora, C.G. Zero-dose children and the immunization cascade: Understanding immunization pathways in low and middle-income countries. *Vaccines* **2021**, *39*, 4564–4570. [CrossRef] [PubMed]
17. Gavi. List of Countries and Economies Eligible Support Under the MICs Approach as of 1 July 2022. Geneva, 2022. Available online: https://www.gavi.org/sites/default/files/programmes-impact/support/Countries-and-economies-eligible-for-support-under-Gavi-MICs-Approach.pdf (accessed on 4 October 2023).
18. Ozawa, S.; Yemeke, T.T.; Evans, D.R.; Pallas, S.E.; Wallace, A.S.; Lee, B.Y. Defining hard-to-reach populations for vaccination. *Vaccine* **2019**, *37*, 5525–5534. [CrossRef] [PubMed]
19. Wonodi, C.; Farrenkopf, B.A. Defining the Zero Dose Child: A Comparative Analysis of Two Approaches and Their Impact on Assessing the Zero Dose Burden and Vulnerability Profiles across 82 Low- and Middle-Income Countries. *Vaccines* **2023**, *11*, 1543. [CrossRef] [PubMed]
20. Bergen, N.; Zhu, G.; Kirkby, K. Reporting immunization coverage inequalities in Pakistan. *East Mediterr. Health J.* **2021**, *27*, 83–89. [CrossRef]
21. Abid, Z.; Castro Delgado, R.; Cernuda Martinez, J.A.; González, P.A. The impact of COVID 19 pandemic lockdown on routine immunization in the province of Laghman, Afghanistan. *Risk Manag. Health Policy* **2022**, *5*, 901–908. [CrossRef] [PubMed]
22. Mashal, T.; Nakamura, K.; Kizuki, M. Impact of conflict on Immunization coverage in Afghanistan, a country wide study 2000–2003. *Int. J. Health Geogr.* **2007**, *6*, 23. [CrossRef]
23. Hogan, D.; Gupta, A. Why Reaching Zero-Dose Children Holds the Key to Achieving the Sustainable Development Goals. *Vaccines* **2023**, *11*, 781. [CrossRef] [PubMed]
24. World health organization. Assessing and Improving the Accuracy of Target Population Estimates for Immunization Coverag. Available online: https://www.who.int/publications/m/item/assessing-and-improving-the-accuracy-of-target-population-estimates-for-immunization-coverage (accessed on 15 January 2024).

Disclaimer/Publisher's Note: The statements, opinions and data contained in all publications are solely those of the individual author(s) and contributor(s) and not of MDPI and/or the editor(s). MDPI and/or the editor(s) disclaim responsibility for any injury to people or property resulting from any ideas, methods, instructions or products referred to in the content.

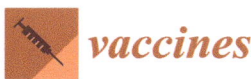

Review

Of Money and Men: A Scoping Review to Map Gender Barriers to Immunization Coverage in Low- and Middle-Income Countries

Anna Kalbarczyk [1,*], Natasha Brownlee [2] and Elizabeth Katz [2,3]

1. Department of International Health, Johns Hopkins Bloomberg School of Public Health, Baltimore, MD 21205, USA
2. Global Center for Gender Equality, Washington, DC 20036, USA; natasha.brownlee@gcfge.org (N.B.); egkatz@usfca.edu (E.K.)
3. Department of Economics, University of San Francisco, San Francisco, CA 94117, USA
* Correspondence: akalbarc@jhu.edu

Abstract: Among the multiple factors impeding equitable childhood immunization coverage in low- and middle-income countries (LMICs), gender barriers stand out as perhaps the most universal. Despite increasing recognition of the importance of gender considerations in immunization programming, there has not yet been a systematic assessment of the evidence on gender barriers to immunization. We conducted a scoping review to fill that gap, identifying 92 articles that described gender barriers to immunization. Studies documented a range of gender influencers across 43 countries in Africa and South Asia. The barrier to immunization coverage most frequently cited in the literature is women's lack of autonomous decision-making. Access to immunization is significantly impacted by women's time poverty; direct costs are also a barrier, particularly when female caregivers rely on family members to cover costs. Challenges with clinic readiness compound female caregiver's time constraints. Some of the most important gender barriers lie outside of the usual purview of immunization programming but other barriers can be addressed with adaptations to vaccination programming. We can only know how important these barriers are with more research that measures the impact of programming on gender barriers to immunization coverage.

Keywords: gender; immunization coverage; vaccination; LMICs; inequality

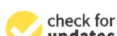

Citation: Kalbarczyk, A.; Brownlee, N.; Katz, E. Of Money and Men: A Scoping Review to Map Gender Barriers to Immunization Coverage in Low- and Middle-Income Countries. *Vaccines* **2024**, *12*, 625. https://doi.org/10.3390/vaccines12060625

Academic Editor: Pedro Plans-Rubió

Received: 29 April 2024
Revised: 22 May 2024
Accepted: 4 June 2024
Published: 5 June 2024

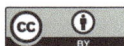

Copyright: © 2024 by the authors. Licensee MDPI, Basel, Switzerland. This article is an open access article distributed under the terms and conditions of the Creative Commons Attribution (CC BY) license (https://creativecommons.org/licenses/by/4.0/).

1. Introduction

Inequality in immunization is normally interpreted to refer to discrepancies in coverage by socioeconomic status, demographic characteristics, and/or geography [1,2]. However, these factors should be understood not only as gradients of vaccine coverage but also as drivers of effective demand for immunization. In other words, inequality is both a cause and a consequence with respect to vaccination.

Among the multiple factors impeding equitable childhood immunization coverage in low- and middle-income countries (LMICs), gender barriers—defined as the ways in which gender roles, norms, and relations impede immunization program performance—stand out as perhaps the most universal [3,4]. This is in large part because, across LMIC geographies, while mothers bear primary responsibility for their children's health, they often lack the resources and/or decision-making authority to access vaccination services [5]. Deepening our understanding of how these barriers operate, and which ones are most salient and pervasive, is key to designing interventions to effectively address them.

But despite increasing recognition of the importance of gender considerations in immunization programming—as evidenced, for example, by the recent WHO publication *Why Gender Matters: Immunization Agenda 2030*—there has not yet been a systematic assessment of the evidence on gender barriers to immunization [6]. This scoping review, funded by the Bill and Melinda Gates Foundation, seeks to fill that gap by documenting the findings of over 90 peer-reviewed research papers and analyzing the results within a coherent conceptual framework. Taken together, the evidence described in this review makes a compelling case that failing to address the significant gender barriers to immunization, particularly routine immunization, will impede progress towards achieving greater equity in vaccine coverage, especially in LMICs.

2. Methods

The research protocol followed the Preferred Items for Systematic Reviews and Meta-analysis extension for Scoping Reviews (PRISMA-ScR) guidelines but was not registered. To identify the published literature on gender barriers to immunization in SSA and South Asia, we conducted a search of three databases, PubMed, Embase, and CINAHL, on 26 September 2023. The search strategy was designed to capture the literature related to the three specific concepts, (1) gender, (2) immunization, and (3) geography (specifically Sub-Saharan Africa (SSA) and South Asia). A complete list of search terms can be found in the supplemental material.

Results from the three databases were downloaded, combined, and deduplicated in Endnote. Unique files were then uploaded to Covidence (www.covidence.org), an online, collaborative scoping review management software. Articles were included if they captured all three concepts and were published in English between 2000 and the date of search. Articles were excluded if they did not meet these inclusion criteria, only discussed vaccine product development, and if the gender analysis was limited to sex disaggregation only.

Title and abstract reviews and full-text reviews followed the same procedures. Two independent reviewers reviewed each and conflicts were resolved by a third, independent reviewer or by team discussion. Systematic and scoping reviews were included so that the references included in them could be reviewed. Additional articles shared by experts were also included and underwent review.

Data were extracted in Covidence and analyzed in Microsoft Excel (https://www.microsoft.com/zh-cn/). The extraction form included questions about the country/region of study, disease/immunization of focus, target population, study design, gender barriers and their relevance along the immunization value chain, gender barrier analysis domains, and other key observations made by reviewers. Descriptive statistics were generated where data could be quantified. Data were initially charted along the immunization value chain, using a gender analysis matrix. This approach seeks to organize data along gender analysis domains (i.e., access to resources; distribution of labor, practices, and roles; norms, values, and beliefs; decision-making power and autonomy; and policies, laws, and institutions). Some manuscripts explicitly named gender barriers using these domains while others were less explicit. The team used their understanding of the influence of gender on health to categorize barriers when needed. Results largely converged in select domains (i.e., decision-making power), requiring an additional lens.

We then used Phillips et al.'s conceptual framework for effective vaccine coverage in LMICs to organize our findings by three principal determinants: (1) Intent to vaccinate, (2) Community Access, and (3) Health Facility Readiness [7]. This framework is specifically designed to be applicable in LMICs and represents a synthesis of multiple previous frameworks, accounting for the nuanced interactions between supply and demand side factors. Gender influencers which had initially been organized using the gender analysis matrix were then grouped into the Intent, Access, or Readiness categories.

3. Results

A total of 3390 references were added to Endnote (version X9), a reference management software, and 845 duplicates were removed. A total of 2545 references were screened during the title and abstract review and an additional 36 duplicates were manually identified during this process; 2359 studies did not meet inclusion criteria. A total of 173 articles were assessed during the full-text review and 63 studies were excluded because there was no full text (n = 9), the article was retracted (n = 1), no focus on gender (n = 36), not related to the immunization value chain (n = 14), analysis was limited to sex disaggregation (n = 2), or was not original research (n = 1). Seven systematic/scoping reviews were also reviewed to identify relevant references; reviews themselves were not included but did support the identification and inclusion of 17 additional references. In total, 92 articles were included in the final analysis which documented gender barriers to immunization. The PRISMA diagram documenting these findings is presented in Figure 1.

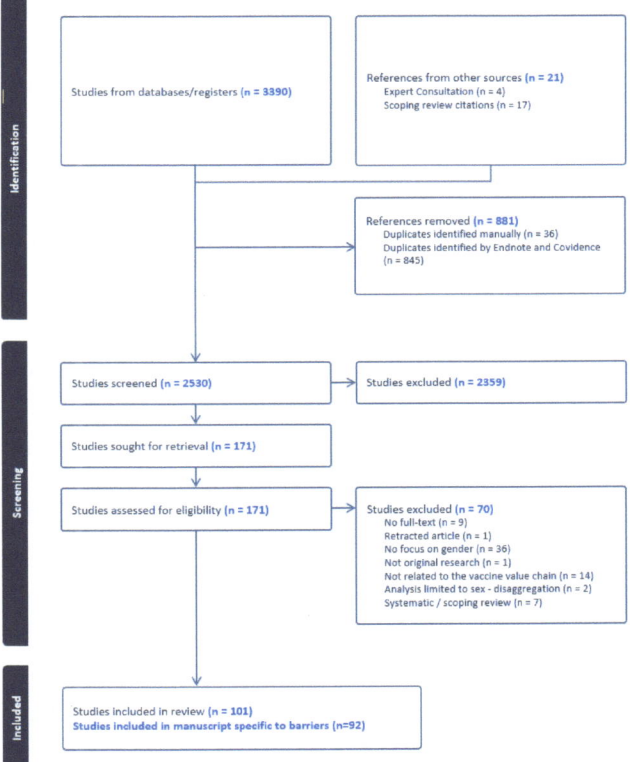

Figure 1. PRISMA diagram.

Most studies assessed barriers to childhood immunizations (n = 63). This was followed by HPV (n = 21), COVID-19 (n = 7), polio (n = 4), maternal vaccines (n = 2), yellow fever (n = 1), and H1N1 (n = 1).

Studies (focused on 25 or fewer countries) documented a range of gender influences of vaccination across 43 countries in Africa and South Asia (see Figure 2). The most frequently studied geographies included Nigeria (n = 21), Ethiopia (n = 12), and Pakistan (n = 10). Three large multi-country studies each contained data from approximately 160 countries. Many studies explored geographic pockets within a country in recognition of the additional and/or specific challenges faced in these unique contexts.

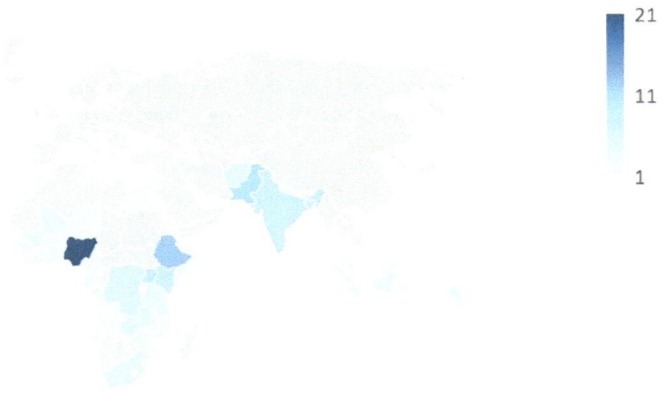

Figure 2. Map of documented gender drivers of immunization.

To assess gender barriers to immunization, studies used quantitative only methods (n = 46), qualitative only methods (n = 39), and mixed methods (n = 8). Of those using quantitative methods, 26 conducted secondary analyses on country Demographic Health Surveys (DHSs). Measurement of immunization coverage varied as well including comparisons between full vs. partial vs. zero dose and hesitancy, readiness, acceptance, and awareness. Measures of gender inequity varied even more widely; nine quantitative studies used gender scores including SWPER Global [8,9], Gender Inequality Ratio (GIR) [10], Gender Development Index (GDI) [11], Gender Inequality Index (GII) [11], and proxies/indexes for empowerment, decision-making power, and autonomy [12–16].

Along the immunization value chain, most studies documented barriers related to demand for immunization and local-level vaccine delivery; very few assessed those barriers influenced by cross-cutting market dynamics such as the supply chain or representation in leadership (see Table 1). Results from the gender barriers analysis are presented by Intent, Access, and Readiness domains, recognizing overlap and intersections.

Table 1. A comprehensive overview of the gender barriers documented.

	Gender Influencers on Immunization	Sub-Theme	Key Points	Geographies/References
Intent—the demand for vaccines that would result in vaccination in the absence of other barriers.				
1.	Women's autonomous decision making	Lack of decision-making over health	-In many settings women rely on their husband's or an elder's permission to seek healthcare services including immunization. -Women with high household decision-making are more likely to have fully immunized children. -Women who make decision jointly with their husbands are more likely to have fully immunized children than when husbands make decision alone. -Some women who oppose their husband's decision face increased risk of intimate partner violence.	Africa (n = 37) South Asia (n = 16) Cross-country (n = 3) [8,12,17–59]

Table 1. Cont.

Gender Influencers on Immunization		Sub-Theme	Key Points	Geographies/References
Intent—the demand for vaccines that would result in vaccination in the absence of other barriers.				
2.	Past experiences with the health system	Negative Experiences	-Some women reported being shamed/bullied by health workers if they missed a prior appointment, forgot the child's vaccine card, or if they or their child appeared dirty and/or malnourished. -Caregivers were not always provided with complete information about the vaccination, including likely side effects and how best to alleviate those side effects. -Caregivers who experience disrespectful treatment are least likely to return to the health system.	Burkina Faso, DRC, Ethiopia Gabon, Nigeria, Mozambique, Pakistan, Timor-Leste, Uganda (n = 8) [25,38,55,60–64]
		Engagement with ANC	Women who attend ANC are more likely to have fully immunized children than women who do not.	Afghanistan, Ethiopia, Nepal, Senegal (n = 8) [16,27,50,65–69]
3.	Gendered myths, misconceptions	Fears of infertility	-Caregivers and health workers expressed concerns that vaccines (including HPV, COVID-19, H1N1, and childhood immunizations) could cause infertility.	Burkina Faso, Kenya, Malawi, Morocco, Tanzania, Zambia (n = 7) [18–20,24,30,60,70]
		Promotion of earlier/increased sexual activity	-Caregivers feared that HPV immunization would result in earlier sexual debut/increased sexual activity for adolescent girls.	Ethiopia, Ghana, India, Malawi, Papua New Guinea, South Africa, Zimbabwe [18,35,54,58,71–73]
Access—ability or inability to successful carry out the transaction of vaccine utilization.				
1.	Time poverty	Competing and gendered demands on time	-Women face competing demands on their time including employment and gendered expectations of caregiving and household labor. This reduces their time for immunizations. -Men's limited contribution in unpaid domestic work exacerbates the demand on women's time.	Burkina Faso, Ethiopia, Nigeria, DRC, Mozambique, Sierra Leone, South Africa, India, Philippines, Somalia, Malaysia, Philippines, Pakistan, Timor-Leste, Uganda, Malawi, Gabon [18,21,23,25,35,40,41,43,44,54,55,60–62,74–77]
		Distance to facilities	-Timing of (schedule) and distance to services can exacerbate this challenge. This effect is worse for low-income women who are socially isolated.	Gabon, Malawi, Nigeria, Malaysia, South Africa, Uganda, Guinea, Malawi, Ethiopia, DRC, Mozambique, Bangladesh [17,25,28,36,61,66,67,74,78–81].
2.	Direct costs	Costs of vaccines, transportation to services, and illicit fees.	-Women reported that the cost of vaccine, transportation costs to access facilities, and illicit fees for services were barriers to immunization.	DRC, Ethiopia, Gabon, Guinea, India, Kenya, Malaysia, Mozambique, Nigeria, Pakistan, Philippines, South Africa, Uganda, Zambia, Zimbabwe [19,23,25,28,29,36,58,61,64,68,70,76,80,82,83]
		Financial Agency	-Women lack financial agency, relying on their husbands to provide the funds and/or approve use of funds for immunization. -Women with their own income and discretion about spending it had increased odds of their children being fully immunized.	DRC, Ethiopia, Gabon, Mozambique, India, Nigeria, Uganda [15,16,25,34,38,61,67,74,79,84]

Table 1. Cont.

Gender Influencers on Immunization	Sub-Theme	Key Points	Geographies/References
Readiness—encompasses the health system's supply of vaccine services to adequately meet demand.			
1. Vaccinators/Health care providers	Lack of women vaccinators/preference for women vaccinators	-A lack of women vaccinators leads to increased coverage inequities, and many men prefer women/daughters are vaccinated by women.	Bangladesh, DRC, Ethiopia, India, Nigeria, Pakistan, Somalia [10,33,43,57,85]
	Women workers' occupational concerns	-Many women health workers experience safety issues, harassment, and low or late remuneration for their services.	Afghanistan, Bangladesh, DRC, Ethiopia, India, Nigeria, [35,86]
2. Health care facilities	Gender unintentional facilities	-Lack of privacy and gender-responsive facilities (i.e., functional and separate washrooms and security for transgender individuals) is a barrier.	Bangladesh, Pakistan [33,64]
	Excessive wait times	-Excessive wait times result in children not receiving immunizations and/or caregivers not being willing to return.	Burkina Faso, DRC, Guinea, Ethiopia, Mozambique, Nigeria, Uganda [25,36,60,63,66,74].
3. Vaccine availability	Vaccine stockouts	-Unavailability of vaccines can lead to pessimism and future nonadherence. -Restrictive vial opening policies result in delayed vaccination and increased frustration among caregivers.	Burkina Faso, Ethiopia, Gabon, Guinea, Nigeria, Papua New Guinea, Tanzania, Uganda [20,36,60–63,72,74].

Intent to vaccinate includes attitudes, perceived norms, and perceived control and represents the demand for vaccines that would result in vaccination in the absence of other barriers.

The most common gender influence on intention is women's **lack of autonomous decision-making** about their health and the health of their children (n = 45) [8,12,17–59]. Across geographies, many women rely on their husband's or an elder's permission to seek healthcare services, including immunization; this was found across Africa (n = 37) and South Asia (n = 16) (note that some studies include more than one country/region). In one study in Nigeria, women with high household decision-making were more likely to have their child fully immunized than women with low decision-making (OR = 1.64, CI: 1.25, 2.14, $p < 0.001$) [48]. Another study in Ethiopia found that mothers who made healthcare decisions jointly with their husbands were 1.88 times (95% CI [1.06–3.34]) more likely to vaccinate their children fully than when decisions were made by the husbands alone. Further, mothers who made healthcare decisions themselves were 4.03 (AOR 95% CI [1.66–9.78]) times more likely to fully vaccinate their children than when decisions were made by husbands alone [49]. Similar results were reported in Bangladesh, where women with more autonomy in healthcare decisions were more likely to have children who were fully vaccinated (86.1%) than those without autonomy (78.8%) (95% CI 1.079–2.317) [51]. Another study in South Africa found that children whose parents were both involved in shared decision making were less likely to have missed opportunities for vaccination than those whose immunization decision-making was not shared (OR = 0.21, 95% CI: 0.07–0.62) [52].

Other decision makers play important roles as well, sometimes interacting or compounding. For example, mothers-in-law were found to have an important influencing effect (n = 4) in Guinea, India, Nigeria, and Uganda [35,36,38,40]. One study in Nigeria explored the nuance of these interactions and noted that men were strongly influenced by their mothers and women valued the direction of fathers-in-law and elders in the community [40]. Dhaliwal et al. described how mothers-in-law use their positions as matriarch to motivate daughters-in-law to vaccinate their children; health workers then leverage this influence when making home visits [35]. Grandparents played a key role in supporting

HPV immunization in South Africa [54] and influencing mothers and fathers for childhood immunization in the Philippines [44] and in Timor-Leste [55]. Both studies in South Asia noted that mothers may play a subsidiary role to maternal and paternal grandparents in decision-making which makes their support critical for childhood immunization [44,55].

Some women who opposed their husbands' decision not to immunize their children faced **intimate partner violence** including emotional, verbal, and physical violence. While this was experienced by a minority of women in one study in Uganda, all female participants reported that they had witnessed or heard about this happening. Adolescent girls and female survivors of IPV sexual violence in Nigeria were found to have higher odds to be vaccine hesitant compared to those who did not face violence [87]. One study in South Africa also reported that child abuse was a problem in their community and women wanted the HPV vaccine for their daughters to reduce the chance of exposure to HPV if they were forced to have unprotected sex [54].

Gendered myths and misconceptions were also identified as barriers to immunization. Some caregivers and healthcare workers feared that different vaccinations might cause infertility for both boys and girls (n = 7). This emerged for a variety of vaccines including HPV (n = 4), COVID (n = 1), H1N1 (n = 1), and childhood vaccinations (n = 1) [18–20,24,30,60,70]. Another important barrier which emerged specifically for HPV was a concern that the vaccine would increase sexual activity among adolescent girls (n = 7) [18,35,54,58,71–73]. Similar concerns were not expressed about boys.

All studies that measured **empowerment** found a positive association between women's empowerment and immunization coverage (n = 10) [8,9,12,13,38,65,74,88–90]. Empowerment was measured in different ways, usually by combining constructs of decision-making power, enabling resources, independence and agency, and attitudes towards GBV and IPV to generate a score or index. Two studies used the Survey-based Women's emPowERment (SWPER) Global Index to measure the influence of women's empowerment on immunization across 50–52 countries [8,9]. Wendt et al. found that the social independence domain of this index presented more consistent associations with no-DPT than other domains [8]. Johns et al. further explored social independence and found that DTP3 immunization coverage was 12.3 percentage points higher among the children of women with the highest social independence score compared with the children of women with the lowest score [9]. In other studies, multivariate models showed the intersecting role of wealth and socioeconomic status with empowerment. Because financial resources are needed to obtain vaccinations, sometimes empowerment plays a less important role when women lack the financial resources to offset the cost of vaccinating their child [13,88].

Access is the ability or inability to successfully carry out the transaction of vaccine utilization, representing barriers and facilitators between an individual's intent and the health system's readiness.

At the intersection of intent and access is women's **occupational status** and associated norms, roles, and responsibilities. Formally employed women face additional challenges to immunizing their children such as loss of income and **opportunity costs** [25,38] and **competing priorities** or demands on their time [18,40,55,61]. Women across geographies and regardless of occupation status experienced gendered expectations of their labor resulting in increased household and caregiving demands, thus decreasing time for immunizations [23,25,40,41,55,60,62,74–76]. Seven studies identified a lack of male engagement in the household and in caregiving as a barrier [21,35,43,44,54,62,75] and four additional studies recommended male engagement as an important strategy given their decision-making power [19,20,63,91].

The **timing of/schedule and distance** to services can exacerbate this challenge. Distance to facilities was reported as a key barrier to immunizations services in 12 studies [17,25,28,36,61,66,67,74,78–81]. This effect was made worse for low-income women who were socially isolated [25]. Safety and security were additional concerns documented by five studies which affected women's ability to travel and/or travel without accompaniment [25,36,57,64,92].

Studies reported barriers associated with **direct costs** including the cost of the vaccine [19,23,64,76,80,82,83], transportation costs to access services [19,25,29,36,58,61,68,70], and illicit fees for services or the need to pay health workers [25,36]. One woman in Malaysia reflected, "What's the point of taking my children to a clinic to be vaccinated if I do not have money?" [28]. Seven studies also reported that women did not have decision-making power over financial resources, relying on their husbands to provide the funds and/or approve the use of funds which negatively influenced immunization [15,25,34,38,61,79,84]. Three studies found that women having their own income and discretion about spending it or joint decision-making on earning had increased odds of the children being fully immunized [16,67,74].

Readiness encompasses the health system's supply of vaccine services to adequately meet demand. This includes immunization supplies, human resources, and related systems and structures.

The **vaccinators** themselves, their characteristics, availability, and level of training were all important influences on immunization. One study documented a preference for more experienced health workers, which in this setting, translated to male health workers [60]. Men in the Philippines also preferred to receive the HPV vaccine from male providers, particularly physicians (not nurses) [76]. Alternatively, other studies noted that a lack of female vaccinators leads to increases in coverage inequities [10,57]. In some settings, women cannot be in contact with men who are not related to them [43,57]. Men have also expressed preferences that their daughters and wives be vaccinated by females [33,85]. In India, one study showed that districts with 50% or more Lady Medical Officers compared to those with 50% or less showed improved full immunization of children 12–23 months old (69.7% vs. 63.7%, $p = 0.02$) [85]. Many female health workers, however, face barriers to providing immunization services including feeling unsafe and being harassed by caregivers [35,57,86] and low and late remuneration [57].

The gender sensitivity of **facility** structures was also a barrier. This included lack of privacy [33], lack of gender-segregated facilities, and reduced access for transgender individuals [64]. Excessive wait times were also reported in six studies, resulting in children not receiving immunizations and/or caregivers not willing to return [25,36,60,63,66,74]. This intersects with women's competing demands for time and availability to wait for services.

Studies described the effect of women's prior **experiences with the healthcare system**, both positive and negative, as influencing vaccination coverage. Some women reported experiencing feelings of shame if they missed a prior appointment, forgot the child's vaccine card, or if their children appeared malnourished or dirty [55,60–63]. Poor mothers in Uganda reported being bullied by other women and health workers; in the same setting, a women described a stigma against teenage motherhood which prevented young mothers from seeking care [38]. A study in DRC, Mozambique, and Nigeria found that caregivers who experienced disrespect in the health system were the least likely to return [25]. Members of the transgender community in Pakistan reported harassment and discrimination at COVID-19 vaccination centers which made it difficult for them to receive services during the pandemic [64].

Antenatal care (ANC) attendance/use emerged as an important positive predictor of immunization. This was most consistently reported in Ethiopia (n = 5) [16,66–69] where studies found that children of mothers who attended ANC were more likely to be immunized than those of mothers who did not. This was also reported in Senegal [27], Afghanistan [50], and Nepal, where children of mothers who used antenatal care were 3.31 times as likely to have received all eight vaccinations, 3.87 times as likely to have received all doses of DPT, 3.80 times as likely to have received polio vaccines, and 3.45 times as likely to have received measles vaccine [65].

Further, while few studies assessed supply-side issues, a few (n = 8) mentioned that the availability of vaccines could be an important barrier [20,36,60–63,72,74]. Schwarz et al. noted that the unavailability of vaccines leads to pessimism and future nonadherence [61]. Kagone described the harmful nature of restrictive vial opening policies which discourage health workers from opening multi-dose vials to avoid wastage; this results in delayed vaccination and increased frustration among caregivers [60]. And in one study, a respondent said, "we have become tired of this, which is why we don't bother going there anymore" [74]. Two studies that explored availability of HPV vaccines indicated that supply could be a concern (based on prior experiences) and therefore programs and policies should prioritize only vaccinating girls and not girls and boys [20,72].

Only one study measured outcomes at the leadership level, assessing the impact of women's political representation on child health outcomes using a dataset covering 162 countries over 30 years [93]. This study found a significant positive effect of women's political representation on measles and DPT vaccination coverage particularly in East Asia and the Pacific, Latin America and the Caribbean, the Middle East and North Africa, South Asia, and Sub-Saharan Africa. The authors found that immunization rates are rising faster in countries with gender quota implementation.

4. Discussion

This review has documented a range of gender barriers to immunization, many of which are interdependent and found across geographies. What can we learn from this evidence? First, we learn that some of the most important reasons that women do not bring their children to get vaccinated lie outside of the usual purview of immunization programming. Household decision-making, for example, which is deeply entwined with social norms governing the appropriate roles for men and women within families, is often perceived as being far outside of the scope of the health system. Similarly, the fact that women often face multiple competing demands on their time is not easily addressed by immunization-focused interventions.

However, some of the gender barriers identified in the research are amenable to being addressed with adaptations to existing vaccination programming. For example, training providers on respectful patient treatment could improve women's experiences with the healthcare system, influencing their likelihood to return for immunization services. Women's engagement with ANC emerged as an important predictor of immunization, indicating that strengthened ANC services could help improve maternal and child immunization coverage [94]. Meeting people where they are to enhance access could include constructing more facilities or satellite clinics, providing mobile options, or conducting home visits to particularly marginalized and hesitant groups [95]. A study conducted in the urban slums of Dhaka, Bangladesh, found that extending vaccination service hours increased childhood immunization among children of employed women who could not previously attend the service window [96].

Our review found that while women are largely responsible for health care seeking, men play a critical role through their decision-making power and control of resources. This is also true for community elders and religious leaders who are able to influence men in their communities. These relationships are complex and different family members hold varying degrees of power depending on the context. But men and other family members can be better engaged throughout the immunization process to relieve the caregiving burden that women tend to manage. Equimundo recently launched their State of the World's Fathers 2023 Report which highlights data from 17 countries showing that while fathers feel equally responsible for care work, mothers overall are still doing the majority of caregiving (3 to 7 times as much as men) [97]. But men who say they take care of their emotional selves are two to eight times more likely to care for another family member than those who do not. Given the overwhelming emotional and physical labor that women face, programs that seek to engage men, in the community and/or in places of employment, could focus on self-care and family care.

There is also abundant evidence that offering caregivers, especially those living in poverty, compensation for the direct and opportunity costs of immunization is a highly effective way of putting financial resources into the hands of women, which can enhance their economic independence and be used to vaccinate children [98–100]. This review documented numerous financial barriers to immunization including transportation, costs of the vaccines, giving up paid labor to attend clinics, and even the shame of appearing poor. Putting cash into women's hands could directly ameliorate many of these gender barriers. That said, enhanced demand for immunization services must be met by supply. This review attempted to identify barriers across the immunization value chain, including on the supply side, but very few gender barriers were documented further up the chain. Only one study assessed the impact of women's representation in leadership positions on health, including immunization [93]. However, evidence on the impact of women's leadership on improving health outcomes is growing [101] and this could have positive implications for immunization programming, prioritization, and health systems changes.

4.1. Areas of Future Research

This review highlights important areas for future research on the influence of gender on global partnerships, vaccine procurement, country-led delivery, supply chains, and national vaccine markets. There is a dearth of research that can establish a causal relationship between gender barriers and vaccine outcomes. Intervention research, which seeks to evaluate interventions targeting specific gender barriers to immunization, could help address this gap, and provide much needed data on what works.

4.2. Strengths and Limitations

Most studies included in this review were qualitative or utilized secondary data, specifically DHS, to generate associations. It is therefore difficult to establish which, if any, gender barriers cause changes in immunization coverage. We only included articles that used an explicit gender lens in their data collection and analysis, beyond sex disaggregation, and may have missed articles that presented gender barriers. However, given the depth and breadth of articles included, and the consistency of findings among these articles, it is unlikely that additional articles would have yielded unique insights. This work was funded by the Bill and Melinda Gates Foundation Immunization Team whose portfolio focuses on select antigens, largely focusing on routine childhood vaccines. Search terms designed to meet the needs of this project may have missed vaccines outside this scope but with documented gender barriers.

4.3. Conclusions

This review definitively establishes that gender barriers are highly relevant in many socioeconomic contexts across LMICs. We also know that these gender barriers intersect with other widely known barriers. But women's lack of agency over the decision to vaccinate and the ability to pay the costs to vaccinate seem to be the most common, possibly most important, factors affecting coverage. We can only know how important these barriers are with more research that measures the impact of programming on gender barriers to immunization coverage. Failing to learn about and address gender barriers to immunization is detrimental to public health programs and policies because without the generation, analysis, and synthesis of gender data, coverage will not change.

Supplementary Materials: The following supporting information can be downloaded at: https://www.mdpi.com/article/10.3390/vaccines12060625/s1.

Author Contributions: All authors contributed to the review design, led by A.K. A.K. conducted the search and led the text reviews, extraction, and analysis with support from others. A.K. led the draft of this manuscript with substantial input from E.K. and N.B., particularly on the background, interpretation, and discussion. All authors reviewed the final manuscript. All authors have read and agreed to the published version of the manuscript.

Funding: This work was supported, in whole or in part, by the Bill and Melinda Gates Foundation INV-043797. Under the grant conditions of the Foundation, a Creative Commons Attribution 4.0 Generic License has already been assigned to the Author Accepted Manuscript version that might arise from this submission. The findings and conclusions contained within are those of the authors and do not necessarily reflect positions or policies of the Bill and Melinda Gates Foundation.

Acknowledgments: The work was commissioned by the Immunization Team of the Bill and Melinda Gates Foundation. We would like to thank Judy Rein, Shelby Bourgault, and Jenny Acton, members of the Global Center for Gender Equality (GCfGE) team who supported the research. GCfGE internal review was also completed by Abigail Donner and Angela Hartley. Whitney Walton provided program management support.

Conflicts of Interest: The authors declare no competing interests.

References

1. Restrepo-Méndez, M.C.; Barros, A.J.; Wong, K.L.; Johnson, H.L.; Pariyo, G.; França, G.V.; Wehrmeister, F.C.; Victora, C.G. Inequalities in full immunization coverage: Trends in low- and middle-income countries. *Bull. World Health Organ.* **2016**, *94*, 794–805B. [CrossRef] [PubMed]
2. Nambiar, D.; Hosseinpoor, A.R.; Bergen, N.; Danovaro-Holliday, M.C.; Wallace, A.; Johnson, H.L. Inequality in immunization: Holding on to equity as we "catch up". *Vaccines* **2023**, *11*, 913. [CrossRef] [PubMed]
3. Feletto, M.; Sharkey, A.; Rowley, E.; Gurley, N.; Sinha, A. *A Gender Lens to Advance Equity in Immunization*; ERG Discussion Paper 05; Equity Reference Group for Immunisation: New York, NY, USA, 2018.
4. Feletto, M.; Sharkey, A. The influence of gender on immunisation: Using an ecological framework to examine intersecting inequities and pathways to change. *BMJ Glob. Health* **2019**, *4*, e001711. [CrossRef] [PubMed]
5. Idris, I.B.; Hamis, A.A.; Bukhori, A.B.M.; Hoong, D.C.C.; Yusop, H.; Shaharuddin, M.A.-A.; Fauzi, N.A.F.A.; Kandayah, T. Women's autonomy in healthcare decision making: A systematic review. *BMC Womens Health* **2023**, *23*, 643. [CrossRef] [PubMed]
6. Why Gender Matters: Immunization Agenda 2030 [Internet]. Available online: https://www.who.int/publications/i/item/9789240033948 (accessed on 17 January 2024).
7. Phillips, D.E.; Dieleman, J.L.; Lim, S.S.; Shearer, J. Determinants of effective vaccine coverage in low and middle-income countries: A systematic review and interpretive synthesis. *BMC Health Serv. Res.* **2017**, *17*, 681. [CrossRef] [PubMed]
8. Wendt, A.; Santos, T.M.; Cata-Preta, B.O.; Costa, J.C.; Mengistu, T.; Hogan, D.R.; Victora, C.G.; Barros, A.J.D. Children of more empowered women are less likely to be left without vaccination in low- and middle-income countries: A global analysis of 50 DHS surveys. *J. Glob. Health* **2022**, *12*, 04022. [CrossRef] [PubMed]
9. Johns, N.E.; Santos, T.M.; Arroyave, L.; Cata-Preta, B.O.; Heidari, S.; Kirkby, K.; Munro, J.; Schlotheuber, A.; Wendt, A.; O'Brien, K.; et al. Gender-Related Inequality in Childhood Immunization Coverage: A Cross-Sectional Analysis of DTP3 Coverage and Zero-Dose DTP Prevalence in 52 Countries Using the SWPER Global Index. *Vaccines* **2022**, *10*, 988. [CrossRef] [PubMed]
10. Siddiqi, D.A.; Iftikhar, S.; Siddique, M.; Mehmood, M.; Dharma, V.K.; Shah, M.T.; Setayesh, H.; Chandir, S. Immunization Gender Inequity in Pakistan: An Analysis of 6.2 Million Children Born from 2019 to 2022 and Enrolled in the Sindh Electronic Immunization Registry. *Vaccines* **2023**, *11*, 685. [CrossRef] [PubMed]
11. Vidal Fuertes, C.; Johns, N.E.; Goodman, T.S.; Heidari, S.; Munro, J.; Hosseinpoor, A.R. The Association between Childhood Immunization and Gender Inequality: A Multi-Country Ecological Analysis of Zero-Dose DTP Prevalence and DTP3 Immunization Coverage. *Vaccines* **2022**, *10*, 1032. [CrossRef] [PubMed]
12. Seidu, A.-A.; Ahinkorah, B.O.; Ameyaw, E.K.; Budu, E.; Yaya, S. Women empowerment indicators and uptake of child health services in sub-Saharan Africa: A multilevel analysis using cross-sectional data from 26 countries. *J. Public Health* **2022**, *44*, 740–752. [CrossRef]
13. Porth, J.M.; Wagner, A.L.; Moyer, C.A.; Mutua, M.K.; Boulton, M.L. Women's empowerment and child vaccination in kenya: The modifying role of wealth. *Am. J. Prev. Med.* **2021**, *60* (Suppl. 1), S87–S97. [CrossRef] [PubMed]
14. Muzzamil, M.; Nisa, M.; Raza, S. The survival rate of neonates in Pakistan: Problems in health care access, quality and recommendations. *Health Promot. Perspect.* **2022**, *12*, 355–357. [CrossRef] [PubMed]
15. Malhotra, C.; Malhotra, R.; Østbye, T.; Subramanian, S.V. Maternal autonomy and child health care utilization in India: Results from the National Family Health Survey. *Asia Pac. J. Public Health* **2014**, *26*, 401–413. [CrossRef] [PubMed]
16. Ebot, J.O. "Girl Power!": The Relationship between Women's Autonomy and Children's Immunization Coverage in Ethiopia. *J. Health Popul. Nutr.* **2015**, *33*, 18. [CrossRef] [PubMed]
17. Adeyanju, G.C.; Sprengholz, P.; Betsch, C.; Essoh, T.-A. Caregivers' Willingness to Vaccinate Their Children against Childhood Diseases and Human Papillomavirus: A Cross-Sectional Study on Vaccine Hesitancy in Malawi. *Vaccines* **2021**, *9*, 1231. [CrossRef] [PubMed]
18. Adeyanju, G.C.; Betsch, C.; Adamu, A.A.; Gumbi, K.S.; Head, M.G.; Aplogan, A.; Tall, H.; Essoh, T.A. Examining enablers of vaccine hesitancy toward routine childhood and adolescent vaccination in Malawi. *Glob. Health Res. Policy* **2022**, *7*, 28. [CrossRef] [PubMed]
19. Venturas, C.; Umeh, K. Health professional feedback on HPV vaccination roll-out in a developing country. *Vaccine* **2017**, *35*, 1886–1891. [CrossRef] [PubMed]

20. Remes, P.; Selestine, V.; Changalucha, J.; Ross, D.A.; Wight, D.; de Sanjosé, S.; Kapiga, S.; Hayes, R.J.; Watson-Jones, D. A qualitative study of HPV vaccine acceptability among health workers, teachers, parents, female pupils, and religious leaders in northwest Tanzania. *Vaccine* **2012**, *30*, 5363–5367. [CrossRef] [PubMed]
21. Malande, O.O.; Munube, D.; Afaayo, R.N.; Annet, K.; Bodo, B.; Bakainaga, A.; Ayebare, E.; Njunwamukama, S.; Mworozi, E.A.; Musyoki, A.M. Barriers to effective uptake and provision of immunization in a rural district in Uganda. *PLoS ONE* **2019**, *14*, e0212270. [CrossRef]
22. Yamanis, T.; Carlitz, R.; Gonyea, O.; Skaff, S.; Kisanga, N.; Mollel, H. Confronting "chaos": A qualitative study assessing public health officials' perceptions of the factors affecting Tanzania's COVID-19 vaccine rollout. *BMJ Open* **2023**, *13*, e065081. [CrossRef]
23. Wong, L.P.; Alias, H.; Seheli, F.N.; Zimet, G.D.; Hu, Z.; Lin, Y. Human papillomavirus (HPV) vaccination intent and its associated factors: A study of ethnically diverse married women aged 27 to 45 in Malaysia, a Southeast Asian country. *Hum. Vaccin. Immunother.* **2022**, *18*, 2076525. [CrossRef] [PubMed]
24. Vermandere, H.; Naanyu, V.; Mabeya, H.; Vanden Broeck, D.; Michielsen, K.; Degomme, O. Determinants of acceptance and subsequent uptake of the HPV vaccine in a cohort in Eldoret, Kenya. *PLoS ONE* **2014**, *9*, e109353. [CrossRef] [PubMed]
25. Shearer, J.C.; Nava, O.; Prosser, W.; Nawaz, S.; Mulongo, S.; Mambu, T.; Mafuta, E.; Munguambe, K.; Sigauque, B.; Cherima, Y.J.; et al. Uncovering the Drivers of Childhood Immunization Inequality with Caregivers, Community Members and Health System Stakeholders: Results from a Human-Centered Design Study in DRC, Mozambique and Nigeria. *Vaccines* **2023**, *11*, 689. [CrossRef] [PubMed]
26. Shafiq, Y.; Khowaja, A.R.; Yousafzai, M.T.; Ali, S.A.; Zaidi, A.; Saleem, A.F. Knowledge, attitudes and practices related to tetanus toxoid vaccination in women of childbearing age: A cross-sectional study in peri-urban settlements of Karachi, Pakistan. *J. Infect. Prev.* **2017**, *18*, 232–241. [CrossRef] [PubMed]
27. Sarker, A.R.; Akram, R.; Ali, N.; Chowdhury, Z.I.; Sultana, M. Coverage and Determinants of Full Immunization: Vaccination Coverage among Senegalese Children. *Medicina* **2019**, *55*, 480. [CrossRef] [PubMed]
28. Salleh, H.; Avoi, R.; Abdul Karim, H.; Osman, S.; Dhanaraj, P.; Ab Rahman, M.A.I. A Behavioural-Theory-Based Qualitative Study of the Beliefs and Perceptions of Marginalised Populations towards Community Volunteering to Increase Measles Immunisation Coverage in Sabah, Malaysia. *Vaccines* **2023**, *11*, 1056. [CrossRef] [PubMed]
29. Monguno, A.K. Socio cultural and geographical determinants of child immunisation in borno state, nigeria. *J. Public Health Afr.* **2013**, *4*, e10. [CrossRef] [PubMed]
30. Lohiniva, A.-L.; Barakat, A.; Dueger, E.; Restrepo, S.; El Aouad, R. A qualitative study of vaccine acceptability and decision making among pregnant women in Morocco during the A (H1N1) pdm09 pandemic. *PLoS ONE* **2014**, *9*, e96244. [CrossRef] [PubMed]
31. Limaye, R.J.; Sara, A.B.; Siddique, A.R.; Vivas, C.; Malik, S.; Omonoju, K. Interpersonal and community influences affecting childhood vaccination decision-making among Nigerian caregivers: Perceptions among frontline workers in Nigeria. *J. Child. Health Care* **2019**, *23*, 403–414. [CrossRef]
32. Khan, M.D. Toward creating equity in access to COVID-19 vaccination for female population in Multan, Punjab, Pakistan. *Health Care Women Int.* **2021**, 1–10. [CrossRef]
33. Jalloh, M.F.; Bennett, S.D.; Alam, D.; Kouta, P.; Lourenço, D.; Alamgir, M.; Feldstein, L.R.; Ehlman, D.C.; Abad, N.; Kapil, N.; et al. Rapid behavioral assessment of barriers and opportunities to improve vaccination coverage among displaced Rohingyas in Bangladesh, January 2018. *Vaccine* **2019**, *37*, 833–838. [CrossRef] [PubMed]
34. Etokidem, A.; Nkpoyen, F.; Ekanem, C.; Mpama, E.; Isika, A. Potential barriers to and facilitators of civil society organization engagement in increasing immunization coverage in Odukpani Local Government Area of Cross River State, Nigeria: An implementation research. *Health Res. Policy Syst.* **2021**, *19* (Suppl. 2), 46. [CrossRef] [PubMed]
35. Dhaliwal, B.K.; Chandrashekhar, R.; Rattani, A.; Seth, R.; Closser, S.; Jain, A.; Bloom, D.E.; Shet, A. Community perceptions of vaccination among influential stakeholders: Qualitative research in rural India. *BMC Public Health* **2021**, *21*, 2122. [CrossRef] [PubMed]
36. Bell, J.; Lartey, B.; Spickernell, G.; Darrell, N.; Salt, F.; Gardner, C.; Richards, E.; Fasakin, L.; Egbeniyi, S.; Odongo, E.; et al. Applying a social-ecological model to understand factors impacting demand for childhood vaccinations in Nigeria, Uganda, and Guinea. *SSM Qual. Res. Health* **2022**, *2*, 100180. [CrossRef] [PubMed]
37. Bell, J.; Lartey, B.; Fernandez, M.; Darrell, N.; Exton-Smith, H.; Gardner, C.; Richards, E.; Akilo, A.; Odongo, E.; Ssenkungu, J.; et al. A structural equation modelling approach to understanding the determinants of childhood vaccination in Nigeria, Uganda and Guinea. *PLOS Glob. Public Health* **2023**, *3*, e0001289. [CrossRef] [PubMed]
38. Babirye, J.N.; Rutebemberwa, E.; Kiguli, J.; Wamani, H.; Nuwaha, F.; Engebretsen, I.M. More support for mothers: A qualitative study on factors affecting immunisation behaviour in Kampala, Uganda. *BMC Public Health* **2011**, *11*, 723. [CrossRef] [PubMed]
39. Ali, R.F.; Arif Siddiqi, D.; Mirza, A.; Naz, N.; Abdullah, S.; Kembhavi, G.; Tam, C.C.; Offeddu, V.; Chandir, S. Adolescent girls' recommendations for the design of a human papillomavirus vaccination program in Sindh, Pakistan: A qualitative study. *Hum. Vaccin. Immunother.* **2022**, *18*, 2045856. [CrossRef] [PubMed]
40. Akwataghibe, N.N.; Ogunsola, E.A.; Broerse, J.E.W.; Popoola, O.A.; Agbo, A.I.; Dieleman, M.A. Exploring Factors Influencing Immunization Utilization in Nigeria-A Mixed Methods Study. *Front. Public Health* **2019**, *7*, 392. [CrossRef] [PubMed]

41. Ahmed, K.A.; Grundy, J.; Hashmat, L.; Ahmed, I.; Farrukh, S.; Bersonda, D.; Shah, M.A.; Yunus, S.; Banskota, H.K. An analysis of the gender and social determinants of health in urban poor areas of the most populated cities of Pakistan. *Int. J. Equity Health* **2022**, *21*, 52. [CrossRef]
42. Abad, N.; Uba, B.V.; Patel, P.; Barau, D.N.; Ugochukwu, O.; Aliyu, N.; Ayanleke, H.B.; Franka, R.; Waziri, N.E.; Bolu, O. A rapid qualitative assessment of barriers associated with demand and uptake of health facility-based childhood immunizations and recommendations to improve immunization service delivery in Sokoto State, Northwest Nigeria, 2017. *Pan Afr. Med. J.* **2021**, *40* (Suppl. 1), 10.
43. Abdullahi, M.F.; Stewart Williams, J.; Sahlèn, K.-G.; Bile, K.; Kinsman, J. Factors contributing to the uptake of childhood vaccination in Galkayo District, Puntland, Somalia. *Glob. Health Action.* **2020**, *13*, 1803543. [CrossRef]
44. Wachinger, J.; Reñosa, M.D.C.; Endoma, V.; Aligato, M.F.; Landicho-Guevarra, J.; Landicho, J.; Bravo, T.A.; McMahon, S.A. Bargaining and gendered authority: A framework to understand household decision-making about childhood vaccines in the Philippines. *BMJ Glob. Health* **2022**, *7*, e009781. [CrossRef]
45. Siddiqui, M.; Khan, A.A.; Varan, A.K.; Esteves-Jaramillo, A.; Sultana, S.; Ali, A.S.; Zaidi, A.K.M. Intention to accept pertussis vaccine among pregnant women in Karachi, Pakistan. *Vaccine* **2017**, *35*, 5352–5359. [CrossRef]
46. Babalola, S. Determinants of the uptake of the full dose of diphtheria-pertussis-tetanus vaccines (DPT3) in Northern Nigeria: A multilevel analysis. *Matern. Child Health J.* **2009**, *13*, 550–558. [CrossRef] [PubMed]
47. Antai, D. Gender inequities, relationship power, and childhood immunization uptake in Nigeria: A population-based cross-sectional study. *Int. J. Infect. Dis.* **2012**, *16*, e136–e145. [CrossRef]
48. Singh, K.; Haney, E.; Olorunsaiye, C. Maternal autonomy and attitudes towards gender norms: Associations with childhood immunization in Nigeria. *Matern. Child Health J.* **2013**, *17*, 837–841. [CrossRef]
49. Darebo, T.D.; Oshe, B.B.; Diro, C.W. Full vaccination coverage and associated factors among children aged 12 to 23 months in remote rural area of Demba Gofa District, Southern Ethiopia. *PeerJ* **2022**, *10*, e13081. [CrossRef] [PubMed]
50. Shenton, L.M.; Wagner, A.L.; Carlson, B.F.; Mubarak, M.Y.; Boulton, M.L. Vaccination status of children aged 1–4 years in Afghanistan and associated factors, 2015. *Vaccine* **2018**, *36*, 5141–5149. [CrossRef] [PubMed]
51. Boulton, M.L.; Carlson, B.F.; Power, L.E.; Wagner, A.L. Socioeconomic factors associated with full childhood vaccination in Bangladesh, 2014. *Int. J. Infect. Dis.* **2018**, *69*, 35–40. [CrossRef]
52. Nnaji, C.A.; Wiysonge, C.S.; Adamu, A.A.; Lesosky, M.; Mahomed, H.; Ndwandwe, D. Missed Opportunities for Vaccination and Associated Factors among Children Attending Primary Health Care Facilities in Cape Town, South Africa: A Pre-Intervention Multilevel Analysis. *Vaccines* **2022**, *10*, 785. [CrossRef]
53. Limaye, R.J.; Singh, P.; Paul, A.; Fesshaye, B.; Lee, C.; Zavala, E.; Wade, S.; Ali, H.; Rahman, H.; Akter, S.; et al. COVID-19 vaccine decision-making among pregnant and lactating women in Bangladesh. *Vaccine* **2023**, *41*, 3885–3890. [CrossRef]
54. Francis, S.A.; Katz, M.L. The HPV vaccine: A comparison of focus groups conducted in South Africa and Ohio Appalachia. *Matern. Child Health J.* **2013**, *17*, 1222–1229. [CrossRef]
55. Amin, R.; De Oliveira, T.J.C.R.; Da Cunha, M.; Brown, T.W.; Favin, M.; Cappelier, K. Factors limiting immunization coverage in urban Dili, Timor-Leste. *Glob. Health Sci. Pract.* **2013**, *1*, 417–427. [CrossRef]
56. Ariyo, T.; Jiang, Q. Mothers' Healthcare Autonomy, Maternal-Health Utilization and Healthcare for Children under-3 Years: Analysis of the Nigeria DHS Data (2008–2018). *Int. J. Environ. Res. Public Health* **2020**, *17*, 1816. [CrossRef]
57. Kalbarczyk, A.; Rao, A.; Adebayo, A.; Decker, E.; Gerber, S.; Morgan, R. The influence of gender dynamics on polio eradication efforts at the community, workplace, and organizational level. *Glob. Health Res. Policy* **2021**, *6*, 19. [CrossRef]
58. Crann, S.E.; Barata, P.C.; Mitchell, R.; Mawhinney, L.; Thistle, P.; Chirenje, Z.M.; Stewart, D.E. Healthcare providers' perspectives on the acceptability and uptake of HPV vaccines in Zimbabwe. *J. Psychosom. Obs. Gynaecol.* **2016**, *37*, 147–155. [CrossRef]
59. Ambe, J. Perceptions, beliefs and practices of mothers in sub-urban and rural areas towards measles and measles vaccination in Northern Nigeria. *Trop. Dr.* **2001**, *31*, 89–90. [CrossRef]
60. Kagoné, M.; Yé, M.; Nébié, E.; Sié, A.; Müller, O.; Beiersmann, C. Community perception regarding childhood vaccinations and its implications for effectiveness: A qualitative study in rural Burkina Faso. *BMC Public Health* **2018**, *18*, 324. [CrossRef]
61. Schwarz, N.G.; Gysels, M.; Pell, C.; Gabor, J.; Schlie, M.; Issifou, S.; Lell, B.; Kremsner, P.G.; Grobusch, M.P.; Pool, R. Reasons for non-adherence to vaccination at mother and child care clinics (MCCs) in Lambaréné, Gabon. *Vaccine* **2009**, *27*, 5371–5375. [CrossRef] [PubMed]
62. Zewdie, A.; Letebo, M.; Mekonnen, T. Reasons for defaulting from childhood immunization program: A qualitative study from Hadiya zone, Southern Ethiopia. *BMC Public Health* **2016**, *16*, 1240. [CrossRef] [PubMed]
63. Kajungu, D.; Muhoozi, M.; Stark, J.; Weibel, D.; Sturkenboom, M.C.J.M. Vaccines safety and maternal knowledge for enhanced maternal immunization acceptability in rural Uganda: A qualitative study approach. *PLoS ONE* **2020**, *15*, e0243834. [CrossRef] [PubMed]
64. Khan, M.D. Access to COVID-19 vaccination for transgender community in Multan, Punjab, Pakistan. *Health Care Women Int.* **2023**, *44*, 824–837. [CrossRef] [PubMed]
65. Pandey, S.; Lee, H.N. Determinants of child immunization in Nepal: The role of women's empowerment. *Health Educ. J.* **2012**, *71*, 642–653. [CrossRef]
66. Tefera, Y.A.; Wagner, A.L.; Mekonen, E.B.; Carlson, B.F.; Boulton, M.L. Predictors and Barriers to Full Vaccination among Children in Ethiopia. *Vaccines* **2018**, *6*, 22. [CrossRef] [PubMed]

67. Wado, Y.D.; Afework, M.F.; Hindin, M.J. Childhood vaccination in rural southwestern Ethiopia: The nexus with demographic factors and women's autonomy. *Pan Afr. Med. J.* **2014**, *17* (Suppl. 1), 9. [CrossRef] [PubMed]
68. Dheresa, M.; Dessie, Y.; Negash, B.; Balis, B.; Getachew, T.; Mamo Ayana, G.; Merga, B.T.; Regassa, L.D. Child vaccination coverage, trends and predictors in eastern ethiopia: Implication for sustainable development goals. *J. Multidiscip. Healthc.* **2021**, *14*, 2657–2667. [CrossRef] [PubMed]
69. Legesse, E.; Dechasa, W. An assessment of child immunization coverage and its determinants in Sinana District, Southeast Ethiopia. *BMC Pediatr.* **2015**, *15*, 31. [CrossRef] [PubMed]
70. Limaye, R.J.; Paul, A.; Gur-Arie, R.; Zavala, E.; Lee, C.; Fesshaye, B.; Singh, P.; Njagi, W.; Odila, P.; Munyao, P.; et al. A socio-ecological exploration to identify factors influencing the COVID-19 vaccine decision-making process among pregnant and lactating women: Findings from Kenya. *Vaccine* **2022**, *40*, 7305–7311. [CrossRef] [PubMed]
71. Shitu, B.F.; Atnafu, D.D.; Agumas, Y. Public school adolescents had increased odds of being willing to uptake HPV vaccinations owing to sociodemographic and healthcare access features in bahir dar city, ethiopia. *Biomed. Res. Int.* **2023**, *2023*, 2663815. [CrossRef]
72. Kelly-Hanku, A.; Newland, J.; Aggleton, P.; Ase, S.; Aeno, H.; Fiya, V.; Vallely, L.M.; Toliman, P.J.; Mola, G.D.; Kaldor, J.M.; et al. HPV vaccination in Papua New Guinea to prevent cervical cancer in women: Gender, sexual morality, outsiders and the de-feminization of the HPV vaccine. *Papillomavirus Res.* **2019**, *8*, 100171. [CrossRef]
73. Coleman, M.A.; Levison, J.; Sangi-Haghpeykar, H. HPV vaccine acceptability in Ghana, West Africa. *Vaccine* **2011**, *29*, 3945–3950. [CrossRef]
74. Cockcroft, A.; Usman, M.U.; Nyamucherera, O.F.; Emori, H.; Duke, B.; Umar, N.A.; Andersson, N. Why children are not vaccinated against measles: A cross-sectional study in two Nigerian States. *Arch. Public Health* **2014**, *72*, 48. [CrossRef]
75. Kulkarni, S.; Ishizumi, A.; Eleeza, O.; Patel, P.; Feika, M.; Kamara, S.; Bangura, J.; Jalloh, U.; Koroma, M.; Sankoh, Z.; et al. Using photovoice methodology to uncover individual-level, health systems, and contextual barriers to uptake of second dose of measles containing vaccine in Western Area Urban, Sierra Leone, 2020. *Vaccine* **2023**, *14*, 100338. [CrossRef]
76. Young, A.M.; Crosby, R.A.; Jagger, K.S.; Casquejo, E.; Pinote, L.; Ybañez, P.; Casquejo, L.; Estorgio, D.; Pinote, L. Influences on HPV vaccine acceptance among men in the Philippines. *J. Men's Health* **2011**, *8*, 126–135. [CrossRef]
77. Babirye, J.N.; Engebretsen, I.M.S.; Makumbi, F.; Fadnes, L.T.; Wamani, H.; Tylleskar, T.; Nuwaha, F. Timeliness of childhood vaccinations in Kampala Uganda: A community-based cross-sectional study. *PLoS ONE* **2012**, *7*, e35432. [CrossRef] [PubMed]
78. Ports, K.A.; Reddy, D.M.; Rameshbabu, A. Barriers and facilitators to HPV vaccination: Perspectives from Malawian women. *Women Health* **2013**, *53*, 630–645. [CrossRef] [PubMed]
79. Oluwadare, C. The social determinants of routine immunisation in ekiti state of nigeria. *Stud. Ethno-Med.* **2009**, *3*, 49–56. [CrossRef]
80. Francis, S.A.; Battle-Fisher, M.; Liverpool, J.; Hipple, L.; Mosavel, M.; Soogun, S.; Mofammere, N.A. A qualitative analysis of South African women's knowledge, attitudes, and beliefs about HPV and cervical cancer prevention, vaccine awareness and acceptance, and maternal-child communication about sexual Health. *Vaccine* **2011**, *29*, 8760–8765. [CrossRef] [PubMed]
81. Hanifi, S.M.A.; Ravn, H.; Aaby, P.; Bhuiya, A. Where girls are less likely to be fully vaccinated than boys: Evidence from a rural area in Bangladesh. *Vaccine* **2018**, *36*, 3323–3330. [CrossRef]
82. Mabeya, H.; Odunga, J.; Broeck, D.V. Mothers of adolescent girls and Human Papilloma Virus (HPV) vaccination in Western Kenya. *Pan Afr. Med. J.* **2021**, *38*, 126. [CrossRef]
83. Krupp, K.; Marlow, L.A.V.; Kielmann, K.; Doddaiah, N.; Mysore, S.; Reingold, A.L.; Madhivanan, P. Factors associated with intention-to-recommend human papillomavirus vaccination among physicians in Mysore, India. *J. Adolesc. Health* **2010**, *46*, 379–384. [CrossRef] [PubMed]
84. Agarwal, S.; Srivastava, A. Social determinants of children's health in urban areas in India. *J. Health Care Poor Underserved.* **2009**, *20* (Suppl. 4), 68–89. [CrossRef] [PubMed]
85. Bhan, N.; McDougal, L.; Singh, A.; Atmavilas, Y.; Raj, A. Access to women physicians and uptake of reproductive, maternal and child health services in India. *EClinicalMedicine* **2020**, *20*, 100309. [CrossRef] [PubMed]
86. Kalbarczyk, A.; Closser, S.; Hirpa, S.; Cintyamena, U.; Azizatunnisa, L.; Agrawal, P.; Rahimi, A.O.; Akinyemi, O.O.; Mafuta, E.M.; Deressa, W.; et al. A light touch intervention with a heavy lift-gender, space and risk in a global vaccination programme. *Glob. Public Health* **2022**, *17*, 4087–4100. [CrossRef]
87. Folayan, M.O.; Arije, O.; Enemo, A.; Sunday, A.; Muhammad, A.; Nyako, H.Y.; Abdullah, R.M.; Okiwu, H.; Lamontagne, E. Associations between COVID-19 vaccine hesitancy and the experience of violence among women and girls living with and at risk of HIV in Nigeria. *Afr. J. AIDS Res.* **2022**, *21*, 306–316. [CrossRef]
88. Wirawan, G.B.S.; Gustina, N.L.Z.; Pramana, P.H.I.; Astiti, M.Y.D.; Jonathan, J.; Melinda, F.; Wijaya, T. Women's Empowerment Facilitates Complete Immunization in Indonesian Children: A Cross-sectional Study. *J. Prev. Med. Public Health* **2022**, *55*, 193–204. [CrossRef] [PubMed]
89. Muzammil, M.; Zafar, S.; Aziz, S.; Usman, M.; Amir-Ud-Din, R. Maternal Correlates of Poliomyelitis Vaccination Uptake: Evidence from Afghanistan, Pakistan, and Nigeria. *Am. J. Trop. Med. Hyg.* **2021**, *105*, 1301–1308. [CrossRef]
90. Khan, M.T.; Zaheer, S.; Shafique, K. Maternal education, empowerment, economic status and child polio vaccination uptake in Pakistan: A population based cross sectional study. *BMJ Open* **2017**, *7*, e013853. [CrossRef]

91. Larson Williams, A.; McCloskey, L.; Mwale, M.; Mwananyanda, L.; Murray, K.; Herman, A.R.; Thea, D.M.; MacLeod, W.B.; Gill, C.J. "When you are injected, the baby is protected:" Assessing the acceptability of a maternal Tdap vaccine based on mothers' knowledge, attitudes, and beliefs of pertussis and vaccinations in Lusaka, Zambia. *Vaccine* **2018**, *36*, 3048–3053. [CrossRef]
92. Watson-Jones, D.; Mugo, N.; Lees, S.; Mathai, M.; Vusha, S.; Ndirangu, G.; Ross, D.A. Access and Attitudes to HPV Vaccination amongst Hard-To-Reach Populations in Kenya. *PLoS ONE* **2015**, *10*, e0123701. [CrossRef]
93. Rustagi, N.; Akter, S. The impact of women's political representation on child health outcomes during 1990–2020: Evidence from a global dataset. *Soc. Sci. Med.* **2022**, *312*, 115366. [CrossRef] [PubMed]
94. Vouking, M.Z.; Tadenfok, C.N.; Ekani, J.M.E. Strategies to increase immunization coverage of tetanus vaccine among women in Sub Saharan Africa: A systematic review. *Pan Afr. Med. J.* **2017**, *27* (Suppl. 3), 25. [CrossRef] [PubMed]
95. Machado, A.A.; Edwards, S.A.; Mueller, M.; Saini, V. Effective interventions to increase routine childhood immunization coverage in low socioeconomic status communities in developed countries: A systematic review and critical appraisal of peer-reviewed literature. *Vaccine* **2021**, *39*, 2938–2964. [CrossRef] [PubMed]
96. Uddin, M.J.; Larson, C.P.; Oliveras, E.; Khan, A.I.; Quaiyum, M.A.; Saha, N.C. Child immunization coverage in urban slums of Bangladesh: Impact of an intervention package. *Health Policy Plan.* **2010**, *25*, 50–60. [CrossRef] [PubMed]
97. State of the World's Fathers 2023 | Equimundo [Internet]. Available online: https://www.equimundo.org/resources/state-of-the-worlds-fathers-2023/ (accessed on 14 April 2024).
98. Owusu-Addo, E.; Cross, R. The impact of conditional cash transfers on child health in low- and middle-income countries: A systematic review. *Int. J. Public Health* **2014**, *59*, 609–618. [CrossRef] [PubMed]
99. Duch, R.; Asiedu, E.; Nakamura, R.; Rouyard, T.; Mayol, A.; Barnett, A.; Roope, L.; Violato, M.; Sowah, D.; Kotlarz, P.; et al. Financial incentives for COVID-19 vaccines in a rural low-resource setting: A cluster-randomized trial. *Nat. Med.* **2023**, *29*, 3193–3202. [CrossRef]
100. Impact of Conditional Cash Transfers on Routine Childhood Immunizations | IDinsight [Internet]. Available online: https://www.idinsight.org/publication/impact-of-conditional-cash-transfers-on-routine-childhood-immunizations-evidence-from-north-west-nigeria/ (accessed on 21 March 2024).
101. Coscieme, L.; Fioramonti, L.; Mortensen, L.F.; Pickett, K.E.; Kubiszewski, I.; Lovins, H.; McGlade, J.; Ragnarsdottir, K.V.; Roberts, D.; Costanza, R.; et al. Women in power: Female leadership and public health outcomes during the COVID-19 pandemic. *medRxiv* **2020**. [CrossRef]

Disclaimer/Publisher's Note: The statements, opinions and data contained in all publications are solely those of the individual author(s) and contributor(s) and not of MDPI and/or the editor(s). MDPI and/or the editor(s) disclaim responsibility for any injury to people or property resulting from any ideas, methods, instructions or products referred to in the content.

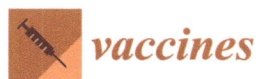 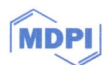

Perspective

Measuring Zero-Dose Children: Reflections on Age Cohort Flexibilities for Targeted Immunization Surveys at the Local Level

Gustavo C. Corrêa [1,*], Md. Jasim Uddin [2], Tasnuva Wahed [2], Elizabeth Oliveras [3], Christopher Morgan [3], Moses R. Kamya [4,5], Patience Kabatangare [4], Faith Namugaya [4], Dorothy Leab [6], Didier Adjakidje [6], Patrick Nguku [7], Adam Attahiru [7], Jenny Sequeira [8], Nancy Vollmer [9] and Heidi W. Reynolds [1]

1. Gavi, The Vaccine Alliance, Chemin du Pommier 40, Le Grand Saconnex, 1218 Geneva, Switzerland
2. International Centre for Diarrhoeal Disease Research, Bangladesh, 68 Shaheed Tajuddin Ahmed Sarani, Mohakhali, Dhaka 1212, Bangladesh; tasnuva.wahed@icddrb.org (T.W.)
3. Jhpiego, The Johns Hopkins University Affiliate, 1615 Thames Street, Baltimore, MD 21231, USA; christopher.morgan@jhpiego.org (C.M.)
4. Infectious Diseases Research Collaboration (IDRC), Kampala P.O. Box 7475, Uganda; mkamya@idrc-uganda.org (M.R.K.); faithsentongo@gmail.com (F.N.)
5. Department of Medicine, Makerere University, Kampala P.O. Box 7072, Uganda
6. GaneshAID, 143 Doc Ngu, Lieu Giai, Ba Dinh, Hanoi 152860, Vietnam
7. African Field Epidemiology Network (AFENET), 50 Haile Selassie St, Asokoro, Abuja 900103, Nigeria
8. The Geneva Learning Foundation (TGLF), Av. Louis-Casaï 18, 1209 Geneva, Switzerland
9. JSI Research & Training Institute, Inc. (JSI), 2733 Crystal Dr 4th Floor, Arlington, VA 22202, USA; nancy_vollmer@jsi.com
* Correspondence: gcorrea@gavi.org

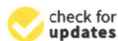

Citation: Corrêa, G.C.; Uddin, M.J.; Wahed, T.; Oliveras, E.; Morgan, C.; Kamya, M.R.; Kabatangare, P.; Namugaya, F.; Leab, D.; Adjakidje, D.; et al. Measuring Zero-Dose Children: Reflections on Age Cohort Flexibilities for Targeted Immunization Surveys at the Local Level. *Vaccines* **2024**, *12*, 195. https://doi.org/10.3390/vaccines12020195

Academic Editors: Ahmad Reza Hosseinpoor, M. Carolina Danovaro, Nicole Bergen, Devaki Nambiar, Ciara Sugerman and Hope L. Johnson

Received: 10 January 2024
Revised: 6 February 2024
Accepted: 8 February 2024
Published: 14 February 2024

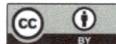

Copyright: © 2024 by the authors. Licensee MDPI, Basel, Switzerland. This article is an open access article distributed under the terms and conditions of the Creative Commons Attribution (CC BY) license (https:// creativecommons.org/licenses/by/ 4.0/).

Abstract: Zero-dose (ZD) children is a critical objective in global health, and it is at the heart of the Immunization Agenda 2030 (IA2030) strategy. Coverage for the first dose of diphtheria–tetanus–pertussis (DTP1)-containing vaccine is the global operational indicator used to estimate ZD children. When surveys are used, DTP1 coverage estimates usually rely on information reported from caregivers of children aged 12–23 months. It is important to have a global definition of ZD children, but learning and operational needs at a country level may require different ZD measurement approaches. This article summarizes a recent workshop discussion on ZD measurement for targeted surveys at local levels related to flexibilities in age cohorts of inclusion from the ZD learning Hub (ZDLH) initiative—a learning initiative involving 5 consortia of 14 different organizations across 4 countries—Bangladesh, Mali, Nigeria, and Uganda—and a global learning partner. Those considerations may include the need to generate insights on immunization timeliness and on catch-up activities, made particularly relevant in the post-pandemic context; the need to compare results across different age cohort years to better identify systematically missed communities and validate programmatic priorities, and also generate insights on changes under dynamic contexts such as the introduction of a new ZD intervention or for recovering from the impact of health system shocks. Some practical considerations such as the potential need for a larger sample size when including comparisons across multiple cohort years but a potential reduction in the need for household visits to find eligible children, an increase in recall bias when older age groups are included and a reduction in recall bias for the first year of life, and a potential reduction in sample size needs and time needed to detect impact when the first year of life is included. Finally, the inclusion of the first year of life cohort in the survey may be particularly relevant and improve the utility of evidence for decision-making and enable its use in rapid learning cycles, as insights will be generated for the population being currently targeted by the program. For some of those reasons, the ZDLH initiative decided to align on a recommendation to include the age cohort from 18 weeks to 23 months, with enough power to enable disaggregation of key results across the two different cohort years. We argue that flexibilities with the age cohort for inclusion in targeted surveys at the local level may be an important principle to be considered. More research is needed to better understand in which contexts improvements in timeliness of DTP1 in the first year of life will translate to improvements in ZD results in the age cohort of 12–23 months as defined by the global DTP1 indicator.

Keywords: zero-dose; equity; immunization; targeted surveys; measurement

1. Introduction

The Immunization Agenda 2030 (IA2030) places missed communities at the heart of its current strategy [1]. Those missed communities under multiple deprivations are considered clusters of zero-dose (ZD) children, systematically not reached by immunization programs. IA2030 defines ZD children as those who did not receive their first dose of a diphtheria–tetanus–pertussis (DTP1)-containing vaccine, and it uses DTP1 coverage to estimate ZD numbers [2]. The rationale for this indicator is that DTP1 is universally used in routine immunization programs across different countries and is usually administered at the first point of contact of communities with the health system, being recommended for infants as early as 6 weeks of age [3]. Gavi, the Vaccine Alliance supports countries to reach those ZD objectives and uses the same ZD definitions and indicators for its current strategy [4,5].

To track annual DTP1 coverage progress, global organizations rely on the World Health Organization (WHO) and United Nations International Children's Emergency Fund (UNICEF) Estimates of National Immunization Coverage (WUENIC). WUENIC relies on country data officially reported to WHO and UNICEF by Member States. Data for WUENIC is generally sourced from administrative systems and surveys conducted at the national level [6].

In many countries, it can be challenging to have reliable coverage estimates based on administrative data. When administrative systems are used, DTP1 coverage is generally calculated by dividing the number of children receiving the vaccine during their first year of life by the estimated number of children who survived their first year of life. However, there are multiple data quality issues that can impact both the numerator and the denominator in this formula. Errors in numerators can be caused by suboptimal data collection and system tools, poor documentation practices, intentional falsification, and lack of reporting from non-governmental providers and there is also much uncertainty on denominators projections [7]. Both errors in numerators and denominators may be aggravated in systematically missed communities with high numbers of ZD children.

Probability-based household surveys may provide an alternative data source for coverage estimation, and WUENIC also relies on national survey data to estimate DTP1 coverage in many countries. For better comparability with administrative data, the estimate is generally based on the report of an annual cohort of children. Usually, surveys based DTP1 coverage estimates rely on information reported from caregivers of children aged 12–23 months, which is also the standard definition used for DTP1 coverage estimation from widely used global survey methodologies, such as the Demographic and Health Survey (DHS) [8] and the Multiple Indicator Cluster Survey (MICS) [9] methods. The main reason why DTP1 coverage estimates start from 12 months of life is because immunization coverage surveys ask about all antigens in the vaccination schedule which should be given by the time a child turns 1 year old. Therefore, measurement of DTP1 coverage starts with children 12 months of age and older, up to 23 months. This way, all children included in the survey cohort would have had the opportunity to receive all age-appropriate vaccinations across all antigens in the first year of life. Following the same logic, a second cohort of children aged 24–35 months may also be surveyed for measuring coverage of antigens administered during the second year of life, but this second cohort is generally not used to measure DTP1 coverage.

Having a clear international definition for measuring ZD children both from administrative systems and from surveys enables the use of existing data in a standardized way to track progress at a portfolio level for global programs. It also enables a common understanding of global level drivers and helps inform activities designed to improve health information system adjustments with key indicators in mind. It simplifies messages used in global communication materials and enables alignment of advocacy efforts, providing a clear direction to the global community. Indeed, national level surveys using DTP1 coverage estimates based on the 12–23-month age cohort have been very important for learning about ZD children distribution, association with multiple deprivations, and drivers at the global level [10–15].

Beyond those global use cases, learning and operational needs at the country level may require different measurement approaches and, where relevant, feasible, and affordable, targeted surveys at the local level may be particularly well placed to identify and gather relevant information on critical equity-related issues. They may be especially useful when targeted to selected communities under multiple deprivations, such as those living in urban slums, in hard-to-reach areas, who are nomadic, refugees or who have been displaced, or belong to ethnic minorities or religious closed communities, among many others.

Because they are targeted, they can offer critical insights on multiple deprivations affecting specific communities and highlight key enablers and drivers to immunization programs with a robustness that cannot be easily achieved with surveys powered at the national or regional level. This type of targeted evidence can be very useful to inform approaches towards other missed communities facing similar contexts.

They may also be a good method to validate the selection of missed communities to be prioritized by the immunization program. A critical assumption of the ZD agenda is that countries should target systematically missed communities and bring them towards full immunization and other primary healthcare services, but it may not be simple to ascertain if communities are systematically missed. The missed communities identified by the program may have never been registered in the local area administrative system, but they may have a different health seeking behavior and they could, for example, be immunized through health services in another area or through other private providers not reporting to the local administrative system. In those cases, they would not be systematically missed, just not registered by the local area health system and targeted surveys can generate clear evidence on this topic where administrative data may fail.

They can also be critical to support monitoring and evaluate programmatic impact in local areas, supplementing routinely collected data while relevant activities to improve data collection and quality in missed communities are rolled out. This may generate critical early evidence to inform adjustments in programmatic interventions and policies with key communities under multiple vulnerabilities in sight [16].

The ZD Learning Hub (ZDLH)—a ZD learning initiative engaging 5 different consortia of partners across 4 countries (Bangladesh, Mali, Nigeria, and Uganda) and at the global level and involving 14 different organizations [17], had a comprehensive discussion on how to better measure ZD children when targeted surveys are used at local level to respond to specific learning needs in a recent workshop. Targeted surveys at the local level have been proposed for the four ZDLH countries. Different methodologies and approaches, adapted to local contexts are proposed and will help answer contextually relevant research questions, but with some commonalities. Firstly, country ZDLH propose to assess the magnitude of the ZD problem in some local communities that have already been prioritized through a national level exercise using secondary data analysis and stakeholder consultations. Well-designed surveys using random sampling frames in some key areas are suggested to validate the country prioritization of key communities. Secondly, targeted surveys at the local level are proposed to better understand ZD drivers affecting childhood immunization in those missed communities to better tailor programmatic activities. Although drivers of ZD children can often be extracted from national level surveys, information on drivers affecting specific communities with higher numbers of ZD children may be inadequate or unavailable. In addition, indicators on other types of drivers using novel and useful tools, such as the behavioral and social driver (BeSD) tools [18], are often not included in traditional surveys among other specific components that can provide insights on specific demand-related barriers affecting specific communities. Finally, measuring the impact of specific interventions designed to reach ZD children in those specific communities is also an objective across countries. This is most often proposed to be achieved with the implementation of at least two rounds of surveys at the same area with trends over time.

All those objectives could be achieved with the traditional approach of using DTP1 coverage estimates from surveys based on the 12 to 23 months age cohort, but this approach can also bring some important gaps. In this article, we synthesize the discussions from the ZDLH group related to age cohort of inclusion in targeted surveys at the local level with the general objective of generating insights to improving methodological approaches for those surveys. We make the case that flexibility with operational definitions of ZD children—particularly related to the age cohort of inclusion across the first years of life—is an important principle to respond to local learning agendas needs. The ZDLH initiative has decided to align on a general recommendation to expand the age cohort for its targeted survey from 18 weeks to 23 months to better respond to key project objectives and research questions, and we also synthesize the reasons for this decision.

2. Key Considerations for Flexibilities of Age Cohort of Inclusion in Targeted Local Surveys

2.1. The Case for the Inclusion of Other Age Cohorts in the First Years of Life

Different countries may have different key concerns related to communities missed by immunization programs. Some may be more focused on reaching children with immunization in a timely manner and others will be concentrating efforts to reach children that may have been missed during a previous period of crisis, such as the COVID-19 pandemic.

Immunization coverage surveys following international standards collect and report DTP1 data from an annual cohort of children aged 12–23 months. This standard age range enables identification of systematically missed communities such as those who were not reached at the end of their first year of life tend to never be reached. However, it usually does not incorporate and generate insights on other relevant principles for children across other age cohorts.

One such relevant principle related to the first year of life is the concept of immunization timeliness. It refers to receiving vaccinations at the earliest appropriate age to confer optimal immunological protection to the child. For DTP1, WHO recommends vaccines from as early as 6 weeks of age and for the third dose of DTP vaccine (DTP3) the recommendation is as early as 14 weeks [3]. The timeliness concept is critical in the first year of life for multiple reasons. After a child is born, transplacental immunity quickly decreases, putting the infant at risk of death and disability from vaccine preventable disease at a time when they are particularly vulnerable [19]. If vaccines are provided too early or too closely spaced, it may not generate an adequate immunological response and reduce duration of protection. When vaccines are delayed, it increases the number of individuals susceptible to specific diseases, reducing herd immunity and exposing the community to circulating vaccine preventable diseases, also putting individuals with medical contraindications and reduced immunity at risk [20].

Generally, administrative data systems do not record the age by which the child has been immunized, thus not allowing the generation of insights on timeliness of immunization. Surveys, in most countries are the only available option when programs need to assess the first year of life. International survey methodologies such as DHS [8] and MICS [9] typically record the age of vaccine administration and, although their standard indicators do not include the immunization timeliness concept, they can and have been used to retrospectively estimate immunization timeliness in the first year of life at the national level across different studies [21,22]. However, in specific communities with high numbers of ZD children, assessing timeliness based on household surveys may be challenging as home-based records (HBR) tend not to be available, making it difficult to retrieve specific dates for vaccine administration and making it inadequate to retrospectively assess it. When the first-year cohort is included in a targeted local survey, it may enable the generation of more reliable and timely insights on immunization timeliness. It may also enable to focus on specific communities with higher number of ZD children, to understand key drivers for untimely immunization, which could be, in some cases, easily actioned by the program.

In addition to the first year of life, countries may also have the need to gather insights about older children and that may be particularly true in the current global context of post-pandemic recovery. There has been clear documentation that the COVID-19 pandemic affected health systems in many countries, which had different recovery speeds [23]. According to the most recent WUENIC release, some countries have not yet fully recovered [24]. WHO, UNICEF, Gavi, and IA2030 recently launched "The Big Catch Up" initiative to intensify efforts to catch up missed children during the pandemic at the global level [25], but there is poor evidence on the local impact of the pandemic in specific communities, what the key local drivers were, and what could work to address the situation. A targeted local survey that includes older age cohorts—beyond 23 months—could also provide good information to support interpretation of the COVID-19 reminiscent impact on ZD, understand recovery trends, and better inform programs in their current catch-up efforts.

2.2. The Case for Comparison of Different Age Cohorts in the Same Targeted Local Survey

Including multiple age cohorts in a single targeted local survey offers the possibility of comparisons of results and key ZD drivers across different cohort years. This may be relevant because each different age cohort will represent a different year of exposure to programmatic activities. Because most vaccines are administered in the first year of life, there is generally a linear correlation of a child's age and the timing of program reach. In other words, the first year of life tends to represent results of the current programmatic year, the second year of life tends to represent results from a year ago, and so forth. Comparing those different age cohorts enables a better understanding of programmatic trends of coverage and drivers in targeted communities to better identify when children are systematically missed and also provides insights on how to better reach them. This may be especially useful to understand communities in dynamic contexts, such as when communities are submitted to a health system shock or on the introduction of a new intervention.

Understanding the immunization results across multiple years in communities is a key need of ZD programming, but focusing on a single cohort year may also not be enough to identify a systematic failure to reach them. A poor immunization performance in one programmatic year could be an outlier—the result of a specific health system shock that was atypical and will not be sustained over time. There are many reasons a community could be affected by time-bound health system shocks. Those could be localized shocks such as a local stock out of vaccines, a key cold chain equipment breakage, an outbreak of infectious disease, a natural disaster, an atypical severe weather event blocking road access, or a local conflict deflagration, among many others. They could also be the result of a national shock such as events of political instability, or a global shock such as global shortages of vaccines or the recent COVID-19 pandemic. If surveys are designed with multiple cohort years, they may be a powerful tool to support the identification of systematically missed communities, or those not affected only by time-bound shocks.

Once a community has been confirmed as systematically missed, there may still be a need to compare results and how the ZD drivers may be shifting across different cohort years. Surveys can measure coverage and also include questions about critical drivers and qualitative components across age cohorts, and this can highlight how well communities are reached and how determinants have changed over time. This may be a critical objective of the implementation research.

Including comparisons of results for the first year of life with other age cohorts in targeted local surveys may be particularly helpful for new ZD interventions. As programs are designed to reach systematically missed communities and as they get better in this objective, we should expect significant shifts in the determinants of ZD children in those communities in a very short timeframe. What could be mostly due to a chronic lack of access can quickly become a demand issue only some months after the introduction of an intervention, and this may have important implications for program adaptation.

The same logic applies to older age cohorts when health systems are recovering from time-bound shocks or crises. Comparing the results and drivers from older age cohorts, at a period when a crisis was hitting hard, with more recent ones when things have been more stable may provide convincing proof of the crisis impact in immunization results for a given community and provide insights on its recovery speed, building evidence for the potential relevance of targeted catch-up efforts. It can also generate useful insights into the design of those catch-up efforts, as it can better demonstrate how prevalent shock-related barriers have been and may still be present, and which programs may need to adjust current activities to better address them. In addition, it may generate evidence for other new interventions to increase the health system resiliency and ensure these crisis-related barriers will not have the same weight in future crisis events.

2.3. Practical Considerations

There are also a number of practical considerations that may need to be carefully dealt with when flexibilities with the age cohort of inclusion are being contemplated in targeted local surveys.

Firstly, when comparison of results and ZD drivers across cohort years using a single survey or when precise estimates for specific cohort years are critical objectives, there will likely be implications for sample size calculations and fieldwork planning.

The study will need to ensure that results for each cohort year are sufficiently reliable to enable meaningful statistical comparisons and conclusions. In those cases, a targeted local survey may need to have enough power to enable disaggregation and comparisons of the data by each relevant age cohort included in the original research questions. To achieve this objective, sample size calculations may need to be separately performed for each cohort year included but allowing simultaneous data collection using the same logistical structure. The lowest number of individuals to be included in the study sample must enable answering the research question that requires a larger sample size, focusing on few critical primary objectives.

WHO has developed useful guidance focused on clustered surveys, indicating methods for sample size calculation for different research questions and objectives that researchers can already build upon [26]. There is also sampling guidance for Lot Quality Assurance Sampling (LQAS) surveys, mainly for the integration of data from different programs in a single survey [27]. The calculation of sample sizes for local targeted surveys focused on ZD children, which tend to be non-clustered and, to use a single indicator across different cohort years, will likely make the task simpler regardless of the survey method.

Despite of the need for a higher sample size in those cases, expanding to a larger age cohort and responding to different research questions or comparing age cohorts using a single survey may also simplify fieldwork, as it may require a substantially lower number of household visits to find eligible children; that is, those matching the wider age range for inclusion. The higher probability of finding children in the eligible age range in any single household visit would reduce the number of household visits required to fulfil the sample size needs.

Secondly, adding other age cohort years in the survey will have implications on recall bias which may affect data reliability and validity.

Generally, when immunization surveys are conducted, the vaccination history is preferably captured from documented evidence sources, such as HBR—and less often from health facility-based records (FBR). Very frequently, it will be based on survey respondent memory recall, especially when HBR are not available [28].

HBR are generally considered a more reliable source of vaccination history data, despite running some risks of containing errors such as incomplete recording, mis-recording or mismatch between children being surveyed and the card presented by the caregiver. However, in many countries with high numbers of ZD children, HBR are often not available [29] and FBR may be of very poor quality. This situation may be aggravated for surveys targeting missed communities with highest numbers of ZD children. In those settings, it is likely that vaccination history will often rely in recall.

Recall data are sometimes not correlated with HBR data and, in general, may have poor agreement with other sources [30]. Memory bias is frequent, as caregivers tend to over-report coverage due to social desirability bias, or they simply may be unable to remember the vaccination history with details. This concern may be intensified due to the growing complexity of the vaccination schedule.

When multiple age cohort years are included in a targeted survey focused on missed communities, researchers should pay special attention to the risk of memory bias from recall, which may affect different age cohorts in dissimilar ways. DTP1 coverage and the ZD concept may itself be less subject to memory bias than other later doses, as the caregiver will have a lower risk of not remembering a first dose of vaccine for a child than to be precise about the number of doses received across the schedule. However, it is reasonable to assume memory bias may play a larger role for older age groups as there will be a larger amount of time elapsed from the time the vaccine has been received and it will be less important for the first year of life as less time may have elapsed from the vaccine dose to the survey inquiry.

In addition, when repeated surveys are considered for estimating the impact of ZD interventions, it is also likely that DTP1 coverage may be overestimated in the first round due to recall bias and underestimated in the second round, assuming ZD interventions are rolled out and those missed communities are finally reached and HBR become more available as part of the intervention. This pattern of coverage overestimation being observed from recall and under estimation from HBR has been recently suggested by a recent and comprehensive systematic review [31]. This may reduce the measured treatment effect size and have other implications for survey design, sample size, and analytical plan. Those limitations need to be highlighted and data from those surveys must be interpreted with care.

Thirdly, when an impact assessment is a critical study objective, the inclusion of the first year of life in the age range of a targeted local survey may considerably simplify the study operationalization. In those cases, it may significantly decrease the sample size needed because the estimated treatment effect size will likely be higher. This is especially true in settings where the prevalence of ZD children is relatively low. Importantly, it will also decrease the time needed to detect impact. It may enable a better study match with programmatic learning needs and available budget without compromising robustness.

Sample size calculation for estimating program impact requires an estimation of the treatment effect size. The treatment effect size can be understood as the difference the intervention will generate when compared to a hypothetical counterfactual such as no intervention. A small decrease in the expected treatment effect size usually means a huge increase in the sample size needed [32], and that may have important operational implications for the study operationalization and its overall cost.

The global coverage of DTP1 is estimated to be around 89% [24]. This means that in many countries, which may legitimately be concerned with ZD children in some key communities, a high national coverage level for DTP1 is also expected. Depending on the ZD distribution in the national territory, some countries may find that their key communities with higher numbers of ZD children, may already have reasonably high DTP1 coverage.

Estimating impact of programmatic approaches when the baseline is already high may be statistically challenging, as the estimated treatment effect size will also be low. For example, it may require a significantly lower sample size to statistically estimate impact when we expect an increase in coverage from 20% to 80% as compared to an increase from 70% to 80%. By including the first-year age cohort in a survey and on the ZD operational definition, we would have an increased expected treatment effect size, because the baseline would definitely be much lower. Unfortunately, untimely vaccination is much more common than missing immunization at 12 months in most settings. This may have important feasibility implications for program impact studies using targeted surveys at local levels, especially in communities with a relatively high baseline DTP1 value.

In addition to a reduced sample size need, incorporating a first-year age cohort in the survey will also have important implications related to the time it takes to demonstrate the impact of an intervention. That is because when a new immunization-related intervention is introduced, researchers may need to wait a significant amount of time to ensure the intervention will be operationally stable and the targeted population will be fully covered. It will also take some time for the results of the new program to start to appear and be adequately measured. Often, there is also uncertainty in terms of precisely when the intervention will be operationalized which may add additional delays in the study workplan. In practice, in a traditional 12–23-month cohort survey, that would mean a 3-year waiting period for measuring impact with at least 2 stable years of implementation to properly enable its documentation. That time may fall outside the evaluation funding window or the programmatic evidence need.

The addition of the first-year age cohort in these cases will enable a reduction in the time needed to follow up programmatic impact by at least one year. The detection of early effects on DTP1 coverage will be already meaningful and it will very likely translate into an effective ZD reduction later on. Although the correlation between improvements in DTP1 coverage in the first year of life and improvements in ZD results is not yet established across different contexts, it makes theoretical sense, and it is likely that DTP1 coverage in the first year of life may serve as a proxy for broader ZD impact. If the first 2 years of life are included and multiple rounds of surveys are performed, the study could also demonstrate how well reaching ZD children in a timely manner in targeted missed communities will finally translate into ZD programmatic results as defined by the global community, contributing to strengthening the evidence on measuring DTP1 immunization timeliness as a proxy indicator for ZD children. This may be a clear priority for ZD research in the coming years.

2.4. The Most Critical Consideration Is an Improved Utility of Evidence for Decision-Making in Rapid Learning Cycles

Finally, the overall objective of implementation research is to generate useful evidence and support decision-making of key stakeholders to improve program implementation and impact in a timely way. The inclusion of different age cohorts in the same survey may enable strengthening of this critical use case.

It will enable researchers to generate timely and meaningful insights on ZD determinants and on different issues such as timeliness of vaccination, COVID-19 impact, and dynamic shifting contexts. In particular, when the first year of life is included, it may significantly reduce the time needed from program operationalization to evidence on its impact. Through rapid learning cycles, it may equip local and national policy-makers and practitioners on current determinants communities may be facing to make timely and adequate decisions. Although less useful for international comparisons, it still could provide insights on ZD children following international standards if data can be disaggregated by different age cohorts.

Understanding coverage and determinants in the first year of life will certainly not be as useful to establish systematically missed communities or to compare with other surveys or local administrative data, but covering this age range may be critical to generate insights on the population currently being targeted by the program and how different they may be from previous cohorts. This information will better link to programmatic decision-making and enable the program to perform fine adjustments as activities are being rolled out and that could not be accomplished with a more traditional age cohort selection.

3. Key Decisions on Targeted Local Surveys from the ZDLH Initiative

In the case of the ZDLH initiative, the decision was made to include the age cohort from 18 weeks to 23 months, effectively including a large part of the first year of life and with a recommendation to enable disaggregation of the data across cohort years in the analysis plan. Eighteen weeks was selected as a starting date because it enables the detection of clear delays on DTP1 vaccines—for at least 12 weeks—and enables the detection of early—2 weeks—delays in DTP3. The hope is that this first-year cohort may generate early insights on ZD children and enable initial calculations of DTP drop-out rates. Twenty-three months was selected as the end date to enable comparisons with international surveys.

Among the key reasons for the ZDLH initiative to include the first year of life included the ability to generate insights on timeliness of immunization, the ability to better identify systematically missed communities, the ability to understand programmatic performance and shifts in ZD determinants across years, and the ability to estimate program impact at an earlier stage, so that all those pieces of information can be linked to program adaptation in a timely way. Other practical reasons considered were a reduction in the sample size and time needed to estimate impact and operational simplification to answer some key questions and the associated costs for countries with higher DTP1 coverage in those communities.

Considerations was also given to including later age cohort years, especially in the context of "The Big Catch-Up initiative", but the ZDLH group decided not to, mainly because key local questions were generally not related to this initiative, but also because some insights on COVID-19 recovery on those communities could already be generated by analyzing data from the 12–23-month cohort. Including later age cohorts was thought to significantly increase the sample size needed and the project budget without a clear use case.

4. Conclusions

Even though the global operational and strategic definition of ZD children for surveys is the lack of DPT1 among children aged 12–23 months, there are many reasons why different age cohorts should be included in targeted local surveys. The inclusion of the first year of life cohort may be relevant to generate useful insights on immunization timeliness, minimize recall bias, and may potentially enable the reduction in sample size and time needed to detect impact, when this is a critical research question. It may significantly improve the utility of evidence for decision-making, as insights will be generated for the population being currently targeted by the program. The inclusion of older age cohorts in the survey may also be relevant to generate insights and inform catch-up activities for older groups, but may increase recall bias. The inclusion of multiple age cohorts in the same survey may enable comparison of results across different age cohort years and support a better identification of systematically missed communities, supporting the validation of set programmatic priorities. It may also generate insights on changes in enablers and barriers to immunization under dynamic contexts such as the introduction of a new ZD intervention or when recovering from the impact of health system shocks. Including multiple age cohorts may require larger sample sizes if results need to be disaggregated by cohort years, but may enable a potential reduction in the need for household visits to find eligible children.

We believe that the approaches laid out in this article may enable better evidence and greatly contribute to improve inequalities in immunization. We think that flexibilities on the age cohort of inclusion in targeted surveys at the local level is an important principle to be considered to improve monitoring of inequalities and to respond to local ZD learning agendas needs. Rather than generating misalignments with the international definition, we think this approach may enable better, more timely and complementary data for ZD learning agendas and critically, it may position implementation research to enhance monitoring and answer learning needs in rapid learning cycles. In this sense, aligning the survey age cohort with international definitions may not be feasible or desirable. Researchers and program managers may need to consider those aspects in their decision-making when surveys are planned.

More research is needed to better understand the specific contexts where improvements in timeliness of DTP1 immunization in the first year of life will translate to improvements in DTP1 coverage in the cohort of 12–23 months as defined by the global ZD indicator.

Author Contributions: Survey methods conceptualization: M.J.U., T.W., E.O. and C.M.; workshop participation, G.C.C., M.J.U., T.W., E.O., M.R.K., P.K., F.N., D.L., D.A., P.N., A.A., J.S., N.V. and H.W.R.; manuscript conceptualization: G.C.C. and H.W.R.; validation, G.C.C., M.J.U., T.W., E.O., C.M., M.R.K., P.K., F.N., D.L., D.A., P.N., A.A., J.S., N.V. and H.W.R.; writing—original draft preparation, G.C.C.; writing—review and editing, G.C.C., H.W.R., M.J.U., T.W., E.O., M.R.K., F.N., J.S. and N.V. All authors have read and agreed to the published version of the manuscript.

Funding: The Zero-Dose Learning Hub is funded by Gavi, the Vaccine Alliance and implemented through agreements with AFENET, icddr,b, IDRC, GaneshAID, and JSI. The APC was funded by Gavi, the Vaccine Alliance.

Institutional Review Board Statement: Not applicable.

Informed Consent Statement: Not applicable.

Acknowledgments: We would like to thank Dan Hogan from Gavi, the Vaccine Alliance, and Jessica Shearer from PATH for their reviews and relevant contributions on earlier versions of this manuscript.

Conflicts of Interest: G.C.C. and H.W.R. are employed by Gavi who sponsored the workshop where this discussion took place. They had total freedom to express their views which do not necessarily reflect those of Gavi, the Vaccine Alliance. Other authors M.J.U., T.W., E.O., C.M., M.R.K., P.K., F.N., D.L., D.A., P.N., A.A., J.S., and N.V. are engaged in the Zero-Dose Learning Hub initiative and receive funds from Gavi. They declare that this article was written in the absence of any commercial or financial relationships that could be construed as a potential conflict of interest.

References

1. Immunization Agenda 2030. Available online: https://www.immunizationagenda2030.org/ (accessed on 25 August 2023).
2. IA2030 Scorecard for Immunization Agenda 2030. Available online: https://scorecard.immunizationagenda2030.org/ig2.1 (accessed on 25 August 2023).
3. WHO Recommendations for Routine Immunization—Summary Tables. Available online: https://www.who.int/teams/immunization-vaccines-and-biologicals/policies/who-recommendations-for-routine-immunization---summary-tables (accessed on 25 August 2023).
4. Zero-Dose Children and Missed Communities. Available online: https://www.gavi.org/our-alliance/strategy/phase-5-2021-2025/equity-goal/zero-dose-children-missed-communities (accessed on 25 August 2023).
5. 2021–2025 Indicators. Available online: https://www.gavi.org/programmes-impact/our-impact/measuring-our-performance/2021-2025-indicators (accessed on 25 August 2023).
6. Burton, A.; Monasch, R.; Lautenbach, B.; Gacic-Dobo, M.; Neill, M.; Karimov, R.; Wolfson, L.; Jones, G.; Birmingham, M. WHO and UNICEF Estimates of National Infant Immunization Coverage: Methods and Processes. *Bull. World Health Organ.* **2009**, *87*, 535–541. [CrossRef] [PubMed]
7. Scobie, H.M.; Edelstein, M.; Nicol, E.; Morice, A.; Rahimi, N.; MacDonald, N.E.; Carolina Danovaro-Holliday, M.; Jawad, J. Improving the Quality and Use of Immunization and Surveillance Data: Summary Report of the Working Group of the Strategic Advisory Group of Experts on Immunization. *Vaccine* **2020**, *38*, 7183–7197. [CrossRef] [PubMed]
8. Croft, T.N.; Marshall, M.J.M.; Allen, C.K. *Guide to DHS Statistics*; ICF: Rockville, MD, USA, 2018.
9. United Nations Children's Fund (UNICEF). Multiple Indicator Cluster Surveys (MICS) 6 Tools. MICS6 Indicators and Definitions (3 March 2021). Available online: https://mics.unicef.org/tools?round=mics6 (accessed on 15 November 2023).
10. Johns, N.E.; Santos, T.M.; Arroyave, L.; Cata-Preta, B.O.; Heidari, S.; Kirkby, K.; Munro, J.; Schlotheuber, A.; Wendt, A.; O'Brien, K.; et al. Gender-Related Inequality in Childhood Immunization Coverage: A Cross-Sectional Analysis of DTP3 Coverage and Zero-Dose DTP Prevalence in 52 Countries Using the SWPER Global Index. *Vaccines* **2022**, *10*, 988. [CrossRef] [PubMed]
11. Wigley, A.; Lorin, J.; Hogan, D.; Utazi, C.E.; Hagedorn, B.; Dansereau, E.; Tatem, A.J.; Tejedor-Garavito, N. Estimates of the Number and Distribution of Zero-Dose and under-Immunised Children across Remote-Rural, Urban, and Conflict-Affected Settings in Low and Middle-Income Countries. *PLoS Glob. Public Health* **2022**, *2*, e0001126. [CrossRef] [PubMed]
12. Wendt, A.; Santos, T.M.; Cata-Preta, B.O.; Arroyave, L.; Hogan, D.R.; Mengistu, T.; Barros, A.J.D.; Victora, C.G. Exposure of Zero-Dose Children to Multiple Deprivation: Analyses of Data from 80 Low- and Middle-Income Countries. *Vaccines* **2022**, *10*, 1568. [CrossRef] [PubMed]

13. Santos, T.M.; Cata-Preta, B.O.; Wendt, A.; Arroyave, L.; Hogan, D.R.; Mengistu, T.; Barros, A.J.D.; Victora, C.G. Religious Affiliation as a Driver of Immunization Coverage: Analyses of Zero-Dose Vaccine Prevalence in 66 Low- and Middle-Income Countries. *Front. Public Health* **2022**, *10*, 977512. [CrossRef] [PubMed]
14. Bergen, N.; Cata-preta, B.O.; Schlotheuber, A.; Santos, T.M.; Danovaro-holliday, M.C.; Mengistu, T.; Sodha, S.V.; Hogan, D.R.; Barros, A.J.D.; Hosseinpoor, A.R. Economic-Related Inequalities in Zero-Dose Children: A Study of Non-Receipt of Diphtheria–Tetanus–Pertussis Immunization Using Household Health Survey Data from 89 Low- and Middle-Income Countries. *Vaccines* **2022**, *10*, 633. [CrossRef] [PubMed]
15. Utazi, C.E.; Pannell, O.; Aheto, J.M.K.; Wigley, A.; Tejedor-Garavito, N.; Wunderlich, J.; Hagedorn, B.; Hogan, D.; Tatem, A.J. Assessing the Characteristics of Un- and under-Vaccinated Children in Low- and Middle-Income Countries: A Multi-Level Cross-Sectional Study. *PLoS Glob. Public Health* **2022**, *2*, e0000244. [CrossRef] [PubMed]
16. FHI 360. Use of Targeted Surveys to Monitor Immunization Programming for Zero-Dose Children and Missed Communities: Evidence on Pro-Equity Interventions to Improve Immunization Coverage for Zero-Dose Children and Missed Communities. Available online: https://zdlh.gavi.org/sites/default/files/2023-09/4._evidence_brief_targeted_surveys.pdf (accessed on 31 January 2024).
17. Zero-Dose Learning Hub: Evidence in Action for Immunization Equity. Available online: https://zdlh.gavi.org/ (accessed on 30 January 2024).
18. World Health Organization (WHO). *Behavioural and Social Drivers of Vaccination: Tools and Practical Guidance for Achieving High Uptake*; World Health Organization (WHO): Geneva, Switzerland, 2022.
19. Dirirsa, K.; Makuria, M.; Mulu, E.; Deriba, B.S. Assessment of Vaccination Timeliness and Associated Factors among Children in Toke Kutaye District, Central Ethiopia: A Mixed Study. *PLoS ONE* **2022**, *17*, e0262320. [CrossRef] [PubMed]
20. Noh, J.W.; Kim, Y.M.; Akram, N.; Yoo, K.B.; Cheon, J.; Lee, L.J.; Kwon, Y.D.; Stekelenburg, J. Determinants of Timeliness in Early Childhood Vaccination among Mothers with Vaccination Cards in Sindh Province, Pakistan: A Secondary Analysis of Cross-Sectional Survey Data. *BMJ Open* **2019**, *9*, 028922. [CrossRef] [PubMed]
21. Masters, N.B.; Wagner, A.L.; Boulton, M.L. Vaccination Timeliness and Delay in Low- and Middle-Income Countries: A Systematic Review of the Literature, 2007–2017. *Hum. Vaccines Immunother.* **2019**, *15*, 2790–2805. [CrossRef] [PubMed]
22. Wariri, O.; Utazi, C.E.; Okomo, U.; Sogur, M.; Murray, K.A.; Grundy, C.; Fofanna, S.; Kampmann, B. Timeliness of Routine Childhood Vaccination among 12–35 Months Old Children in The Gambia: Analysis of National Immunisation Survey Data, 2019–2020. *PLoS ONE* **2023**, *18*, e0288741. [CrossRef] [PubMed]
23. Shet, A.; Carr, K.; Danovaro-Holliday, M.C.; Sodha, S.V.; Prosperi, C.; Wunderlich, J.; Wonodi, C.; Reynolds, H.W.; Mirza, I.; Gacic-Dobo, M.; et al. Impact of the SARS-CoV-2 Pandemic on Routine Immunisation Services: Evidence of Disruption and Recovery from 170 Countries and Territories. *Lancet Glob. Health* **2022**, *10*, e186–e194. [CrossRef] [PubMed]
24. Progress and Challenges with Achieving Universal Immunization Coverage: 2022 WHO/UNICEF Estimates of National Immunization Coverage. Available online: https://www.who.int/publications/m/item/progress-and-challenges-with-achievinguniversal-immunization-coverage (accessed on 25 August 2023).
25. O'Brien, K.L.; Lemango, E. The Big Catch-up in Immunisation Coverage after the COVID-19 Pandemic: Progress and Challenges to Achieving Equitable Recovery. *Lancet* **2023**, *402*, 510–512. [CrossRef] [PubMed]
26. World Health Organization (WHO). *Vaccination Coverage Cluster Surveys: Reference Manual*; World Health Organization (WHO): Geneva, Switzerland, 2018.
27. CORE Group. *Protocol for Parallel Sampling: Using Lot Quality Assurance to Collect Rapid CATCH Information*; CORE Group, Inc.: Washington, DC, USA, 2008.
28. World Health Organization (WHO). *Harmonizing Vaccination Coverage Measures in Household Surveys: A Primer*; World Health Organization (WHO): Washington, DC, USA, 2019.
29. Brown, D.W.; Gacic-Dobo, M. Home-Based Record Prevalence among Children Aged 12–23 Months from 180 Demographic and Health Surveys. *Vaccine* **2015**, *33*, 2584–2593. [CrossRef] [PubMed]
30. Dansereau, E.; Brown, D.; Stashko, L.; Danovaro-Holliday, M.C. A Systematic Review of the Agreement of Recall, Home-Based Records, Facility Records, BCG Scar, and Serology for Ascertaining Vaccination Status in Low and Middle-Income Countries. *Gates Open Res.* **2019**, *3*, 923. [CrossRef] [PubMed]
31. Miles, M.; Ryman, T.K.; Dietz, V.; Zell, E.; Luman, E.T. Validity of Vaccination Cards and Parental Recall to Estimate Vaccination Coverage: A Systematic Review of the Literature. *Vaccine* **2013**, *31*, 1560–1568. [CrossRef] [PubMed]
32. Serdar, C.C.; Cihan, M.; Yücel, D.; Serdar, M.A. Sample Size, Power and Effect Size Revisited: Simplified and Practical Approachin Pre-Clinical, Clinical and Laboratory Studies. *Biochem. Med.* **2021**, *31*, 1–27. [CrossRef] [PubMed]

Disclaimer/Publisher's Note: The statements, opinions and data contained in all publications are solely those of the individual author(s) and contributor(s) and not of MDPI and/or the editor(s). MDPI and/or the editor(s) disclaim responsibility for any injury to people or property resulting from any ideas, methods, instructions or products referred to in the content.

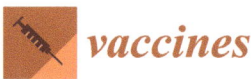

Project Report

Building Data Triangulation Capacity for Routine Immunization and Vaccine Preventable Disease Surveillance Programs to Identify Immunization Coverage Inequities

Audrey Rachlin [1,*], Oluwasegun Joel Adegoke [1], Rajendra Bohara [2], Edson Rwagasore [3], Hassan Sibomana [3], Adeline Kabeja [3], Ines Itanga [3], Samuel Rwunganira [4], Blaise Mafende Mario [5], Nahimana Marie Rosette [6], Ramatu Usman Obansa [7], Angela Ukpojo Abah [7], Olorunsogo Bidemi Adeoye [8], Ester Sikare [1], Eugene Lam [1], Christopher S. Murrill [1] and Angela Montesanti Porter [1]

1. Global Immunization Division, Centers for Disease Control and Prevention, Atlanta, GA 30333, USA
2. World Health Organization, Dhaka 1212, Bangladesh
3. Rwanda Biomedical Centre, Ministry of Health, Kigali P.O. Box 7162, Rwanda
4. African Field Epidemiology Network, Kigali, Rwanda
5. Health Information Systems Program (HISP), Kigali, Rwanda; mafendeblaise@hisprwanda.org
6. World Health Organization, Kigali P.O. Box 1324, Rwanda
7. National Stop Transmission of Polio (NSTOP) Program, African Field Epidemiology Network (AFENET), Abuja 900103, Nigeria
8. Division of Global Health Protection, Centers for Disease Control and Prevention, Atlanta, GA 30329, USA
* Correspondence: rhu0@cdc.gov

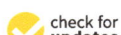

Citation: Rachlin, A.; Adegoke, O.J.; Bohara, R.; Rwagasore, E.; Sibomana, H.; Kabeja, A.; Itanga, I.; Rwunganira, S.; Mafende Mario, B.; Rosette, N.M.; et al. Building Data Triangulation Capacity for Routine Immunization and Vaccine Preventable Disease Surveillance Programs to Identify Immunization Coverage Inequities. *Vaccines* **2024**, *12*, 646. https://doi.org/10.3390/vaccines12060646

Academic Editors: Giuseppe La Torre, Ahmad Reza Hosseinpoor, M. Carolina Danovaro, Devaki Nambiar, Hope L. Johnson, Ciara Sugerman and Nicole Bergen

Received: 24 April 2024
Revised: 30 May 2024
Accepted: 6 June 2024
Published: 11 June 2024

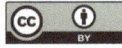

Copyright: © 2024 by the authors. Licensee MDPI, Basel, Switzerland. This article is an open access article distributed under the terms and conditions of the Creative Commons Attribution (CC BY) license (https://creativecommons.org/licenses/by/4.0/).

Abstract: The Expanded Programme on Immunization (EPI) and Vaccine Preventable Disease (VPD) Surveillance (VPDS) programs generate multiple data sources (e.g., routine administrative data, VPD case data, and coverage surveys). However, there are challenges with the use of these siloed data for programmatic decision-making, including poor data accessibility and lack of timely analysis, contributing to missed vaccinations, immunity gaps, and, consequently, VPD outbreaks in populations with limited access to immunization and basic healthcare services. Data triangulation, or the integration of multiple data sources, can be used to improve the availability of key indicators for identifying immunization coverage gaps, under-immunized (UI) and un-immunized (zero-dose (ZD)) children, and for assessing program performance at all levels of the healthcare system. Here, we describe the data triangulation processes, prioritization of indicators, and capacity building efforts in Bangladesh, Nigeria, and Rwanda. We also describe the analyses used to generate meaningful data, key indicators used to identify immunization coverage inequities and performance gaps, and key lessons learned. Triangulation processes and lessons learned may be leveraged by other countries, potentially leading to programmatic changes that promote improved access and utilization of vaccination services through the identification of UI and ZD children.

Keywords: data visualization; capacity building; immunization; surveillance; health equity

1. Background

The Immunization Agenda 2030 (IA2030), a global immunization strategy endorsed by the World Health Assembly in 2020, envisions a world "where everyone, everywhere, at every age, fully benefits from vaccines" [1]. The strategy emphasizes "data-guided" decision-making as a fundamental component of any successful immunization program, necessary to direct strategies to achieve program targets. Greater data use can lead to better-quality data and ultimately contribute to improved immunization program performance by identifying and targeting those who are eligible for vaccination [2,3]. Improved data quality and use are also critical for measuring progress towards achieving the Sustainable Development Goals (SDGs) and Universal Health Coverage (UHC) targets [2,4,5], and for identifying underserved populations for vaccination to achieve measurable reductions in mortality and morbidity from targeted vaccine preventable diseases (VPDs), as highlighted in the U.S. Centers for Disease Control and Prevention Global Health Equity Strategy 2022–2027 [6].

The COVID-19 pandemic affected immunization programs worldwide and highlighted equity issues in immunization coverage, including outreach services commonly used in many low- and middle-income countries with inadequate access to health facilities [7]. In 2021, the number of infants who did not receive the first dose of the diphtheria-tetanus-pertussis-containing vaccine (DTPcv1) was 37% (18.2 million) higher than in 2019 (13.3 million) [8]. In the push to leave no one behind with immunization services, there is a growing need to reach "zero-dose children", those who have not received any routine vaccinations (measured by the lack of DTPcv1), as well as "under-immunized children" (defined as those missing the third dose of DTPcv (DTPcv3)) [1]. These children often have limited access to primary healthcare and social services, limited economic and educational opportunities, and limited political representation [9–11]. Zero-dose and under-immunized children are at an increased risk during disease outbreaks and also often lack access to other basic services. Providing these children with immunization services can connect them to other health services and the associated economic and social benefits [9]. Even in countries with high vaccination coverage, immunity gaps might occur among people in racial and ethnic minority groups, religious groups, urban settings, remote rural locations, migrant/nomadic communities, or low socioeconomic status [12]. Data to look at these zero-dose and under-immunized communities may not be routinely captured by the immunization program, or there may be challenges with the use of available data for programmatic decision-making, such as poor data accessibility and lack of timely analysis [2,3].

One approach that is being increasingly recognized as effective in improving data use and quality for decision-making in public health programs is data triangulation, or the synthesis of multiple datasets [13–15]. Data triangulation integrates data sources to identify data quality and immunization program performance gaps, including immunization-coverage inequities. The results can be used to guide programmatic action in communities that are often missed across the spectrum of essential health services [12]. In 2019, the Strategic Advisory Group of Experts (SAGE) Working Group on Immunization and Surveillance Data Quality and Use suggested that data triangulation should be the standard for public health analyses and that, even in the absence of perfect data, combining many pieces of weaker evidence through triangulation can form a strong basis for more informed decision-making [2,3]. As a result, the World Health Organization (WHO), UNICEF, and the U.S. Centers for Disease Control and Prevention (U.S. CDC) developed global guidance titled *Triangulation for Improved Decision-Making in Immunization Programmes* to describe a triangulation process that can be used by Expanded Programme on Immunization (EPI) and Vaccine Preventable Disease Surveillance (VPDS) programs to develop questions, identify data sources, and interpret different data together considering underlying context and limitations [12].

Many data sources are generated within and outside the EPI and VPDS programs (e.g., routine administrative data, VPD case data, coverage surveys, vaccine supply, serosurveys, and population estimates). However, there are challenges with the use of these separate data systems for programmatic decision-making, including poor data accessibility and lack of timely analysis, contributing to immunity gaps and VPD outbreaks in populations with limited access to immunization and basic healthcare services [2,12].

Since 2018, the U.S. CDC, in consultation with immunization experts from the WHO, has supported Ministries of Health (MoH) to build the capacity of the EPI and VPDS workforce in Bangladesh, Rwanda, and Nigeria to perform data triangulation for evidence-based decision-making. Here, we describe the methods, example triangulation indicators, and electronic information systems implemented by these three countries for routine data triangulation in RI and VPD Surveillance (VPDS) programs. We aimed to document how data triangulation activities have improved the availability of key indicators used for identifying

DTPcv, polio, and measles-containing vaccine (MCV) immunization coverage inequities and examine how these triangulation processes may be used to improve immunization program performance, identify coverage gaps, and support the characterization of zero-dose or under-immunized children at all levels of the healthcare system in Bangladesh, Rwanda, and Nigeria.

2. Methods

2.1. Data Sources

A desk review of secondary data sources was conducted in each of the three countries. The data sources reviewed included country-specific VPDS and routine immunization (RI) data sources, electronic reporting systems, data triangulation analyses and dashboards, triangulated indicators, project reports, conference abstracts, and conference and national workshop presentations.

2.2. Data Review and Analysis

A manual thematic content analysis was performed using Microsoft Excel and Microsoft Word (Microsoft 365 MSO, Version 2308) on desk review materials, using themes identified by three reviewers a priori to inform the country-specific approaches to data triangulation activities. These themes examined the approach to data triangulation implementation, including stakeholder engagement and partnerships in each country, the mechanisms of implementation, data sources and processes, and approaches to building capacity for data triangulation. We also examined the results of country-specific data triangulation activities, including data triangulation immunity gap and immunization and VPDS program-performance indicators, data triangulation technologies and projects, visualization of indicators, and current use.

The results were summarized into four key areas based on the identified a priori themes: (1) project conceptualization (development) and partnerships, (2) approach to data triangulation processes and indicator prioritization, (3) data triangulation capacity building efforts, and (4) successes and demonstrated potential for impact. Our findings for each country and the lessons learned from these four key areas are presented below.

3. Results

3.1. Bangladesh

3.1.1. Project Conceptualization and Partnerships

In 2019, the Bangladesh Directorate General of Health Services (DGHS), with funding and technical support from the U.S. CDC, served as the first pilot country to assist in the development of the global guidance for the publication *Triangulation for Improved Decision-Making in Immunization Programmes* [12]. At an initial triangulation concept-development workshop in March 2019, the DGHS prioritized the following topic areas as the biggest challenges in the country's national and subnational immunization programs: (1) measles immunity gaps, (2) program performance, and (3) target-population estimates. The initial workshop resulted in project commitment and participation from the DGHS EPI, Surveillance, and Management Information System units; the Civil Registration and Vital Statistics Division; and the Bangladesh Bureau of Statistics. Additional key technical partners included the WHO and UNICEF Bangladesh offices.

3.1.2. Approach to Triangulation Processes and Indicator Prioritization

During the national workshop, a data-mapping exercise of relevant data sources was completed prior to the development of a triangulation analysis plan to investigate the three identified programmatic areas: (1) measles immunity gaps, (2) program performance, and (3) target-population estimates. The data mapping included the name of the data source, at what administrative level the data are collected, in which information system the data are available, the reporting frequency, and at which administrative levels the data are used. Table 1 summarizes the data sources identified in Bangladesh. From the data inventory, key triangulation indicators for each of the three programmatic areas were prioritized based on the data sources and variables available, key questions of programmatic interest, and expected trends across datasets [12]. A list of example triangulation indicators to identify immunity gaps is summarized in Table 2. These indicators were ultimately incorporated into the triangulation global guidance. The global guidance documents describe each indicator in depth, including the data sources or elements required, potential analysis outputs, and sample visualizations from anonymized countries and publicly available references through collaboration with global subject-matter experts.

Once available data sources were identified and key triangulation indicators were prioritized within an agreed-upon data-analysis plan, datasets from various data sources (e.g., vaccination stock and supply, EPI administrative coverage, serosurveys, etc.) (Table 1) and information systems were exported into Microsoft Excel to allow for necessary data elements to be compiled into one standardized format for analysis. Additionally, the triangulation of data elements within datasets available on the same electronic information system, such as District Health Information System 2 (DHIS2), could be analyzed within the DHIS2 platform. Visualizations of the prioritized triangulation indicators were then presented to key national-level and subnational-level stakeholders for review and interpretation. While WHO Bangladesh and U.S. CDC conducted national- and district-level triangulation analyses between March and December 2019, national partners were instrumental in providing existing program guidance, policies, and access to data. Triangulation visualizations and corresponding interpretations were summarized according to programmatic areas (program performance, immunity gaps, and immunization-program target-population estimates) in a PowerPoint presentation, along with recommended programmatic action items, and presented to key stakeholders at a final dissemination workshop held in Dhaka in December 2019.

More recently, in 2022, Bangladesh assessed zero-dose (ZD) and under-immunized (UI) children by conducting data triangulation of existing data, like those listed in Table 1 [16]. The triangulation analyses of existing data sources conducted to identify communities with ZD and UI children are described in Table 2. Further description of the methodology used to identify missed ZD communities can be found in the report "Country Learning Hub for Immunization Equity in Bangladesh: Findings from Rapid Assessment Bangladesh" [17].

Table 1. Data sources used to conduct triangulation analyses in Bangladesh. Summary of data sources identified in Bangladesh to assess immunization program performance, identify immunity gaps, and assess immunization-program target-population estimates.

Data Source	Dataset Types
Global-population estimates	• World Population Projection (UNDP) [18]
Immunization-program target-population estimates based on census	• M.G.S. Uddin 2014 census projection (commissioned for National EPI program) • G. Feeney 2017 revised census projection (commissioned for National EPI program)
Immunization-program target-population estimates based on microplan	• EPI Annual Microplans (2012–2018)
Civil Registration and Vital Statistics	• Birth and Death Registration Information System (BDRIS), including Civil Registration and Vital Statistics (CRVS)
Bureau of Statistics Data	• BBS Census Projections (2011–2061) [19] • Sample Registration and Vital Statistics Surveys (annual)
Vaccine Stock and Supply	• Stock/supply (vials used, received, and available) • Wastage

Table 1. Cont.

Data Source	Dataset Types
Program Management	• Vaccination sessions held (variable in DHIS2) • Human resources • Stockouts
Vaccination Coverage	• EPI administrative coverage • WHO UNICEF Estimates of National Immunization Coverage (WUENIC) [20] • Coverage surveys, e.g., Demographic Health Surveys, Multiple Indicator Cluster Surveys (MICS), or others • SIA administrative coverage and post-campaign surveys
Surveillance	• Case-based and laboratory databases • Aggregate (passive) reporting systems, e.g., DHIS2 • Disease incidence reported to the Joint Reporting Form (JRF) [21]
Contextual Information	• Vaccination schedule and history of any changes (e.g., vaccine intro) • Major geo-political events (e.g., insecurity, mass migrations, and disasters)
Other data on population immunity or disease burden	• Serosurveys • Modeled estimates of coverage, population immunity, or disease burden

Table 2. Triangulation analyses conducted by Bangladesh to identify communities with ZD and UI children. List of Bangladesh's priority indicators used to identify immunity gaps in 2018 and ZD/UI children in 2022 [12,17].

Analyses Performed to Identify Immunity Gaps	Analyses Performed to Assess Zero-Dose and Under-Immunized Children
• Comparison of administrative coverage, WUENIC, and coverage surveys • Trends in vaccination coverage or immunity by age group/birth cohort • Geographic trends in vaccination coverage across different data sources • Surveillance performance and reported cases/outbreaks at the subnational level • Comparison of vaccination coverage and surveillance data • Measles epidemiology (age and vaccination status of cases) • Immunity gaps in special populations • Outbreaks, vaccine stock, and other contextual information • Vaccination coverage surveys • Serosurveys • Modeling studies	• Ranking of percent ZD (%) for top 10 districts and top 5 urban city corporations (CC) for 2014, 2015, 2016, and 2019 coverage surveys (calculated using DTPcv1 coverage) • Ranking of percent ZD (%) using DHIS2 EPI administrative data from 2019 to 2022 to identify the top 10 health facilities • Comparison of DHIS2 EPI administrative data with monthly EPI reports and microplan target-population estimates of top 10 health facilities with the highest percent ZD • Lot quality assurance sampling (LQAS) to confirm the clusters with a high percentage (>10%) of ZD or UI children according to survey data and DHIS2 data analyses

3.1.3. Approach to Capacity Building

To build triangulation capacity in the country, a final workshop was conducted in December 2019 to present the triangulation findings, provide recommendations based on the findings, and train national and subnational immunization program staff on triangulation methodology. An additional training workshop was conducted for district-level WHO consultants serving as Surveillance and Immunization Medical Officers (SIMOs) to build capacity for frequent and potentially automated analyses of key triangulation indicators related to identifying immunity gaps (see Table 2). The SIMO training included a hands-on workshop that allowed SIMOs to conduct triangulation analyses within DHIS2 by using available data sources within their assigned districts, including immunization coverage and VPD Surveillance. SIMOs were able to disaggregate triangulation indicators by health facility, ultimately identifying data quality issues and potential immunity gaps requiring follow-up in the field. The Bangladesh exercise was paramount in developing and finalizing the global triangulation guidance, which has since been published [12].

3.1.4. Successes and Demonstrated Potential Impact

WHO Bangladesh and the Ministry of Health used recommendations from the final triangulation workshop in 2019 to inform Bangladesh's National Data Improvement Plan required by Gavi, the Vaccine Alliance (Gavi). The following activities were incorporated into their 2019 plan: data triangulation-capacity building for SIMOs, revision of the 2020 microplan guidance for establishing district- and health facility-level target-population estimates, and development of DHIS2 triangulation dashboards to enhance supportive supervision [16].

As a follow-up to the triangulation analyses used to identify communities with the highest number of zero-dose and under-immunized children in 2022, rapid community assessments were conducted to better understand the reason why vaccine doses were not given or missed. A rapid community assessment (RCA) is a process for quickly triangulating existing data to identify missed communities with ZD and UI children. The RCAs also collected vaccination demand-and-supply barrier data, identifiable challenges of ZD and UI children in these communities, and stakeholders' suggestions to reduce ZD and UI children. Targeted interventions were then developed as part of the RCAs to reach these children (Figure 1) [17].

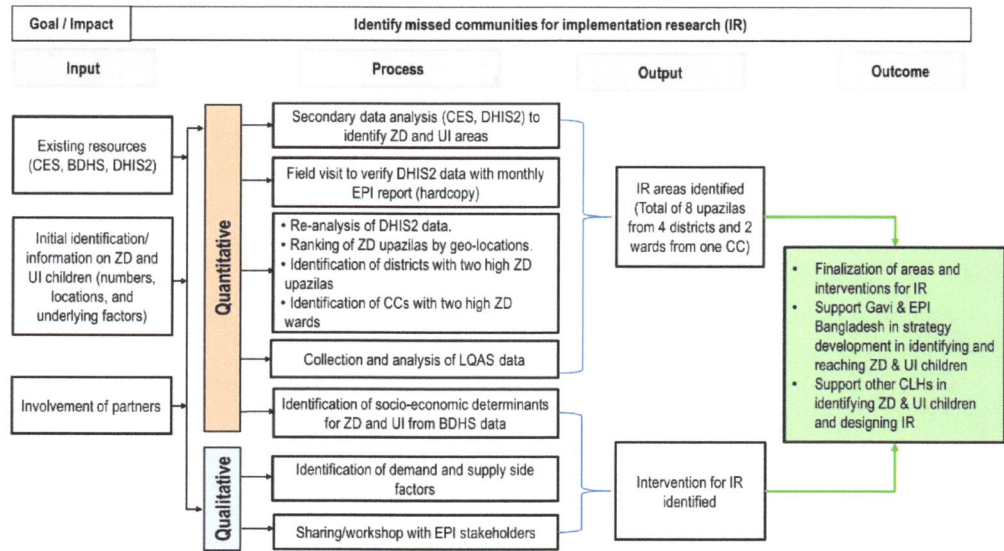

Figure 1. Conceptual framework for the rapid assessment of zero-dose (ZD) and under-immunized (UI) children. The RCA conceptual framework is used for quickly triangulating existing data to identify missed communities and develop more targeted interventions to reach ZD and UI children. Triangulation is an integral part of the quantitative methodology used to identify areas in which to conduct RCAs, with qualitative information also used to develop strategies for identifying and reaching ZD and UI children [17]. Acronyms: BDHS, Bangladesh Demographic and Health Survey; CC, city corporation; CES, Coverage Evaluation Survey; EPI, Expanded Programme on Immunization; IR, implementation research; CLH, Country Learning Hub.

The RCAs were conducted between December 2022 and May 2023 in the missed communities identified through the triangulation of the Coverage Evaluation Survey (CES) and DHIS2 administrative immunization-coverage data. The RCAs identified five rural districts and one urban (city corporation) with zero-dose, under-immunized, and missed communities by utilizing the triangulation indicators listed in Table 2. Findings from the missed communities with high zero-dose and under-immunized children confirmed that the initially identified areas were mainly inhabited by those who lacked access to educational institutions and health centers. The transportation system and household condition of these areas were also inadequate. The most common profession for the head-of-households in these clusters was farmer, followed by service professional, except for the urban clusters where most residents were day laborers [17]. This information, which was identified through the data triangulation process and RCAs, can be used to inform more targeted interventions to reach these communities, such as Friday, evening, or holiday vaccination sessions to reach the children of working mothers or transportation-cost reimbursement for healthcare workers to conduct outreach.

3.2. Rwanda

3.2.1. Project Conceptualization and Partnerships

In 2022, the Rwanda Biomedical Centre (RBC), with funding and technical support from the U.S. CDC, designed a live web-based DHIS2 RI and VPDS data triangulation dashboard. The triangulation dashboard aimed to streamline the integration of data from DHIS2 EPI and VPD Surveillance packages to assess program performance and investigate immunity gaps in Rwanda. The RBC provided leadership on the implementation of data triangulation processes and data and dashboard management, with backend development performed by the Health Information System Programme (HISP) of Rwanda, a global organization supporting DHIS2 implementation. Other technical partners included WHO Rwanda and the University of Oslo (UiO), with further support and coordination from the African Field Epidemiology Network (AFENET).

3.2.2. Approach to Triangulation Processes and Indicator Prioritization

Dashboard customization occurred from November 2022 to July 2023 using an online, publicly available global triangulation dashboard protype designed by UiO in collaboration with the U.S. CDC and WHO [22]. Customization began with mapping the existing DHIS2 data packages for VPDS and RI, including aggregate Integrated Disease Surveillance and Response (IDSR), case-based (individual level) VPDS data, and EPI Electronic Immunization Registry (aggregate and individual).

RBC then adapted key VPDS and RI program indicators to be used for monitoring program performance and immunity gaps for measles, polio, and neonatal tetanus, following the established guidance in the WHO, UNICEF, and U.S. CDC publication, *Triangulation for Improved Decision-Making in Immunization Programmes* [12]. A workshop was held with key national-, provincial-, and district-level stakeholders to prioritize specific indicators that could be compared or analyzed together to provide greater insight into immunization program performance and immunity gaps, at what administrative level this data triangulation process should occur, and what the review processes should look like.

Custom scripts were designed to allow the exchange of data between VPDS and Electronic Immunization Registry data packages (Figure 2). Data elements from the different modules were used to create indicators and design programmatically informative dashboard visualizations. The dashboard underwent external review by global and national stakeholders during May–June 2023. The beta version of the dashboard was deployed at the national level for use by the surveillance and immunization programs in July 2023, with wider dissemination to thirteen districts in October 2023.

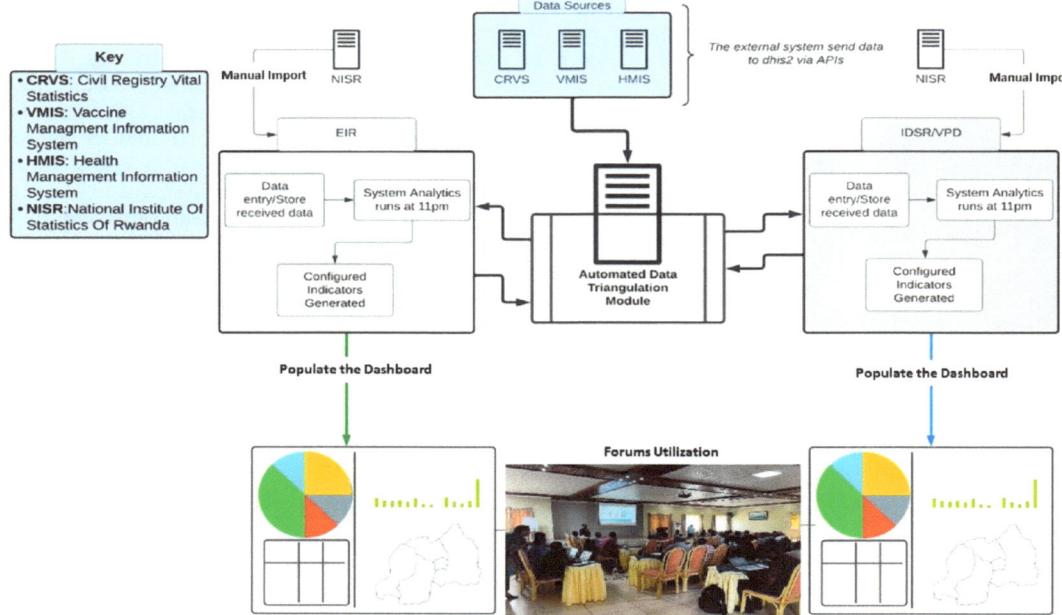

Figure 2. Approach to the triangulation of RI and VPDS data sources in Rwanda. Diagram showing the approach to the triangulation of routine immunization (RI) Electronic Immunization Registry (EIR), and Integrated Disease Surveillance and Response (IDSR)/case-based vaccine preventable disease surveillance (VPDS) data sources within Rwanda's health management information system (HMIS) and external data sources utilized by Rwanda. Integration of the Laboratory Information System (LIS), electronic Civil Registration and Vital Statistics (CRVS), and Vaccine Logistics Management Information System (vLMIS) datasets into the triangulation dashboard is ongoing [23].

A total of 14 immunity-gap and 11 program-performance indicators were ultimately included in the dashboard. Dashboard indicators were designed to permit the disaggregation of data across healthcare administrative levels (e.g., national-level data could be further disaggregated to the district and health-facility levels) and by time (e.g., yearly versus monthly) to tailor indicators to different user levels and data analysis needs.

Key triangulation indicators for the identification of immunity gaps included the vaccination status of VPD cases (including measles and rubella, acute flaccid paralysis (AFP; poliomyelitis), and neonatal tetanus) by age and vaccine eligibility, vaccination dropout rates (e.g., the proportion of infants who begin the vaccination schedule but fail to complete it) for MR, polio and DTP vaccinations, and the number of zero-dose and under-immunized children by administrative level each month.

For immunization program performance, prioritized indicators included the numbers of measles and rubella, AFP, and neonatal tetanus cases reported in the aggregate IDSR system compared to the individual-level, case-based surveillance reporting system. Combining multiple data sources with different aggregation levels in one visualization can facilitate easier identification of data quality issues and issues with reporting. Additional indicators included the access to and utilization of immunization services by district, monthly. Figure 3 shows one of these program-performance visualizations: DTP1 coverage (signifying immunization service access issues) versus DTP1-DTP3 dropout rate (a high rate is indicative of many individuals not utilizing the immunization services offered) by district in Rwanda.

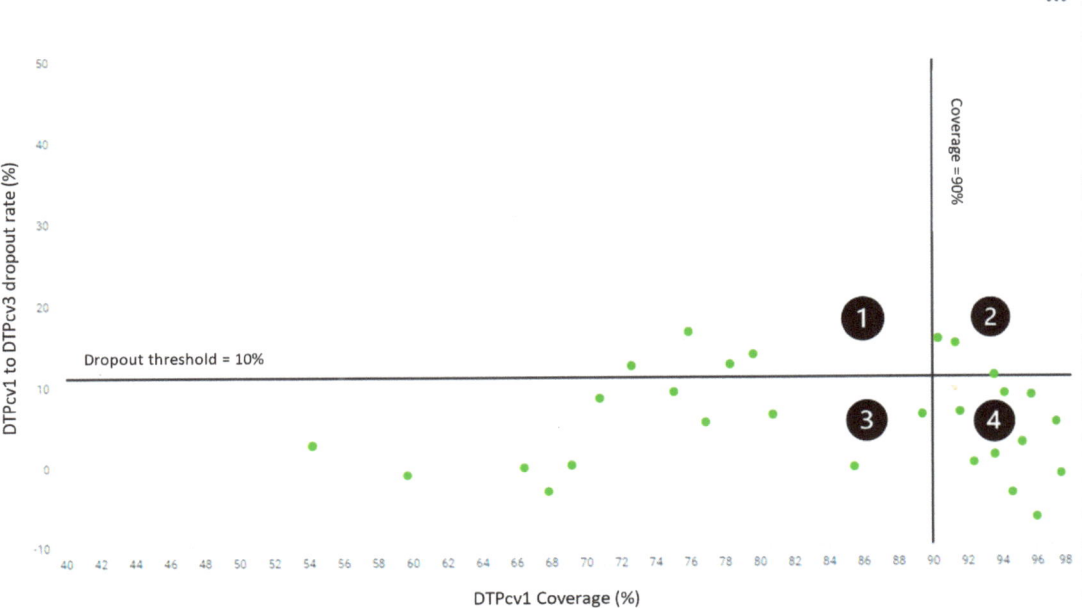

Figure 3. Scatter plot of monthly DTPcv1 coverage (%) versus DTPcv1-DTPcv3 dropout rate by district in Rwanda. (**1**) Low DTPcv1 coverage (<90%) and high dropout (>10%) = access and utilization issues. (**2**) High DTPcv1 coverage but high dropout = utilization issues. (**3**) Low DTPcv1 coverage but low dropout = access issues. (**4**) High DTPcv1 coverage and low dropout = No access and utilization issues. Each green dot is representative of a district in Rwanda.

3.2.3. Approach to Capacity Building

National and international VPDS, immunization, and Health Management Information System (HMIS) experts conducted a series of three-to-five-day data triangulation workshops between July and September 2023, at both national and district levels to promote a clear understanding and effective use of the DHIS2 triangulation dashboard. The training curriculum consisted of didactic materials, including presentations on the basics of data triangulation and triangulation for identifying immunity gaps and program performance challenges, as well as case studies and live demonstrations of the dashboard. Thirty-eight HMIS data managers, IDSR focal persons, and EPI supervisors from 14 of Rwanda's 30 districts participated in these initial workshops (at the time of the training, only these 14 districts were utilizing the DHIS2 case-based module for VPDS). Real-time anonymous feedback was collected during workshops to assess the comprehension of the materials and the usefulness of the dashboard, as well as offer suggestions for improvement and use. In April 2024, mentorship sessions were conducted in the 14 trained districts. Mentors held discussions with district staff, and questionnaires were used to gather feedback regarding their usage frequency and experience with using the dashboard, and examine how the dashboard had assisted in addressing programmatic queries. According to the questionnaire, 43% of surveyed staff reported actively using the dashboard, with 21% reporting weekly use. However, the remainder of those surveyed reported that they were not actively utilizing the dashboard, primarily attributing this to a general lack of understanding of how to interpret dashboard indicators. Based on the user feedback received, a triangulation dashboard self-study guide was created to guide users through dashboard indicators, clarify meanings in their specific context, identify and record data quality issues and immunity gaps, and propose and track corrective actions.

3.2.4. Successes and Demonstrated Potential for Impact

Multiple efforts have been made to improve our understanding and utilization of the DHIS2 data triangulation dashboard through national and subnational workshops and feedback-gathering sessions. One achievement has been the establishment of the Rwanda Immunization Data Technical Working Group (TWG). The TWG provides a forum for HMIS, immunization, and VPD Surveillance representatives from the national, provincial, and district levels to discuss current activities and issues around immunization-related data collection, entry, and analysis and the use of the DHIS2 immunization data triangulation dashboard. Examples of observations made by the TWG using the triangulation dashboard include the identification of the immunization status of measles cases by age group and geographic location during a measles outbreak, indicating which groups to target for vaccination, and multiple data quality discrepancies between case-based and aggregate VPD Surveillance reporting systems for measles. Additional plans by the TWG to ensure the use of the dashboard at the subnational level include incorporating dashboard reviews into supportive supervision and mentorship visits and monthly meetings between Provincial Health Emergency Operation Centers and District hospitals.

3.3. Nigeria

3.3.1. Project Conceptualization and Partnerships

Nigeria's National Primary Health Care Development Agency (NPHCDA) manages the EPI program, and RI data are reported through DHIS2. The national DHIS2 platform is hosted by the Federal Ministry of Health (FMOH). Comparably, the Surveillance Outbreak Response Management and Analysis System (SORMAS) platform, managed by the National Centre for Disease Control (NCDC), is used to report VPDS data. The reporting of immunization and surveillance data through multiple siloed systems and to different responsible agencies has contributed to a lack of data access, sharing, coordination, and use in Nigeria. In 2019, recognizing the need for improved data integration and use, NPHCDA, NCDC, and AFENET staff developed a data triangulation dashboard leveraging the U.S. CDC Growing Expertise in E-Health Knowledge and Skills (GEEKS) traineeship program [24]. The primary objective of the dashboard was to collate, analyze, and visualize RI and VPD Surveillance data from the DHIS2 and SORMAS platforms. Additional technical partners included the HISP of Nigeria, and NIX Technologies—an Information and Communications Technology (ICT) organization that supports NCDC in managing the SORMAS system in Nigeria.

3.3.2. Approach to Triangulation Processes and Indicator Prioritization

A data-mapping exercise was conducted to identify the existing data elements and indicators in the DHIS2 and SORMAS RI and VPDS platforms. During the data-mapping process, indicator calculations, the administrative levels of data collection and use, and the frequency of reporting were reviewed. Stakeholders also reviewed performance indicators extracted from the WHO, UNICEF, and U.S. CDC guidelines on *Triangulation for Improved Decision-Making in Immunization Programmes* [12]. Stakeholders from FMOH, NPHCDA, NCDC, and AFENET created a prioritized list of indicators, analyses, and visualizations to incorporate into the triangulation dashboard. Indicator prioritization was guided by key program issues and relevant questions identified by stakeholders. Based on the programmatic issues identified, immunization coverage reports from multiple survey data conducted since 2013 were also included in the dashboard configuration. The results of the indicator prioritization activity, including the data sources and visualizations initially selected for inclusion in the triangulation dashboard, are shown in Table 3.

Table 3. Triangulation analyses conducted to identify program performance and immunity gaps in Nigeria. Prioritized indicators, data sources, and visualizations included in Nigeria's RI and VPDS data triangulation dashboard.

Indicator	Visualization	Disease	Data Source
Confirmed cases versus admin coverage	Combo chart	Measles/yellow fever/meningitis	DHIS2 and SORMAS
Age group of confirmed cases by vaccination status	Stacked column chart	Measles/yellow fever/meningitis	SORMAS
Vaccine stock analysis and admin coverage	Combo chart	Measles/yellow fever/meningitis	DHIS2
Dropout rate	Combo chart	Measles	DHIS2
Discrepancy between co-administered vaccine doses	Combo chart	Measles/yellow fever/meningitis	DHIS2
Confirmed versus admin coverage	Map	Measles/yellow fever/meningitis	DHIS2 and SORMAS
National measles coverage by different data sources	Combo chart	Measles/yellow fever/meningitis	DHIS2, SORMAS, WHO/UNICEF estimates of national immunization coverage (WUENIC), Standardized Monitoring and Assessment of Relief and Transitions (SMART), Nigeria Demographic and Health Survey (NDHS), Multiple Indicator Cluster Survey (MICS)/National Immunization Coverage Survey (NICS)

The dashboard was configured for four VPDs (measles, yellow fever, meningitis, and diphtheria). The selected indicators were visualized on a web-based dashboard developed using R, R Shiny, Python, and JavaScript (see Figure 4). The dashboard was integrated into the national SORMAS platform and stored in a cloud-based Structured Query Language (SQL) database.

3.3.3. Approach to Capacity Building

The RI/VPDS triangulation dashboard was designed and implemented through the GEEKS Nigeria traineeship program [19]. A one-week onboarding training was provided to all GEEKS fellows, followed by a 12-month dashboard design, customization, and implementation period. Regular mentorship sessions were held bi-weekly between mentors and fellows to build the capacity for data triangulation and on the use of DHIS2, SORMAS, R, Microsoft Suites, and additional relevant areas of data and project management.

3.3.4. Successes and Demonstrated Potential for Impact

Several initiatives have been undertaken to ensure the ongoing use of the RI and VPDS dashboard at both the national and subnational levels in Nigeria. The dashboard has been integrated into SORMAS, and efforts are currently ongoing to embed it within the national DHIS2 platform, meaning that RI and surveillance staff at the national and subnational levels are able to access the dashboard and make use of the data for decision-making. A national TWG has also been established for NPHCDA and NCDC staff to review the dashboard monthly. Additionally, the dashboard has been implemented in two states in Nigeria (Yobe and Jigawa), where it is reviewed by subnational RI and surveillance staff during monthly TWGs to guide programmatic decision-making. Several actions taken by the national TWG based on these triangulated data have included the provision of feedback to state and local government areas (LGAs) on MCV-coverage data quality issues, the identification of geographical areas with measles outbreaks to support more targeted outbreak response and vaccination activities, and the identification of LGAs in need of supportive supervision.

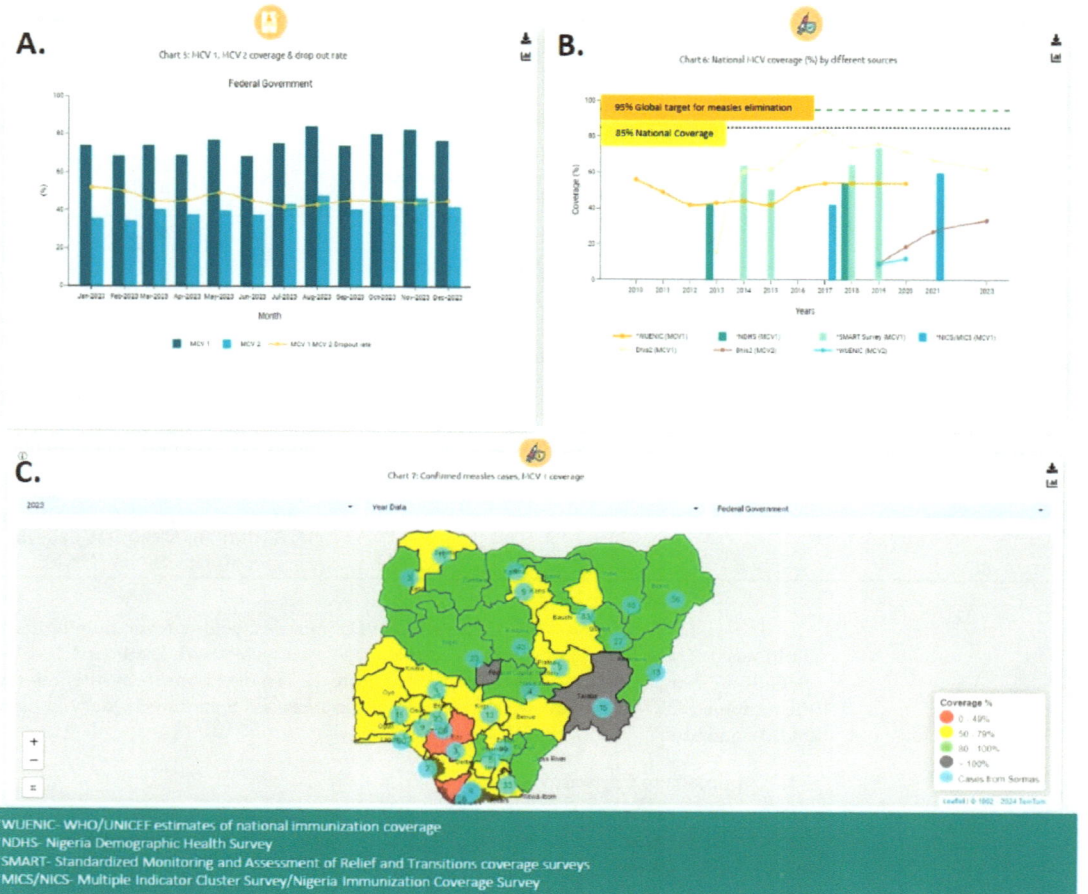

Figure 4. Screenshot displaying Nigeria's R Shiny dashboard for DHIS2 RI, VPD Surveillance data from SORMAS, and vaccination coverage survey data. (**A**) Measles-containing vaccine first-dose (MCV1) and second-dose (MCV2) coverage and dropout rate. (**B**) MCV1 and MCV2 coverage by different data sources between 2010 and 2023 (administrative coverage, Nigeria Demographic Health Survey (NDHS), Multiple Indicator Cluster Survey/Nigeria Immunization Coverage Survey (MICS/NICS), Standardized Monitoring and Assessment of Relief and Transitions (SMART) coverage surveys, and WHO/UNICEF estimates of national immunization coverage (WUENIC)). (**C**) Maps of measles cases verses MCV1 coverage by state.

4. Discussion

If the IA2030 targets to reduce the number of zero-dose children are to be met, immunization programs need to be able to accurately identify those children and take appropriate action [1,4,9,11,25]. In the context of immunization programs, greater data use can result in better quality data and ultimately contribute to improved program performance by better identifying and targeting those who are eligible for vaccination [2,12,26,27].

Here, we described how three countries have taken a data-driven approach to identify immunization coverage inequities and program performance challenges by using triangulation analyses and dashboards for identifying DTPcv, polio, and MCV immunization coverage gaps at all levels of the healthcare system. Even in the absence of perfect data, combining many parts of less robust evidence through triangulation can provide a strong basis for more informed decision-making.

5. Lessons Learned and Recommendations

To further strengthen the use of data triangulation for improving health equity in immunization and VPDS programs, we provide several lessons learned and recommendations based on findings from our four a priori themes.

5.1. Early Engagement and Ongoing Coordination across Programs and Stakeholders at Each Level Is Critical

Since the success of triangulation is contingent on access to and use of many data sources, a high degree of cooperation and buy-in are required from multiple institutions and stakeholders. Triangulation is most effective when stakeholders are involved at all stages, including prioritizing the questions to be answered, identifying the data sources, guiding the analysis and interpretation, and using the results for decision-making in their policies and programs. Collective engagement from national and subnational immunization, VPDS, and HMIS staff early in the development process will help to promote the cross-program prioritization of triangulation indicators and integration into existing program activities to ensure ongoing use and prevent any additional burden on health staff.

5.2. Establish Regular Processes for Reviewing and Using Triangulated Data

Having regular processes and accountability mechanisms in place that support data access, quality, interoperability, and use is important for establishing useful triangulation analyses. In all three countries, establishing triangulation processes with imperfect data allowed stakeholders to work collaboratively and increase their comfort and capacity to use triangulated data to develop targeted interventions and corrective actions. Creating a strong "data-use culture" from the local to the national level can result in better-quality data and ultimately contribute to improved immunization program performance.

5.3. Continued Capacity Building for Triangulation Analysis and Use for Action Are Needed at All Levels, Even after Electronic Tools and Processes Are Established

Dashboards and tools cannot perform all the triangulation analyses and interpretation for the end-user. Data use and critical thinking are required for staff to synthesize and contextualize data into actionable recommendations. Ongoing capacity building for triangulation analysis and data use beyond trainings are required, such as incorporating dashboard reviews into supportive supervision visits, regular review meetings at national and subnational levels, and other accountability mechanisms. These will help to equip both national and subnational staff with the skills they need to make decisions and take actions based on analyses and interpretations to vaccinate under-immunized communities and reach zero-dose children.

5.4. The Greatest Successes and Impact Occur When There Is Collaboration and Utilization of Triangulated Data by Health Staff and Policymakers across Programs and Healthcare Levels

While Bangladesh, Nigeria, and Rwanda were able to conduct data triangulation analyses, develop dashboards, and integrate multiple data sources, the greatest successes were due to the collaboration and utilization of information by health staff and policymakers across programs and healthcare levels. In Rwanda and Nigeria, immunization and VPDS data-use working groups were established to further promote the use of data across stakeholders and programs in order to best address and support targeted vaccination-response activities and areas in need of supportive supervision. In Bangladesh, triangulation was used to identify missed communities with high zero-dose and under-immunized children, which led to targeted rapid convenience assessments to identify barriers to reaching them so that effective and targeted interventions could be developed. To further optimize the impact, triangulation analyses and interpretation could be included in existing regular periodic activities where analysis is already performed, such as monthly data-review meetings, annual desk reviews, National Immunization Technical Advisory Group (NITAG) meetings, or National Committees for certifying polio eradication or verifying measles and rubella elimination.

6. Considerations and Limitations

This manuscript describes data triangulation processes in only three countries. The results are not generalizable to all settings and unique country challenges. Apart from the limited capacity for conducting and interpreting triangulation analyses, many reasons may exist for not effectively using data, from data-access challenges to the lack of a supportive "data-use culture". Triangulation is not a singular solution to these larger problems. However, actions increasing data access, use, and understanding may lead to gradual improvements over time.

Additionally, it is important to consider local knowledge and contextual information to further interpret the available data, including explanatory causes, and develop targeted program-improvement efforts. Unexpected or contradictory findings may emerge. However, local and contextual knowledge can provide additional insights into the reasons behind data discrepancies or conflicting evidence, leading to a more nuanced understanding of the programmatic question.

Lastly, since no formal assessments or evaluations of RI and VPDS triangulation activities have been conducted in these three countries since triangulation tools and processes have been established, it is not yet possible to measure the extent to which their implementation has directly impacted data use and quality, or how triangulated data have been used for programmatic action. Such evaluations to measure data triangulation outcomes and document impact more formally are needed.

7. Future Directions and Needs

Additional initiatives to support WHO Regional Offices and countries at both the national and subnational levels to incorporate triangulation sessions and experience-sharing into existing data workshops and trainings are needed. These should involve stakeholders across multiple programs where possible (e.g., immunization, surveillance, HMIS, national statistics offices, birth/civil registration offices, and other relevant organizations) which would help to promote immunization program coordination. It is critical that any new data triangulation initiatives for identifying zero-dose and under-immunized children be integrated with larger, multi-sectoral efforts to improve overall immunization performance.

Likewise, an increasing number of low- and middle-income countries are leveraging the availability of new electronic information technologies for immunization and VPDS data management, including electronic immunization registries (EIRs), electronic Logistics Management Information Systems (eLMISs), and the DHIS2 VPD CBS package, which have the potential to improve the quality, timeliness, and use of data [2,28–30]. However, these new electronic systems are not magic solutions to more systemic problems, and they are unlikely to lead to lasting programmatic improvements unless other factors are considered, such as infrastructure, strong national governance and coordination, and workforce capacity [29,30]. Additionally, the integration and interoperability of newly introduced systems are crucial to ensuring that all available data can be leveraged. By enhancing integration and interoperability, the exchange, access, and utilization of data can be significantly improved. Additional efforts to support the interoperability between data systems for easier triangulation analyses and integration of these systems, such as VPD CBS with laboratory information systems, will be critical. At the country-level, planning across programs to ensure the integration and interoperability of any newly introduced tools within the existing information system should also be prioritized.

8. Conclusions

In order to address inequities in immunization coverage and protect zero-dose and under-immunized children against VPDs, sustainable improvements in data quality and use are needed at all levels. Here, we described how data triangulation was used by three countries to identify immunity gaps, detect zero-dose and under-immunized children, and assess program performance at all levels of the healthcare system. Triangulation methodologies and processes, as well as lessons learned, may be leveraged by different country contexts and incorporated into routine RI and VPDS data analyses, potentially leading to programmatic changes that promote improved access to vaccination services.

Author Contributions: Conceptualization, A.R., O.J.A., E.S., E.L., C.S.M., and A.M.P.; methodology, A.R., O.J.A., E.S., A.M.P., E.L., and C.S.M.; software, A.R., O.J.A., and A.M.P.; validation, A.R., O.J.A., and A.M.P.; formal analysis, A.R., O.J.A., and A.M.P.; investigation, A.R., O.J.A., and A.M.P.; resources, A.R., O.J.A., E.S., E.L., C.S.M., and A.M.P.; data curation, R.B., E.R., H.S., A.K., I.I., S.R., B.M.M., N.M.R., R.U.O., A.U.A., and O.B.A.; writing—original draft preparation, A.R., O.J.A., E.L., C.S.M., and A.M.P.; writing—review and editing, E.S., E.L., C.S.M., R.B., E.R., H.S., A.K., I.I., S.R., B.M.M., N.M.R., R.U.O., A.U.A., and O.B.A.; visualization, A.R., O.J.A., A.M.P., R.B., E.R., H.S., A.K., I.I., S.R., B.M.M., N.M.R., R.U.O., A.U.A., and O.B.A.; supervision, A.R., O.J.A., E.L., C.S.M., and A.M.P.; project administration, A.R., O.J.A., E.L., C.S.M., A.M.P., S.R., R.B., and O.B.A.; funding acquisition, A.R., O.J.A., E.L., C.S.M., and A.M.P. All authors have read and agreed to the published version of the manuscript.

Funding: Data triangulation projects and this work were funded by the U.S. Centers for Disease Control and Prevention.

Institutional Review Board Statement: This activity was reviewed by CDC and was conducted consistent with applicable federal law and CDC policy (45 C.F.R. part 46.102(l)(2), 21 C.F.R. part 56; 42 U.S.C. 145 Sect. 241(d); 5 U.S.C. Sect. 552a; 44 U.S.C. Sect. 3501 et seq). Triangulation projects in each country were additionally reviewed and approved by the relevant Ministries of Health.

Informed Consent Statement: Not applicable.

Data Availability Statement: No new data were created as part of this report. Data sharing is not applicable to this article.

Acknowledgments: We would like to thank the Ministries of Health of Bangladesh, Rwanda, and Nigeria; all country staff who supported this work; and the WHO Geneva staff, who supported the development of the immunization triangulation global guidance. We are also grateful to Heather Scobie and Michelle Morales for their significant contribution to the triangulation global guidance.

Conflicts of Interest: The authors declare no conflict of interest. The findings and conclusions in this report are those of the authors and do not necessarily represent the official position of the U.S. Centers for Disease Control and Prevention or any institutions they are affiliated with.

References

1. World Health Organization. Immunization Agenda 2030: A Global Strategy to Leave No One Behind. 2020. Available online: https://www.who.int/publications/m/item/immunization-agenda-2030-a-global-strategy-to-leave-no-one-behind (accessed on 18 January 2024).
2. Scobie, H.M.; Edelstein, M.; Nicol, E.; Morice, A.; Rahimi, N.; MacDonald, N.E.; Danovaro-Holliday, M.C.; Jawad, J. Improving the quality and use of immunization and surveillance data: Summary report of the Working Group of the Strategic Advisory Group of Experts on Immunization. *Vaccine* **2020**, *38*, 7183–7197. [CrossRef]
3. World Health Organization. Meeting of the Strategic Advisory Group of Experts on Immunization, April 2019—Conclusions and Recommendations. *Wkly. Epidemiol. Rec.* **2019**, *94*, 261–280. Available online: https://www.who.int/publications/i/item/WER9422 (accessed on 22 January 2024).
4. United Nations. *The Sustainable Development Goals Report 2016*; United Nations: New York, NY, USA, 2016. Available online: https://desapublications.un.org/publications/sustainable-development-goals-report-2016 (accessed on 20 February 2024).
5. World Health Organization. *Universal Health Coverage (UHC)*; World Health Organization: Geneva, Switzerland, 2014. Available online: https://www.who.int/data/monitoring-universal-health-coverage (accessed on 24 February 2024).

6. U.S. Centers for Disease Control and Prevention. *Global Health Equity Strategy 2022–2027*; U.S. Centers for Disease Control and Prevention: Atlanta, GA, USA, 2022. Available online: https://www.cdc.gov/global-health-equity/media/pdfs/ghe_strategy_2022_2027.pdf (accessed on 26 February 2024).
7. Kaur, G. Routine Vaccination Coverage—Worldwide, 2022. *MMWR Morb. Mortal. Wkly. Rep.* **2023**, *72*, 1155–1161. [CrossRef] [PubMed]
8. Rachlin, A.; Danovaro-Holliday, M.C.; Murphy, P.; Sodha, S.V.; Wallace, A.S. Routine Vaccination Coverage—Worldwide, 2021. *Morb. Mortal. Wkly. Rep.* **2022**, *71*, 1396. [CrossRef]
9. Hogan, D.; Gupta, A. Why Reaching Zero-Dose Children Holds the Key to Achieving the Sustainable Development Goals. *Vaccines* **2023**, *11*, 781. [CrossRef] [PubMed]
10. Hosseinpoor, A.R.; Bergen, N.; Schlotheuber, A.; Grove, J. Measuring health inequalities in the context of sustainable development goals. *Bull. World Health Organ.* **2018**, *96*, 654. [CrossRef] [PubMed]
11. Gavi, the Vaccine Alliance. The Zero-Dose Child: Explained. 2021. Available online: https://www.gavi.org/vaccineswork/zero-dose-child-explained (accessed on 11 February 2024).
12. World Health Organization; U.S Centers for Disease Control and Prevention. Triangulation for Improved Decision-Making in Immunization Programmes 2020. 2022. Available online: https://www.technet-21.org/media/com_resources/trl/6616/multi_upload/0_Triangulation_CoverOrientation_DRAFT_27Jul2020.pdf (accessed on 28 February 2024).
13. World Health Organization; UNAIDS; Global Fund to Fight AIDS, Tuberculosis and Malaria. HIV Triangulation Resource Guide: Synthesis of Results from Multiple Data Sources for Evaluation and Decision-Making. 2009. Available online: https://iris.who.int/handle/10665/44107 (accessed on 12 February 2024).
14. Rutherford, G.W.; McFarland, W.; Spindler, H.; White, K.; Patel, S.V.; Aberle-Grasse, J.; Sabin, K.; Smith, N.; Taché, S.; Calleja-Garcia, J.M.; et al. Public health triangulation: Approach and application to synthesizing data to understand national and local HIV epidemics. *BMC Public Health* **2010**, *10*, 447. [CrossRef] [PubMed]
15. Denzin, N.K. *Sociological Methods: A Sourcebook*; Routledge: London, UK, 2017. [CrossRef]
16. Bangladesh Expanded Programme on Immunization. *Data Improvement Plan 2022–2025*; Bangladesh Expanded Programme on Immunization: Dhaka, Bangladesh, 2022.
17. Chowdhury, M.E.A.N.; Sarker, B.K.; Das, H.; Shiblee, S.I.; Jannat, Z.; Rahman, M.; Ali, M.W.; Rahman, M.M.; Rahim, M.A.; Oliveras, E.; et al. Country Learning Hub for Immunization Equity in Bangladesh: Findings from Rapid Assessment Bangladesh. 2023. Available online: https://zdlh.gavi.org/resources/country-learning-hub-immunization-equity-bangladesh-findings-rapid-assessment (accessed on 24 February 2024).
18. United Nations. World Population Prospects 2022: United Nations, Department of International, Economic and Social Affairs. 2022. Available online: https://population.un.org/wpp/ (accessed on 21 March 2024).
19. Bangladesh Bureau of Statistics. Bangladesh Statistics 2020. Statistics and Informatics Division, Ministry of Planning, 2020. Available online: https://bbs.portal.gov.bd/sites/default/files/files/bbs.portal.gov.bd/page/a1d32f13_8553_44f1_92e6_8ff80a4ff82e/2021-06-30-09-23-c9a2750523d19681aecfd3072922fa2c.pdf (accessed on 19 March 2024).
20. World Health Organization. *WHO/UNICEF Estimates of National Immunization Coverage*; WHO: Geneva, Switzerland, 2022. Available online: https://www.who.int/news-room/questions-and-answers/item/who-unicef-estimates-of-national-immunization-coverage (accessed on 22 March 2024).
21. World Health Organization. *WHO/UNICEF Joint Reporting Process*; WHO: Geneva, Switzerland. Available online: https://www.who.int/teams/immunization-vaccines-and-biologicals/immunization-analysis-and-insights/global-monitoring/who-unicef-joint-reporting-process (accessed on 28 May 2024).
22. University of Oslo. DHIS2 Documentation: Immunization Triangulation Dashboard. 2022. Available online: https://docs.dhis2.org/en/implement/health/immunization/immunization-triangulation-dashboard/design.html (accessed on 18 January 2024).
23. DHIS2 Data Triangulation for Immunization and Vaccine Preventable Diseases: A Roadmap for Implementation and Early Findings. In Proceedings of the DHIS2 Annual Conference, Oslo, Norway, 12-15 June 2023.
24. Rachlin, A.; Adegoke, O.J.; Sikare, E.; Adeoye, O.B.; Dagoe, E.; Adeyelu, A.; Tolentino, H.; MacGregor, J.; Obasi, S.; Adah, G.; et al. Lessons learned from early implementation of the Growing Expertise in E-health Knowledge and Skills (GEEKS) program in Nigeria, 2019–2021. *Pan Afr. Med. J.* **2023**, *46*, 81. [CrossRef]
25. Wigley, A.; Lorin, J.; Hogan, D.; Utazi, C.E.; Hagedorn, B.; Dansereau, E.; Tatem, A.J.; Tejedor-Garavito, N. Estimates of the number and distribution of zero-dose and under-immunised children across remote-rural, urban, and conflict-affected settings in low and middle-income countries. *PLoS Glob. Public Health* **2022**, *2*, e0001126. [CrossRef] [PubMed]
26. Dabbagh, A.; Eggers, R.; Cochi, S.; Dietz, V.; Strebel, P.; Cherian, T. A new global framework for immunization monitoring and surveillance. *Bull World Health Organ* **2007**, *85*, 904–905. [CrossRef]
27. The Pan American Health Organization; PATH. Immunization Data: Evidence for Action, A Realist Review of What Works to Improve Data Use for Immunization, Evidence from Low-and Middle-Income Countries Seattle: PATH. 2019. Available online: https://www3.paho.org/hq/index.php?option=com_docman&view=download&alias=48126-march-2019&category_slug=paho-articles-published-to-gin-8836&Itemid=270&lang=en (accessed on 22 February 2024).
28. Danovaro-Holliday, M.C.; Contreras, M.P.; Pinto, D.; Molina-Aguilera, I.B.; Miranda, D.; García, O.; Velandia-Gonzalez, M. Assessing electronic immunization registries: The Pan American Health Organization experience. *Rev. Panam. Salud Publica* **2019**, *43*, e28. [CrossRef] [PubMed]

29. World Health Organization. *WHO Guideline Recommendations on Digital Interventions for Health System Strengthening*; World Health Organization: Geneva, Switzerland, 2019. Available online: https://www.who.int/publications/i/item/9789241550505 (accessed on 12 February 2024).
30. World Health Organization. *Strategy for Optimizing National Routine Health Information Systems: Strengthening Routine Health Information Systems to Deliver Primary Health Care and Universal Health Coverage*; World Health Organization: Geneva, Switzerland, 2023. Available online: https://www.who.int/publications/i/item/9789240087163 (accessed on 12 February 2024).

Disclaimer/Publisher's Note: The statements, opinions and data contained in all publications are solely those of the individual author(s) and contributor(s) and not of MDPI and/or the editor(s). MDPI and/or the editor(s) disclaim responsibility for any injury to people or property resulting from any ideas, methods, instructions or products referred to in the content.

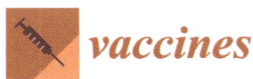

Article

Geospatial Analyses of Recent Household Surveys to Assess Changes in the Distribution of Zero-Dose Children and Their Associated Factors before and during the COVID-19 Pandemic in Nigeria

Justice Moses K. Aheto [1,2,*], Iyanuloluwa Deborah Olowe [1], Ho Man Theophilus Chan [1,3], Adachi Ekeh [4], Boubacar Dieng [5], Biyi Fafunmi [6], Hamidreza Setayesh [7], Brian Atuhaire [7], Jessica Crawford [7], Andrew J. Tatem [1] and Chigozie Edson Utazi [1,3,8]

1. WorldPop, School of Geography and Environmental Science, University of Southampton, Southampton SO17 1BJ, UK; i.d.olowe@soton.ac.uk (I.D.O.); hmtc1u18@soton.ac.uk (H.M.T.C.); a.j.tatem@soton.ac.uk (A.J.T.); c.e.utazi@soton.ac.uk (C.E.U.)
2. Department of Biostatistics, School of Public Health, College of Health Sciences, University of Ghana, Accra P.O. Box LG13, Ghana
3. School of Mathematical Sciences, University of Southampton, Southampton SO17 1BJ, UK
4. Sydani Group, Abuja, Nigeria; adachi.ekeh@sydani.org
5. Gavi, The Vaccine Alliance, Abuja, Nigeria; bdieng@gmail.com
6. National Bureau of Statistics, Abuja, Nigeria; biyifafunmi@nigerianstat.gov.ng
7. Gavi, The Vaccine Alliance, Geneva, Switzerland; hsetayesh@gmail.com (H.S.); batuhaire@gavi.org (B.A.); jcrawford@gavi.org (J.C.)
8. Department of Statistics, Nnamdi Azikiwe University, Awka PMB 5025, Nigeria
* Correspondence: j.m.k.aheto@soton.ac.uk; Tel.: +44-7551563348

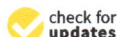

Citation: Aheto, J.M.K.; Olowe, I.D.; Chan, H.M.T.; Ekeh, A.; Dieng, B.; Fafunmi, B.; Setayesh, H.; Atuhaire, B.; Crawford, J.; Tatem, A.J.; et al. Geospatial Analyses of Recent Household Surveys to Assess Changes in the Distribution of Zero-Dose Children and Their Associated Factors before and during the COVID-19 Pandemic in Nigeria. *Vaccines* 2023, *11*, 1830. https://doi.org/10.3390/vaccines11121830

Academic Editors: Pedro Plans-Rubió, Ahmad Reza Hosseinpoor, M. Carolina Danovaro, Nicole Bergen, Devaki Nambiar, Ciara Sugerman and Hope L. Johnson

Received: 26 October 2023
Revised: 25 November 2023
Accepted: 1 December 2023
Published: 8 December 2023

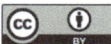

Copyright: © 2023 by the authors. Licensee MDPI, Basel, Switzerland. This article is an open access article distributed under the terms and conditions of the Creative Commons Attribution (CC BY) license (https://creativecommons.org/licenses/by/4.0/).

Abstract: The persistence of geographic inequities in vaccination coverage often evidences the presence of zero-dose and missed communities and their vulnerabilities to vaccine-preventable diseases. These inequities were exacerbated in many places during the coronavirus disease 2019 (COVID-19) pandemic, due to severe disruptions to vaccination services. Understanding changes in zero-dose prevalence and its associated risk factors in the context of the COVID-19 pandemic is, therefore, critical to designing effective strategies to reach vulnerable populations. Using data from nationally representative household surveys conducted before the COVID-19 pandemic, in 2018, and during the pandemic, in 2021, in Nigeria, we fitted Bayesian geostatistical models to map the distribution of three vaccination coverage indicators: receipt of the first dose of diphtheria-tetanus-pertussis-containing vaccine (DTP1), the first dose of measles-containing vaccine (MCV1), and any of the four basic vaccines (bacilli Calmette-Guerin (BCG), oral polio vaccine (OPV0), DTP1, and MCV1), and the corresponding zero-dose estimates independently at a 1 × 1 km resolution and the district level during both time periods. We also explored changes in the factors associated with non-vaccination at the national and regional levels using multilevel logistic regression models. Our results revealed no increases in zero-dose prevalence due to the pandemic at the national level, although considerable increases were observed in a few districts. We found substantial subnational heterogeneities in vaccination coverage and zero-dose prevalence both before and during the pandemic, showing broadly similar patterns in both time periods. Areas with relatively higher zero-dose prevalence occurred mostly in the north and a few places in the south in both time periods. We also found consistent areas of low coverage and high zero-dose prevalence using all three zero-dose indicators, revealing the areas in greatest need. At the national level, risk factors related to socioeconomic/demographic status (e.g., maternal education), maternal access to and utilization of health services, and remoteness were strongly associated with the odds of being zero dose in both time periods, while those related to communication were mostly relevant before the pandemic. These associations were also supported at the regional level, but we additionally identified risk factors specific to zero-dose children in each region; for example, communication and cross-border migration in the northwest. Our findings can help guide tailored strategies to reduce zero-dose prevalence and boost coverage levels in Nigeria.

Keywords: MCV1 coverage; DTP1 coverage; composite coverage; zero-dose prevalence; Demographic and Health Surveys; Multiple Indicator Cluster Survey; Bayesian geostatistical modelling; Bayesian multilevel modelling

1. Introduction

Vaccination is often regarded as one of the most successful and cost-effective public health interventions, saving millions of lives each year and guaranteeing global wellbeing and development [1]. Despite this, many children, especially those living in low- and middle-income countries (LMICs), continue to miss out on life-saving vaccines even though there have been increased efforts globally to improve vaccination coverage and reduce zero-dose prevalence [2]. Before the pandemic in 2019, 18.4 million children globally did not receive all three recommended doses of the DTP vaccine, and of those, 70% (12.9 million) were zero-dose children, defined as those who did not receive any dose of the DTP vaccine [2]. In 2020, these figures increased to 22 million children and 73% (16 million), respectively, due to the disruptions to immunization services caused by the coronavirus disease 2019 (COVID-19) pandemic [2–4]. These disruptions continued in 2021, resulting in 24 million being under-vaccinated and about 18 million being zero dose, with about 62% [5,6] of the estimated zero-dose children found to be living in 10 LMICs, including Nigeria. However, in 2022, a partial recovery in global DTP vaccination coverage was recorded, with the number of zero-dose children decreasing to 14.3 million, evidencing concerted efforts within countries to reach zero-dose children [2].

Zero-dose children often live in marginalized or underserved communities characterised by poverty, a lack of access to basic health services, overcrowding, poor sanitation practices, and conflict [7–10]. These characteristics, combined with other health-related, socioeconomic, demographic, and gender-related factors, cause substantial disparities in the distribution of zero-dose children within countries [8]. Reaching these at-risk populations, therefore, requires a timely and accurate evidence base regarding their sizes, geographic distribution, and other characteristics, to support country-tailored strategies and interventions. Also, with recovery from the pandemic being uneven and much slower in LMICs [11], understanding any changes in vulnerabilities due to disruptions to both routine immunization and vaccination campaigns can help with planning effective mitigation strategies and strengthening immunization services to reach zero-dose children. Administrative data are regularly collected in many LMICs through platforms such as the District Health Information System version 2 (DHIS2) [12,13]. However, due to limitations such as numerator and denominator errors (e.g., incomplete reporting, inaccurate the aggregation of numerators, and mismatches between numerator and denominator estimates due to migration and the bypassing of health facilities), these often have coverage values that cannot reliably inform spatially detailed heterogeneities in the coverage and identification of zero-dose children. Household surveys, on the other hand, tend to produce more reliable estimates of coverage, but these are usually designed to be representative at coarse spatial scales, necessitating the use of geospatial modelling approaches to produce coverage estimates at fine spatial scales and for operationally relevant areas, e.g., districts, which are then integrated with population data to assess zero-dose prevalence [14–16]. Moreover, survey questionnaires include several modules that assess different characteristics of the participants, making the data ideal for evaluating correlates of non-vaccination to further inform targeted interventions. Undoubtedly, addressing zero-dose prevalence is critical to achieving the WHO's Immunisation Agenda 2030 target of a 50% reduction in zero-dose children by 2030 and promises to "leave no one behind", as well as targets within the Sustainable Development Goals [7,17] and Gavi, the Vaccine Alliance's 2021–2025 Strategy [7,18].

Nigeria has one of the largest cohorts of un- and under-vaccinated children globally, with 2.3 million and 3 million children estimated to not have received any dose of the DTP and MCV vaccines, respectively, in 2022 [2]. Before the pandemic in 2019, the routine coverage of essential vaccines such as DTP1 and MCV1 was estimated to be 72% and 58%, respectively. In 2022, although global coverage levels showed some recovery following the pandemic, routine coverage remained suboptimal in Nigeria, standing at 70% and 60%, respectively, for both basic vaccines [2]. As a result, Nigeria has continued to experience measles outbreaks, with a resurgence of diphtheria outbreaks in 2023 [19]. Utazi et al. [20] found that despite repeated measles vaccination campaigns, measles' incidence was related to routine immunization (RI) coverage. Over the years, there has been a persistent north–south divide in the vaccination coverage in Nigeria, with the northern regions having poorer coverage levels and often higher rates of disease incidence [20,21]. Many studies have also identified several demand- and supply side factors such as low rates of maternal education, belonging to certain religious groups, poor maternal access to and utilization of health services, the poor attitude of health workers, staff shortages, poor conditions at health facilities and vaccine stockouts [22–25], and geographic factors such as remoteness and living in an urban slum [7,26], as being responsible for poor vaccine uptake and heterogeneities in the distribution of vaccination coverage within the country. The first case of the SARS-CoV-2 virus was recorded on 27 February 2020 [27] in Lagos State, Nigeria, following which the government launched a response to the pandemic, including a lockdown from 30 March to 15 May 2020 [28]. COVID-19 vaccination began on 5 March 2021, which saw significant shifts of priorities and resources from vaccination services to the COVID-19 response [29]. These and other interventions are also thought to have further impacted immunization services negatively in the form of reduced access to vaccination, decreases in vaccine demand and uptake, the cessation of outreach services, and the postponement of vaccination campaigns [3,20,30–32]. These challenges call for innovative approaches and intensified efforts to identify and reach zero-dose children in Nigeria.

Against this backdrop, our study aimed to estimate changes in the spatial distribution of zero-dose children and the associated risk factors before and during the COVID-19 pandemic in Nigeria, with a view to assessing the impact of the pandemic on immunization service delivery in the country, which can help consolidate mitigation and other strategies required to boost coverage beyond pre-pandemic levels. We analyzed three outcomes/indicators using data from two household surveys implemented before and during the COVID-19 pandemic in Nigeria. We defined a zero-dose child for each outcome as a child aged 12–23 months who had not received DTP1 (i.e., DTP or PENTA zero dose) or MCV1 (MCV zero dose) or any dose of the four basic vaccines—BCG, OPV0, DTP1, and MCV1—(composite zero dose). Due to data constraints, our study considered only demand-side factors or reasons for non-vaccination.

2. Materials and Methods

2.1. Data and Sources

We utilized data from two recent household surveys conducted in Nigeria, namely the 2018 Demographic and Health Survey (DHS) [33] and the 2021 Multiple Indicator Cluster Survey—National Immunization Coverage Survey (MICS-NICS) [34]. We also assembled geospatial covariate data obtained from various sources and relevant geospatial population data. To ensure respondent confidentiality, the cluster-level geographical coordinates were displaced up to 2 km in urban areas and up to 5 km in rural areas. We present detailed descriptions of these data sources in this section.

2.1.1. 2018 Nigeria Demographic and Health Survey (DHS)

The 2018 Nigeria DHS was conducted between August and December 2018. The survey was designed to be representative at the national, zonal, and state levels (including the Federal Capital Territory) and for urban and rural areas. It employed a two-stage stratified sampling design with stratification achieved by separating each of the 36 states and the Federal Capital Territory (FCT) into urban and rural areas. The first and second stages of the sampling design involved the selection of enumeration areas (EAs) or survey clusters with a probability proportional to their size from each stratum, using a national sampling framework and the selection of households at random from household lists within the selected clusters. Detailed information on the methods employed in the survey is published elsewhere [33].

The survey was implemented in a total of 1389 clusters, with 11 of the 1400 clusters selected initially dropped due to security reasons. Also, in Borno State, only 11 of the 27 local government areas were considered in the survey due to high insecurity. Data on children between age 12–23 months were extracted for this study. Information on routine vaccination coverage obtained from both home-based records (or vaccination cards) and through maternal/caregiver recall were included in our study, as in previous studies [7,23].

2.1.2. 2021 Nigeria Multiple Indicator Cluster Survey—National Immunization Coverage Survey (MICS-NICS)

UNICEF implements MICS surveys to collect globally comparable data on several indicators relating to the situation of women and children within countries. On the other hand, the NICS surveys are implemented by the Nigerian government to provide reliable estimates of the indicators of vaccination coverage used to evaluate the performance of the vaccination program. The MICS survey was integrated with NICS for the first time in Nigeria during its 5th round in 2016–2017, paving the way for the joint implementation of both surveys in the current round in 2021.

Field work for the 2021 MICS-NICS took place between September and December 2021. Similar to the 2018 NDHS, the survey had a two-stage stratified sampling design and was also representative at the national, zonal, and state levels and for urban and rural areas. Details of the sampling methodology are provided in the survey report [34]. The MICS had a target sample size of 1850 clusters. A supplemental sample of 337 clusters was selected for the NICS to increase the combined sample of children and the precision of the vaccination coverage indicators, resulting in a total of 2187 clusters for the MICS-NICS. About 128 of the combined sampled clusters were inaccessible and could not be visited during the survey. Also, in Borno State, sampling took place in only 7 (out of 27) accessible local government areas, in which 29% of the total population of the state resided. As with the 2018 DHS, we extracted all relevant information on routine vaccination coverage for our study for children aged 12–23 months.

As we show in Supplementary Figure S1, children aged 12–23 months in the MICS-NICS survey were born between September 2019 and September 2020. Among these, those born after January 2020 became eligible to receive BCG, OPV0, and DTP1 vaccinations during the pandemic, whereas the entire birth cohort became eligible to receive MCV1 within the pandemic period. Also, the first and second waves of the pandemic, which peaked in July 2020 and February 2021, respectively, overlapped considerably with the time intervals during which the MICS-NICS birth cohort became eligible for all four vaccines included in our study. This demonstrates that the analysis carried out using the 2021 MICS-NICS is ideal for assessing the impact of the COVID-19 pandemic on immunization service delivery within the country. Also, since data collection for the 2018 DHS took place before the pandemic, that survey is suitable for assessing the performance of the vaccination program before the pandemic. However, because both surveys were implemented independently and not as rolling/repeated surveys, there could be sampling and other methodological differences that could impact the comparisons between both surveys, which is a potential limitation of our study.

2.1.3. Outcome Indicators of Zero-Dose Children Included in the Study

To assess the changes in zero-dose prevalence and the associated risk factors before and during the pandemic in Nigeria, our study considered binary indicators of the receipt of DTP1 (PENTA1) (yes = 1, no = 0), receipt of MCV1 (yes = 1, no = 0), and receipt of any of the four basic vaccines—BCG, OPV0, DTP1, and MCV1—as a composite coverage indicator (yes = 1, no = 0) among children aged 12–23 months. We note that both BCG and OPV0 are birth doses, while DTP1 and MCV1 are administered at the age of 6 weeks and from the age of 9 months, respectively, according to Nigeria's immunization schedule [35]. For all the 3 indicators, we extracted data on 5459 children and 6393 children aged 12–23 months from the 2021 MICS and the 2018 DHS, respectively, for our analysis.

At the cluster level, we aggregated the individual level data to produce the numbers of children surveyed, numbers vaccinated, and empirical proportions of children vaccinated. In each case, we obtained the (displaced) geographical (i.e., longitude and latitude) coordinates of the survey clusters. These cluster-level data are displayed in Figure 1 for both surveys.

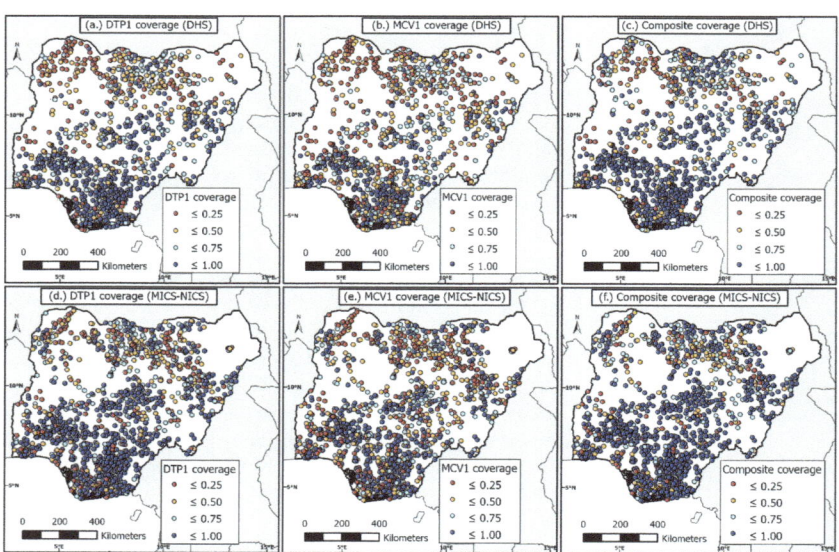

Figure 1. Survey cluster locations and observed vaccination coverage for children aged 12–23 months for both the 2018 DHS (**top** panels) and 2021 MICS-NICS (**bottom** panels).

2.1.4. Independent Variables and Geospatial Covariate Data

Following previous studies [7,23], we included the individual child, mother, household, and community characteristics as risk factors for being zero-dose [7,23]. These are the sex of the child, skilled birth attendance, mother's receipt of tetanus toxoid vaccination, mother's antenatal care visits, maternal age and mother's marital status, maternal education, religion, access to media and phone/internet, land ownership, health insurance, ethnicity, sex of household head, and household wealth. Other covariates considered are maternal access to a bank account, household size and length of stay, and place (urban/rural) and region of residence. These variables were considered due to their data availability in both the 2018 DHS and 2021 MICS-NICS surveys. Detailed definitions of the variables are provided in Supplementary Table S1.

The geospatial covariates considered include travel time to the nearest health facility, distance to conflict areas, poverty index, number of wet days, daytime land surface temperature, livestock density index, slope, enhanced vegetation index (EVI), distance to coastline, distance to the edge of cultivated areas, proximity to national borders, and proximity to protected areas. Consideration of these covariates was informed by their use in previous studies [15,20,36] to model and predict various indicators of vaccination coverage. These covariates were processed as detailed in previous work [15,20,36,37] to produce 1×1 km raster layers and cluster-level data using the geographical coordinates from each of the surveys. Some of these covariate layers are displayed in Supplementary Figure S2 and detailed descriptions are provided in Supplementary Table S2. The classifications of the cluster-level values of some of the covariates, for use in the multilevel analyses, are also shown in Supplementary Figure S3.

Furthermore, for our multilevel analyses (see model (1)) using each survey, we calculated the tertiles of the distribution of the extracted cluster-level data and used these to group the (continuous) values of the covariates into three classes, namely, lower, medium, and higher, which were used in the analyses (see Supplementary Table S1 and Figure S3) together with the survey-derived covariates discussed previously. However, for the geospatial models, the included covariates were on their original continuous scale (except where these were log-transformed prior to model-fitting). As in previous studies [16,36,37], for each survey and indicator, we implemented a detailed covariate selection process to determine the best combination of the geospatial covariates to be included in the geospatial analyses, using model (2). The covariate selection process involved various steps to check the relationships between the geospatial covariates and the coverage indicators, resolve the problem of multicollinearity and then choose the best set of covariates using stepwise regression (backward elimination based on Akaike Information Criterion (AIC)) in a non-spatial framework. The final step of the covariate selection process involved creating a uniform set of covariates for modelling all the indicators for both time periods to enhance comparability.

2.1.5. Population Data

We obtained 1×1 km estimates of the numbers of children aged under 1 year old in 2017 and 2020 (corresponding to the birth cohorts included in our analyses) from WorldPop [38], adjusted to the United Nations Population Division (UNPD) estimates at the national level for both time periods [39]. These data were used in our work to calculate zero-dose estimates through integration with the coverage maps, and as weighting layers when aggregating grid-level coverage estimates to the administrative level.

2.2. Statistical Analysis

2.2.1. Descriptive and Bivariate Analysis

Descriptive analyses were performed using individual-level data for each survey to estimate the frequencies and corresponding proportions for each indicator at the national level, as a precursor to the multilevel analyses.

2.2.2. Multilevel Model

We fitted Bayesian multilevel random intercept logistic regression models, accounting for individual-, household-, community-, and stratum-level variation, to estimate the relationships between each outcome variable (i.e., odds of DTP1, MCV1 and composite coverage) and the covariates/risk factors for zero dose.

Let i indicate a child aged 12–23 months residing in household j, community/cluster k and stratum l (there were 37 strata in MICS-NICS and 74 in DHS). Also, let x_{ijkl} be a vector of the associated covariates. The multilevel model is given by

$$Y_{ijkl}|p_{ijkl} \sim \text{Binomial}(1, p_{ijkl}), \ i = 1, \ldots, n_{jkl}, \ j = 1, \ldots, n_{kl}, \ k = 1, \ldots, n_l, \ l = 1, \ldots, L,$$

$$\log\left(\frac{p_{ijkl}}{1-p_{ijkl}}\right) = \gamma_0 + x_{ijkl}'\beta + \alpha_{jkl} + v_{kl} + \tau_l, \ \alpha_{jkl} \sim N(0, \sigma_\mu^2), \ v_{kl} \sim N(0, \sigma_v^2), \ \tau_l \sim N(0, \sigma_\tau^2) \quad (1)$$

'where Y_{ijkl} denotes a binary response (or vaccination status; coded as 1—vaccinated and 0—unvaccinated) for child $ijkl$, p_{ijkl} represents the corresponding odds of DTP1, MCV1 or zero-dose vaccination, γ_0 is the overall intercept, β is a vector of the associated regression coefficients for the covariates x_{ijkl}, τ_l is the residual random effect for stratum l, v_{kl} is the residual random effect for community (or survey cluster) k located in stratum l, and α_{jkl} is the random effect of household j within community k located in stratum l. The quantities $\alpha_{jkl}, v_{kl},$ and τ_l are assumed to be identically and independently normally distributed with the zero means and variances σ_α^2, σ_v^2, and σ_τ^2, respectively [40]. We note that the individual level (level 1) residual is assumed to follow standard logistic distribution with variance expressed as $\frac{\pi^2}{3} \cong 3.29$ [41].

We applied model (1) to both surveys to identify the significant associated risk factors for zero dose, using all three indicators at the national level. In addition, we applied the model to examine regional variation in the risk factors associated with zero dose by subsetting the data to the north central, north east, north west and southern regions of the country. The three geopolitical zones in the southern part of the country (i.e., the southeast, south-south, and southwest regions) were combined in the regional analysis due to insufficient sample sizes. Also, a reduced set of risk factors were considered in the regional analyses to increase the samples sizes within the categories of the risk factors in each region.

The Bayesian models were fitted using the integrated nested Laplace approximation (INLA) approach, implemented in the R-INLA package. The default priors in R-INLA were assigned to both the fixed- and random-effect parameters in the models [42]. Following model-fitting, we calculated the adjusted odds ratios and their associated 95% credible intervals to evaluate the significance of the associations between the risk factors and the odds of zero dose.

2.2.3. Geostatistical Model

To predict each of the outcome indicators on a 1×1 km grid, we applied a Bayesian geostatistical model to the aggregated cluster-level data from each survey. Let $Y(s_i)$ denote the number of children who received DTP1, MCV1, or any of the four basic vaccines (BCG, OPV0, DTP1, and MCV1) out of a total of $m(s_i)$ children drawn from each sampled cluster location s_i, $i = 1, 2, \ldots, n$, and $p(s_i)$ represent the corresponding unknown true vaccination coverage. Also, let $\mathbf{x}(s_i)$ denote a vector of the geospatial covariate information for location s_i. The geostatistical model assumes that $Y(s_i)$ follows the binomial probability distribution given by

$$Y(s_i)|p(s_i) \sim \text{Binomial}(m(s_i), p(s_i)),$$

$$\log\left(\frac{p(s_i)}{1 - p(s_i)}\right) = \gamma_0 + \mathbf{x}(s_i)'\boldsymbol{\beta} + \omega(s_i) + \epsilon(s_i) \qquad (2)$$

where γ_0 is an intercept parameter, $\boldsymbol{\beta}$ is a vector of the regression coefficients corresponding to $\mathbf{x}(s_i)$, and $\omega(s_i)$ is a spatially structured random effect and follows a zero-mean Gaussian process with variance σ^2 and a covariance function, Σ_ω. There are various parametric families for Σ_ω [43]. In the current analysis, we assumed the Matérn class of covariance functions [44] given by

$$\Sigma_\omega(s_i, s_j) = \frac{\sigma^2}{2^{v-1}\Gamma(v)}(\kappa||s_i - s_j||)^v K_v(\kappa||s_i - s_j||)$$

where the notation $||.||$ denotes the Euclidean distance between locations s_i and s_j, σ^2 is the variance of the spatial field $\omega(s_i)$ as noted earlier, v is a smoothness parameter, $\kappa > 0$ is a scaling parameter related to the range $r = \frac{\sqrt{8v}}{\kappa}$—the distance at which spatial correlation is negligible or approaches 0.1 and $K_v(.)$ is the modified Bessel function of the second kind and order $v > 0$. The smoothness parameter v was set to 1 for the purpose of identifiability, as recommended [45]. Lastly, $\epsilon(s_i)$ is an iid Gaussian random effect with mean 0 and variance, σ_ϵ^2, capturing non-spatial residual variation.

The geostatistical model was fitted using the Integrated Nested Laplace Approximation—Stochastic Partial Differential Equations (INLA-SPDE) approach, implemented in the R-INLA package [45,46]. The predictive performance of all the fitted models were assessed using approaches discussed in previous work [16].

To aggregate the 1 × 1 km grid-level estimates to the district and other administrative levels, we computed the areal estimates as population-weighted averages of the corresponding indicators (i.e., DTP1, MCV1, or composite coverage) taken over all the grid cells falling within the administrative area, as in previous work [16]. We note that this is a common approach to handling point-to-area misalignment when mapping health and development indicators [16,47].

3. Results

3.1. Outcome Indicators of Vaccination Coverage

The national-level coverage estimates for DTP1, MCV1, and the composite coverage indicator were 64.8% (95% CI: 63.6–66.0%), 53.4% (95% CI: 52.1–54.6%), and 73.8% (95% CI: 72.7–74.8%), respectively, for the 2018 DHS. For the 2021 MICS-NICS, the national-level coverage estimates were 71.0% (95% CI: 69.8–72.2%), 61.1% (95% CI: 59.8–62.4%), and 79.4% (95% CI: 78.3–80.4%), respectively, for DTP1, MCV1, and the composite coverage indicator. Generally, the coverage estimates appeared to be higher for the 2021 MICS-NICS than the 2018 DHS for all the three indicators (Supplementary Table S3).

3.2. 1 km × 1 km Modelled Estimates of Coverage and Associated Uncertainties before and during the Pandemic

Predicted coverage estimates and associated uncertainties for children aged 12–23 months in 2018 and 2021 are presented in Figures 2 and S4 for DTP1, MCV1, and the composite coverage indicator. These maps show broadly similar patterns in coverage in both years, although coverage seemed relatively higher in some areas (e.g., parts of the northwest) in 2021. There are substantial geographical differences in coverage when examining DTP1 and MCV1 coverage, with a clear north–south divide for both vaccines and years. As expected, the coverage of the composite indicator is generally higher than DTP1 and MCV1 and areas of low coverage are also concentrated more in the northern areas for this indicator, as well as some southern coastal areas and some areas in Cross River state. Importantly, there are substantial overlaps in low coverage areas across all three indicators in both time periods, suggesting a persistent lack of access to vaccination services in these areas. These low coverage areas are more pronounced in the Sokoto, Zamfara, Yobe, and Kwara states, and parts of the Bauchi, Gombe, and Taraba states. In both the Sokoto and Zamfara states, the poorest coverage levels were observed in areas such as Tangaza, Sangiwa, Naman Goma, Tureta, Anka, Ramfashi, Maru, Bungudu, Yar-Mahanga, and Maholo, among others, when examining the interactive web-based maps (https://data.worldpop.org/repo/lf/visual/justice/all_indicators_coverage_final/ (accessed on 28 September 2023)).

The corresponding uncertainty maps showed standard deviations less than 0.33 for the predicted vaccination coverage estimates for 2018 DHS and less than 0.36 for the 2021 MICS-NICS, suggesting low uncertainties around the predicted coverage estimates in both years (Supplementary Figure S3).

3.3. District-Level Estimates of the Numbers of Zero-Dose Children before and during the Pandemic

Figure 3 presents district-level estimates of the numbers of zero-dose children for the three coverage/zero-dose indicators before and during the pandemic, in 2018 and 2021, respectively. In general, the spatial distributions of the zero-dose estimates are identical across all three indicators in both time periods. The district-level zero-dose estimates exhibit a clear north–south divide similar to the coverage estimates, with children residing in the northern districts being at higher risk of zero dose for all three indicators compared to their counterparts in the south. However, there are also clusters of districts with relatively higher numbers of zero-dose children in the south (in the Lagos and Ogun states). As expected, there is a substantial overlap between the low coverage areas and areas with higher numbers of zero-dose children, although there are a few exceptions. For example, some districts in the southern coastal areas had lower coverage levels (Supplementary

Figure S5), but these were not densely populated areas, hence the zero-dose estimates were lower relative to some northern districts with similar coverage estimates.

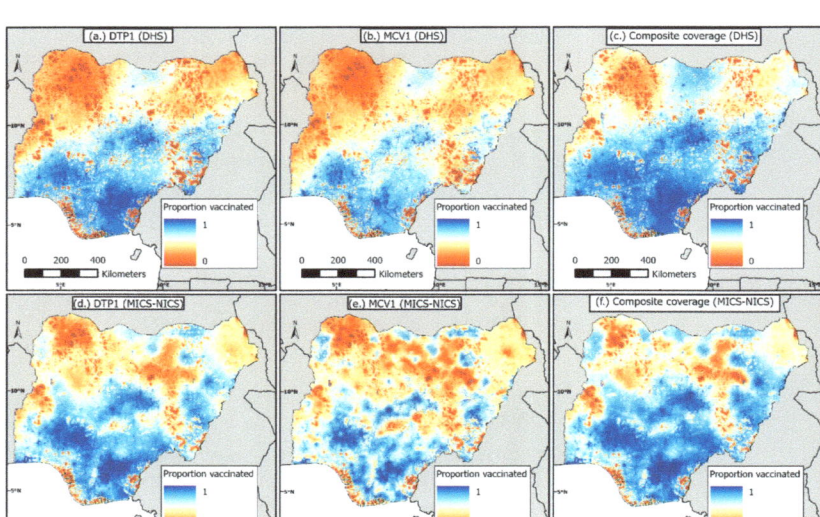

Figure 2. 1 km × 1 km modelled estimates of vaccination coverage for DTP1, MCV1, and composite coverage indicator before the pandemic, produced using the 2018 DHS (**top** panels), and during the pandemic, produced using the 2021 MICS-NICS (**bottom** panels). The associated uncertainty maps are shown in Supplementary Figure S4.

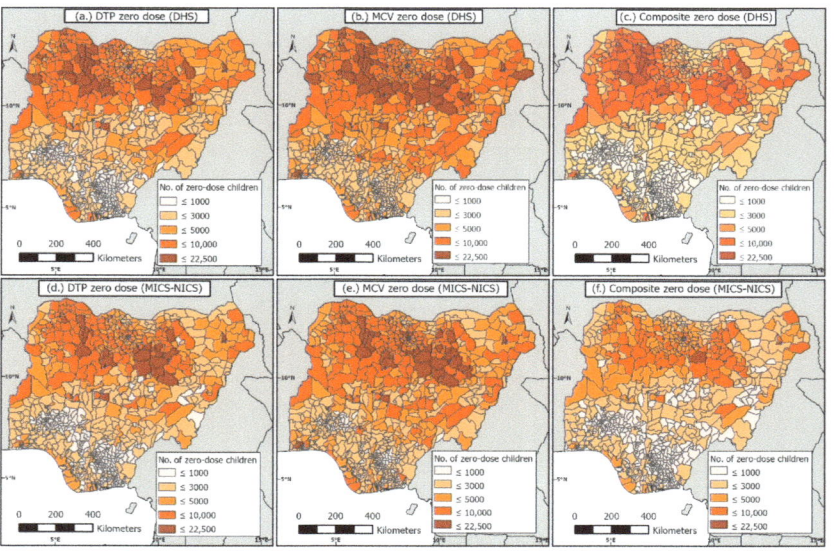

Figure 3. District-level estimates of numbers of DTP, MCV, and composite (i.e., BCG, OPV, DTP, and MCV) zero-dose children during the pre-pandemic period in 2018 (**top** panels) and the pandemic period in 2021 (**bottom** panels). Corresponding coverage estimates are shown in Supplementary Figure S5.

In 2018, the national estimates of DTP, MCV, and composite zero-dose children were 2,364,020, 3,121,156, and 1,703,296, respectively, while in 2021, these were 2,063,375, 2,784,980, and 1,457,068, respectively, indicating no increases in zero-dose prevalence due to the pandemic. The same pattern was generally observed at the district level (Figure 3), where we observed more decreases than increases in zero-dose prevalence (Figure 4). Additionally, we observed no (marked) increases in zero-dose prevalence in districts that had moderate to higher numbers of zero-dose children in 2018 (Figure 4d–f). However, there were a few districts, particularly those in the Lagos (Alimosho), Bauchi (Ningi), Kano (Ugongo, Dala, Tarauni, Kumbotso, Dawakin Tofa, Minjibir, Gwale, etc.), and Borno (Jere) states where considerable increases (>3000 unvaccinated children) were observed relative to the pre-pandemic period (Figure 4a–c). Also, we observed greater increases in zero-dose prevalence for MCV relative to DTP and the composite coverage indicator (Figure 3).

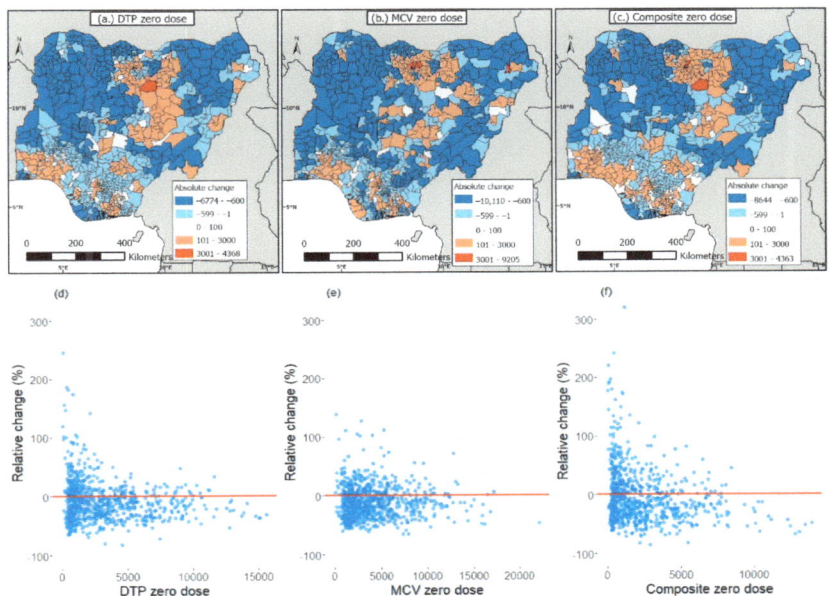

Figure 4. (**a–c**) Absolute changes in estimates of numbers of zero-dose children between 2018 and 2021 (i.e., 2021 estimates minus 2018 estimates) and (**d–f**) 2018 zero-dose estimates versus the relative changes in zero-dose estimates between both time periods.

The districts with the highest numbers of composite zero-dose children (>10,000) were mostly located in Zamfara state (Bungudu, Gusau, Kaura Namoda, Zurmi, Maradun, Maru and Bukkuyum) in 2018, whereas in 2021, these (>9000 zero-dose children) were located in the Bauchi (Ningi, Shira, Ganjuwa), Lagos (Alimosho), Kano (Ugongo), and Sokoto (Dange-Shuni) states, reflecting areas with a lack of access to or poor utilization of vaccination services in both time periods. In Supplementary Figures S6 and S7, we display the zero-dose estimates at the state and regional levels to facilitate comparisons at these administrative levels. These estimates show that the greatest numbers of unvaccinated children were located in the northwestern region in both time periods and across all three indicators, driven by highly populated states such as the Kano and Katsina states.

The zero-dose estimates are also displayed using interactive web-based maps (https://data.worldpop.org/repo/lf/visual/justice/district_number_zero_dose_DHS_MICS/ (accessed on 28 September 2023)) for better visualization.

3.4. Risk Factors Associated with Zero Dose at the National and Regional Levels before and during the Pandemic

The associations between the risk factors (adjusted odds ratios (aORs) and corresponding 95% credible intervals (CIs)) and the odds of vaccination or zero dose are plotted in Figure 5 and Supplementary Figures S8 and S9 at the national level for both time periods. When considering the composite coverage indicator (Figure 5), we observed strong similarities as well as subtle/minor differences in both time periods with respect to the factors associated with zero dose. Factors associated with the odds of zero dose in both time periods include: skilled birth attendance, birth quarter, mother's receipt of tetanus toxoid vaccination status, mother's education, ethnicity, household wealth, and access to bank account. The directions of the estimated relationships were generally the same between both time periods for these factors, except for the birth quarter, suggesting different seasonal patterns in vaccination in both periods. These similarities mostly reflect a lack of changes in the associations between the risk factors characterising maternal access to and utilization of health services, socioeconomic/demographic status, and the odds of zero dose in both time periods. Factors associated with zero dose in the pre-pandemic period in 2018 only include antenatal care attendance, access to media, use of the phone/internet, rural/urban, and travel time to the nearest health facility; while those associated with zero dose in the pandemic period only include marital status, livestock density, distance to coastline, and distance to conflicts. Considering that similar variables were also associated with vaccination in both time periods in most cases, these differences mostly reflect changes in the effect of communication, which was only associated with zero dose before the pandemic, and different characterizations of the effect of remoteness on vaccination in both time periods. We also note that the unexpected direction of the effect of the urban/rural variable before the pandemic is likely due to undetected collinearity or the effect of suppressing variables [7,48]. Detailed results of the estimated odds ratios are provided in the Supplementary Materials (see Figures S8–S13 and Tables S4 and S5).

In Figures 5 and 6, we provide summary plots of the (significant) risk factors that characterized the inequities in vaccination coverage at both the national and regional levels before and during the pandemic. At the national level, we found that the mother's receipt of the tetanus toxoid vaccination, household wealth, access to a bank account, and the mother's education were associated with all three zero-dose indicators in both the pre-pandemic and pandemic periods. Also, the mother's ethnicity, religion, marital status, antenatal care attendance, and skilled birth attendance were associated with the receipt of DTP1 during both time periods, whereas the length of stay, mother's age, and birth quarter were additionally associated with MCV1 in both periods. Additional factors associated with the composite coverage indicator in both periods were ethnicity, birth quarter, and skilled birth attendance. When examining the differences in the risk factors associated with zero dose/vaccination between both time periods, we observed that travel time and phone/internet use were associated with all three outcome indicators before the pandemic, while the distance to coastline was associated with all three outcomes during the pandemic. There were also other factors associated with vaccination in one time period only when examining individual outcome indicators—e.g., additional remoteness variables such as distance to the edge of cultivated areas and distance to conflicts were associated with DTP1 during the pandemic only. Interestingly, the mother's age and length of stay (although with changing patterns for this risk factor) were only associated with MCV1 in both time periods and not associated with any other indicator in either or both time periods, highlighting the importance of both factors for MCV vaccination. Overall, these results agree with our initial conclusions via the composite coverage indicator.

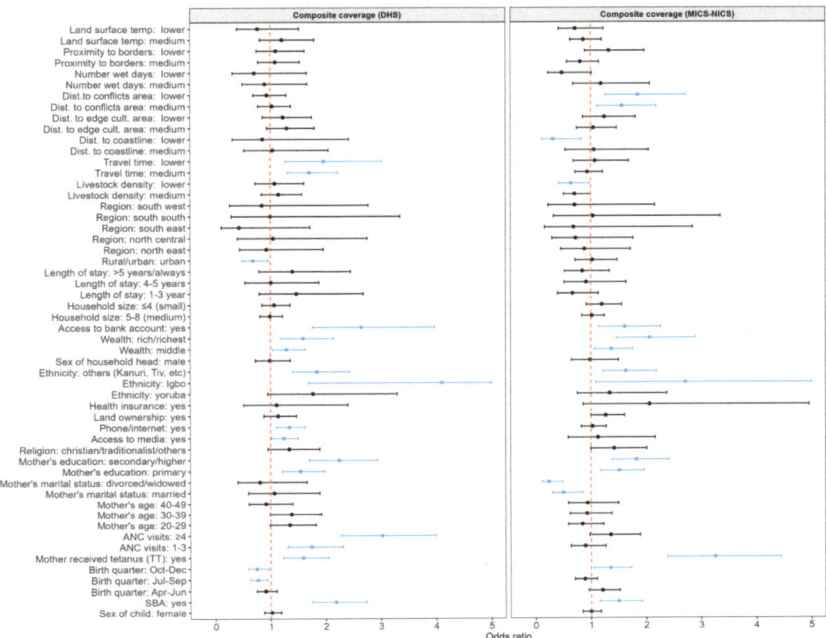

Figure 5. Adjusted odds ratios (aORs) and corresponding 95% credible intervals (95% CI) showing associations between the risk factors and the composite coverage indicator in the pre-pandemic period in 2018 (DHS) and the pandemic period in 2021 (MICS-NICS) at the national level. The vertical dotted red lines mark the odds ratio of 1. Light blue dots and lines show the aORs and 95% CIs of variables that had significant associations with zero dose. The black dots and lines show the aORs and 95% CIs of variables that had no significant associations with zero dose. Some upper CIs have been truncated at a value of 5. The definitions of the risk factors and their reference categories are provided in Supplementary Table S1.

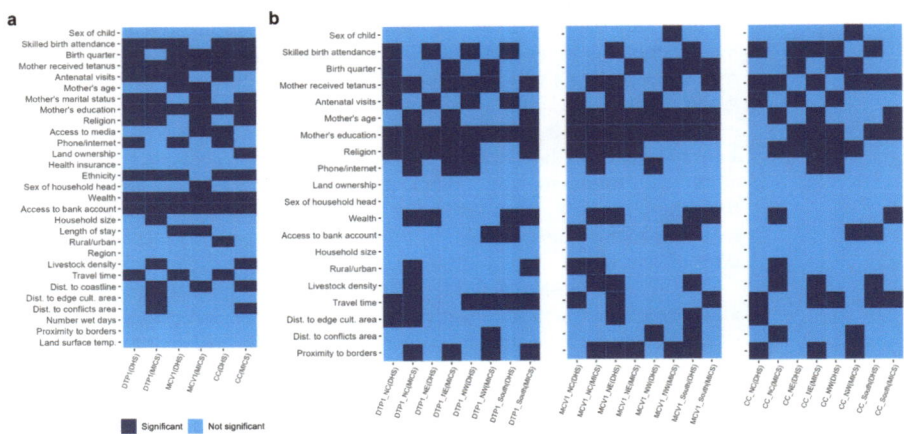

Figure 6. Summary plots showing the risk factors associated with zero dose before the pandemic in 2018 (DHS) and during the pandemic in 2021 (MICS-NICS) at the (**a**) national and (**b**) regional levels, identified using three vaccination coverage indicators, namely DTP1, MCV1, and composite coverage (CC).

At the regional level (Figures 6 and S10–S13), no risk factor was associated with all three indicators in both time periods in all the regions, evidencing greater variation in the associations between the risk factors and vaccination at the regional level, or the effect of the smaller sample sizes available at this level in the analysis (as highlighted previously, these analyses at the regional level were undertaken with a reduced set of risk factors due to sample size limitations). However, when examining individual indicators, we found that the mother's education was associated with DTP zero dose in all four regions in both time periods. Also, the mother's education and the mother's age were associated with MCV zero dose in all four regions in both time periods. No risk factor was associated with composite zero dose in all four regions and both time periods, although there were strong effects of religion in the northern regions, the mother's education in the northeast and southern regions, and the mother's receipt of the tetanus toxoid vaccination in the north central and southern regions.

In the northwestern region, which had the highest estimates of the numbers of zero-dose children among the six regions, no risk factor was associated with all three indicators in both time periods, although the mother's education was associated with DTP1 and MCV1 in both time periods. Additional factors associated with all three indicators in either of the two time periods were antenatal care attendance (pre-pandemic), phone/internet use (pre-pandemic), access to a bank account (pandemic), and proximity to borders (pandemic). These results additionally evidence changes in the effect of communication between the two periods and the importance of maternal education, as in the national-level results. In the northeast region, the mother's education and religion were associated with all three indicators both before and during the pandemic. Additionally, antenatal care attendance was associated with all three indicators in the pre-pandemic period in this region. No risk factor was consistently associated with all three indicators in one time period only. We note that the estimated associations in both periods for this region are also in agreement with the results obtained at the national level.

In the north central region, no risk factor was associated with all three indicators in both time periods. However, the mother's education and religion were associated with DTP and MCV zero dose in both time periods while the mother's receipt of the tetanus toxoid vaccination was associated with DTP1 and composite coverage in both time periods. Other risk factors associated with all three indicators either before or during the pandemic were antenatal care attendance (pre-pandemic), household wealth (pandemic), livestock density (pandemic), and proximity to borders (pandemic). These results obtained for this region are generally in agreement with the national-level results, but additionally demonstrate the effect of wealth and potential cross-border migration on zero dose. In the southern region, the mother's education was associated with all three indicators in both time periods. Additionally, travel time was associated with DTP and composite coverage zero dose in both time periods. Skilled birth attendance and access to a bank account were also associated with all three indicators before the pandemic. No risk factor was associated with all three indicators in the pandemic period only. These results are also in agreement with the national results and additionally highlight the effect of maternal literacy, remoteness, maternal access to and utilization of health services, and socioeconomic disparities on the odds of zero dose.

In general, these regional-level results, though limited by smaller sample sizes, generally corroborate the findings at the national level and have additionally highlighted the risk factors most important for each region through consistent associations with all three indicators either in one or both of the time periods studied.

4. Discussion

By evaluating recent spatial and temporal trends in the distribution of zero-dose children in the context of the COVID-19 pandemic, our study further strengthens the scientific evidence base for improving childhood immunization in Nigeria.

Our study provided estimates of numbers of unvaccinated children for DTP, MCV, and a composite coverage indicator at different spatial scales during the pre-pandemic and pandemic periods in Nigeria. Interestingly, our 2018 national-level DTP and MCV zero-dose estimates of 2.4 million and 3.1 million are in very good agreement with the (WHO and UNICEF estimates of national immunization coverage) WUENIC zero-dose estimates of 2.2 million and 3.1 million, respectively. Also, our 2021 national-level DTP and MCV zero-dose estimates of 2.1 million and 2.8 million in 2021 are very close to the corresponding WUENIC zero-dose estimates of 2.2 million and 2.9 million children, respectively (WUENIC zero-dose estimates were calculated using 2022 WUENIC coverage estimates and the UNPD estimates 2022 revision). Clearly, the pandemic did not result in any dramatic increases in zero-dose prevalence at the national level, but the persistence of large numbers of unvaccinated children in both time periods means that renewed efforts and novel strategies are needed to reach zero-dose and missed communities in the country. At the district level, no dramatic increases in zero-dose prevalence were found during the pandemic relative to the pre-pandemic era. However, there were some areas with elevated zero-dose estimates (>3000 children) during the pandemic, as highlighted previously. Some of these districts were located in the Kano and Lagos states where either relatively higher COVID-19 cases or deaths [49] were recorded during the study period, which could have also occurred as a result of the larger population sizes of both states [38]. The subnational variation in the effect of the pandemic on zero-dose prevalence in Nigeria has also been reported at the state level in a previous study [31], which focused on the Kano and Kaduna states. We note that the lack of substantial increases in zero-dose prevalence at the national level and in many subnational areas in our study, contrary to expectations, might have been due to modest interruptions or a quick recovery from the disruptions caused by the pandemic [50,51]. Additionally, our study revealed strong geographical disparities and a clear north–south divide in zero-dose prevalence in both time periods and across all three indicators, with districts with higher numbers of zero-dose children concentrated in the northern areas, as corroborated by previous studies [14,15,20,36,52]. However, there were also some districts in the south (e.g., in Lagos state) with higher numbers of zero-dose children. This recurring spatial pattern in the distribution of zero-dose children is a strong indication that targeted RI and campaign strategies, focusing on the most problematic areas, will be needed to achieve substantial reductions in the zero-dose prevalence within the country. Previous studies [20,21] have also revealed higher measles case counts in the north and high correlations between measles case counts and MCV zero-dose estimates, further strengthening the evidence for targeted interventions.

The underlying coverage levels also had similar patterns, revealing persistent areas of low coverage, mostly concentrated in the northeast and northwest regions across all three indicators and for both time periods. There were also persistent pockets of low coverage areas in the south, e.g., some areas in Cross River state and some areas near the coastline. However, we note that there were differences in the problematic areas when examining coverage and the zero-dose estimates at the district level. For example, there were some districts in the Lagos and Ogun states with moderate coverage levels, but which had higher zero-dose estimates. Also, some of the low coverage districts in Cross River state did not have higher zero-dose estimates, likely due to these areas having lower population densities. Hence, efforts aimed at reducing zero-dose prevalence should target areas where higher zero-dose estimates were estimated, whereas strategies to improve the equity in coverage should focus on the low coverage areas. When comparing maps of DTP1 and MCV1 coverage, we observed very similar patterns, with DTP1 coverage being higher in many places, due to the dropouts that often occur between both vaccine doses (and perhaps, the result of the suspension of MCV campaigns during the pandemic in 2021). This is a strong indication that the frequent campaigns conducted in Nigeria for MCV, though an effective temporary measure, have not been successful in boosting coverage beyond RI levels. The targeted strategies advocated earlier should, therefore, focus more on strengthening the country's RI program, as we have also argued elsewhere [20].

Furthermore, when examining maps of the composite coverage indicator, the low coverage areas occurring mostly in the northeast and northwest and overlapping considerably with low coverage areas for MCV1 and DTP1, are strongly indicative of the non-availability of vaccination services and/or vaccine hesitancy. Different strategies would be required in these areas to unravel and address the barriers to vaccination.

When examining the risk factors associated with zero dose, we found that while there were strong similarities between the pre-pandemic and pandemic periods, there were also some minor differences, which appeared more pronounced at the subnational/regional level. These similarities and differences are important for characterising the inequities that exist in the vaccination coverage in both time periods. At the national level, our study revealed consistent associations between each of the socioeconomic status (e.g., maternal literacy, household wealth and access to a bank account) and maternal access to and utilization of health services (e.g., skilled birth attendance) and the odds of zero dose in both time periods. We also found evidence of consistency in the effect of demographic factors (e.g., ethnicity, religion, and the mother's age) and the seasonality of vaccination (e.g., birth quarter) on the odds of zero dose in both time periods. At the regional level (based on a reduced set of risk factors), we found additional evidence supporting the results obtained at the national level. Also, these regional-level analyses revealed the risk factors most relevant to reaching zero-dose and missed communities in each region. These were maternal access to and utilization of health services (all regions), communication (northwest), socioeconomic status (northwest, northcentral, and south), religion (northeast and, to a great extent, north central), cross-border migration (northwest and northcentral), and remoteness (south). Furthermore, at the national level, we did not find any remarkable differences in the associations between the risk factors and the odds of zero dose between both time periods. However, we found that there were changes in the variables characterizing the effect of remoteness on zero dose in both time periods. For example, travel time to the nearest health facility was associated with all three zero-dose indicators before the pandemic, while distance to coastline was associated with all three zero-dose indicators during the pandemic. Also, there was a pronounced positive effect of communication on the odds of vaccination before the pandemic, suggesting reduced communication regarding vaccination services during the pandemic. We did not explore the differences between both time periods at the regional level further due to the smaller sample sizes at this level.

To facilitate the operationalization of these findings, our study produced interactive web-based maps (https://data.worldpop.org/repo/lf/visual/justice/all_indicators_coverage_final/; https://data.worldpop.org/repo/lf/visual/justice/district_number_zero_dose_DHS_MICS/ (accessed on 28 September 2023)) to further assist with the identification of towns, communities, and, potentially, settlements in the problematic areas. Additional analyses can also be undertaken through triangulation with other data sets, e.g., data on public health facilities offering vaccination services, to better understand the costs and/or efforts needed to reach zero-dose children within each district. Furthermore, the multi-temporal analyses presented here are highly relevant to planning effective outbreak response strategies or catch-up vaccination activities. Nigeria is currently experiencing a diphtheria outbreak which, according to reports [19], has been more pronounced in the Kano, Katsina, Yobe, Bauchi, Kaduna, Borno and Jigawa states as of the beginning of October 2023. Interestingly, these states were among the states where we had estimated the highest prevalence of DTP zero-dose children in both 2018 (mostly between 120,000 and 215,000 DTP zero-dose children per state—see Supplementary Figure S6) and 2021 (mostly between 80,000 and 240,000 DTP zero-dose children per state), further corroborating the findings from our study. Also, the occurrence of a considerable proportion (one third) of the confirmed cases of the disease in children aged between 5 and 9 years (as of October 2023), which includes the birth cohort for which we produced zero-dose estimates in 2018 in our study, further evidences the programmatic and operational relevance of our analyses. Specifically, our maps of DTP zero-dose children for both years can be used to determine areas where interventions are needed to fill immunity gaps in both older and younger birth cohorts throughout the country. We also note that our district/LGA-level zero-dose estimates can be further disaggregated to the ward level and health facility catchment areas to enhance field operations if needs be.

Through its Zero-dose Reduction Operational Plan (Z-DROP) programme, Nigeria is continuing to intensify efforts to reach its zero-dose and missed communities. Fundamentally, the Z-DROP programme is one of the strategies for achieving the country's vision of integrated primary health care service delivery [53]. Through a rigorous prioritization exercise led by the National Primary Health Care Development Agency, Gavi, the Vaccine Alliance, and the University of Southampton in August 2022, about 100 LGAs were identified as priority areas where (RI) interventions were urgently needed to reach zero-dose and under-immunized children. About 60 of these LGAs, spread across eight states, are being targeted in the current phase of the Z-DROP programme. The programme employs a bottom-up approach to design and implement interventions in these areas through engagement with local health workers. These interventions include initial catch-up immunization activities planned as part of the 2023 measles campaigns, aiming to administer recommended routine vaccines to identified zero-dose children, and then follow up RI activities to sustain the gains made and to ensure the completion of the immunization schedule. The process of identifying zero-dose children in these LGAs additionally involves the triangulation of coverage survey/zero-dose, surveillance, and outreach services data at the ward and health facility levels to identify, geolocate, and classify (unreached, far-to-reach, hard-to-reach, and never reached) high-priority settlements. These additional analyses also include estimating the target populations and the cost of implementing the required interventions in the identified high-priority settlements to guide resource allocation. The programme also provides a mechanism to document all operational activities for the effective supervision and timely tracking of progress.

Our study is subject to some limitations. Our vaccination coverage estimates were produced using information obtained from both home-based records and maternal/caregiver recall, with the latter being subject to recall bias. The sampling frames used in both the 2018 DHS and 2021 MICS-NICS may have missed important vulnerable populations such as those living in conflict areas in Borno state, as highlighted previously. This may have led to an underestimation of the zero-dose prevalence in some areas. Our analyses included comparisons of the vaccination coverage and zero-dose estimates between the 2018 NDHS and 2021 MICS-NICS to assess the impact of the COVID-19 pandemic on immunization services in Nigeria. Since these surveys were implemented independently and not as repeated or rolling surveys, differences in the survey instruments (e.g., questionnaires), sampling designs, and implementation, could have affected the differences seen in the comparisons. Our analyses utilized displaced cluster-level geographical coordinates to predict coverage levels at a 1×1 km resolution. While this may not matter for coverage and zero-dose estimation at the district level using the 2018 DHS data, since the DHS program often retains the displaced clusters within their original districts [54], the displacement may have affected the district-level estimates produced using the 2021 MICS-NICS, as the initial displacement conducted by the MICS team which was used in our work only preserved the state boundaries. Since completing our analyses, the displacement of the geographical coordinates from the 2021 MICS-NICS has been updated to preserve the district-level boundaries. We carried out some sensitivity analyses (results not presented here) using the updated coordinates, which revealed very minor differences from the results (coverage maps) presented in this work. Furthermore, we did not quantify the uncertainties associated with the zero-dose estimates presented in our work. These uncertainties can arise from both the vaccination coverage and population estimates. In particular, the population estimates used in our work were based on projections from the 2006 Nigeria population and housing census and broad area-level age breakdowns. Also, no uncertainty estimates were available for these estimates since they were produced using the "top-down approach" [38]. However, alternative approaches [55] can be used to produce more accurate population estimates and associated uncertainties when recent input data are available. Also, when uncertainty estimates are available for the population estimates [55,56], these can be combined with the uncertainties from vaccination coverage in a statistical framework to produce uncertainties for the zero-dose estimates. Our analysis of the risk factors associated with zero dose included mainly demand-side factors due to data limitations. The inclusion of supply side factors in future work will likely yield more programmable insights and will further explain any residual variation in the multilevel models for the coverage indicators. Lastly, our exploration of the differences in the risk factors associated with zero dose at the regional level in the pre-pandemic and pandemic periods was limited by the smaller sample sizes. This challenge can be overcome in future work through a pooled data analysis.

As immunization programmes around the world continue to recover from the disruptions to immunization services caused by the COVID-19 pandemic and get back on track to achieving the goals and targets set out in the Immunization Agenda 2030, our study has provided programmatically important insights that can aid policy makers to plan and implement effective strategies to reach zero-dose and missed communities in Nigeria.

Supplementary Materials: The following supporting information can be downloaded at https://www.mdpi.com/article/10.3390/vaccines11121830/s1, Figure S1: Timeline of the 2018 DHS and 2021 MICS-NICS surveys in Nigeria showing the time intervals the 12–23-month birth cohort analysed became eligible to receive the vaccines included in the study. The timeline also shows the history of the COVID-19 pandemic in Nigeria and important related events; Figure S2: Geospatial covariates used in our analyses (top row) and the corresponding cluster-level values (bottom row); Figure S3: Classification of the geospatial covariates included in the multi-level analyses using the tertiles of the distribution of each covariate; Figure S4: Uncertainty estimates associated with the coverage estimates for DTP1 (a), MCV1 (b), and composite coverage (c) for 2018 DHS (top panel) and 2021 MICS-NICS (bottom panel) for DTP1 (d), MCV1 (e) and composite coverage (f) at 1×1 km resolution for Nigeria; Figure S5: District level coverage estimates and associated uncertainties for DTP1, MCV1, and Composite Coverage (CC) for both DHS and MICS-NICS; Figure S6: Estimates of numbers of DTP, MCV and composite zero-dose children at the state level before the pandemic in 2018 (DHS) and during the pandemic in 2021 (MICS-NICS); Figure S7: Estimates of numbers of DTP, MCV and composite zero-dose children at the regional level before the pandemic in 2018 (DHS) and during the pandemic in 2021 (MICS-NICS); Figure S8: Risk factors associated with DTP1, MCV1, and composite coverage before the pandemic in 2018 (DHS) at the national level. The odds ratios and 95% credible intervals for significant risk factors are coloured in blue. Also, the upper limit for Igbo ethnicity is 10.85 for DTP1, 5.6 for MCV1, and 9.94 for composite coverage; Figure S9: Risk factors associated with DTP1, MCV1, and composite coverage during the pandemic in 2021 (MICS-NICS) at the national level. The odds ratios and corresponding 95% credible intervals for significant risk factors are coloured in blue. Also, the upper limit for Igbo ethnicity is 5.21 for DTP1, and 6.77 for composite coverage; Figure S10: Risk factors associated with DTP1, MCV1, and composite coverage before and during the pandemic in 2018 (DHS—top panel) and 2021 (MICS-NICS—bottom panel) in the north central region. The odds ratios and corresponding 95% credible intervals for significant risk factors are coloured in blue; Figure S11: Risk factors associated with DTP1, MCV1, and composite coverage before and during the pandemic in 2018 (DHS—top panel) and 2021 (MICS-NICS—bottom panel) in the northeast region. The odds ratios and corresponding 95% credible intervals for significant risk factors are coloured in blue; Figure S12: Risk factors associated with DTP1, MCV1, and composite coverage before and during the pandemic in 2018 (DHS—top panel) and 2021 (MICS-NICS—bottom panel) in the northwest region. The odds ratios and corresponding 95% credible intervals for significant risk factors are coloured in blue; Figure S13: Risk factors associated with DTP1, MCV1, and composite coverage before and during the pandemic in 2018 (DHS—top panel) and 2021 (MICS-NICS—bottom panel) in the southern region. The odds ratios and corresponding 95% credible intervals for significant risk factors are coloured in blue; Table S1: Description and coding of outcome variables and covariate factors; Table S2: Description and sources of geospatial covariates used in our analyses; Table S3: Distribution of sample characteristics of the study population by receipt of vaccine status for MICS-NICS 2021 and DHS 2018; Table S4: Factors associated with DTP1, MCV1 and composite coverage by region for DHS 2018 using multilevel binary logistic regression models; Table S5: Factors associated with DTP1, MCV1 and composite coverage by region for the 2021 MICS-NICS using multilevel binary logistic regression models.

Author Contributions: Conceptualization, C.E.U., A.J.T. and J.M.K.A.; methodology, C.E.U. and J.M.K.A.; software, C.E.U. and J.M.K.A.; validation, C.E.U. and J.M.K.A.; formal analysis, C.E.U., J.M.K.A. and H.M.T.C.; investigation, C.E.U., J.M.K.A., H.M.T.C., I.D.O., A.J.T., A.E., B.D., B.F., H.S., B.A. and J.C.; resources, C.E.U.; data curation, C.E.U., J.M.K.A., H.M.T.C., I.D.O., A.J.T., A.E., B.D., B.F., H.S., B.A. and J.C.; writing—original draft preparation, C.E.U. and J.M.K.A.; writing—review and editing, C.E.U., J.M.K.A., A.J.T., I.D.O., H.M.T.C., A.E., B.D., B.F., H.S., B.A. and J.C.; visualization, C.E.U., J.M.K.A., I.D.O. and H.M.T.C.; supervision, C.E.U. and A.J.T.; project administration, C.E.U.; funding acquisition, C.E.U. All authors have read and agreed to the published version of the manuscript.

Funding: This research was funded by GAVI, the Vaccine Alliance.

Institutional Review Board Statement: Ethics approval for this study was provided by the University Ethics Committee (ID: 48522.A1), University of Southampton, UK.

Informed Consent Statement: Informed consent was obtained from all subjects involved in the study during the primary data collection by the various survey programs. Only de-identified secondary data were analyzed in this study, and all methods were performed in accordance with the relevant guidelines and regulations.

Data Availability Statement: The data used in this study are available from the DHS (https://dhsprogram.com/data/available-datasets.cfm (accessed on 28 September 2023)) and MICS (https://mics.unicef.org/surveys (accessed on 28 September 2023)) programmes upon request. Other data (i.e., geospatial covariates) are publicly available via the sources referenced in the manuscript. The authors are not allowed to redistribute these datasets.

Conflicts of Interest: B.D., B.A. and J.C. work for GAVI, the Vaccine Alliance. The authors declare no other conflict of interest.

References

1. World Health Organization (WHO). *Global Immunization Coverage 2021*; WHO Estimates of National Immunization Coverage: Geneva, Switzerland, 2021. Available online: https://www.who.int/news-room/fact-sheets/detail/immunization-coverage (accessed on 20 March 2023).
2. World Health Organization (WHO); UNICEF. 2022 WHO/UNICEF Estimates of National Immunization Coverage (WUENIC). WHO and UNICEF. 2023. Available online: https://cdn.who.int/media/docs/default-source/immunization/wuenic-progress-and-challenges.pdf?sfvrsn=b5eb9141_12&download=true (accessed on 21 August 2023).
3. Causey, K.; Fullman, N.; Sorensen, R.J.; Galles, N.C.; Zheng, P.; Aravkin, A.; Danovaro-Holliday, M.C.; Martinez-Piedra, R.; Sodha, S.V.; Velandia-González, M.P.; et al. Estimating global and regional disruptions to routine childhood vaccine coverage during the COVID-19 pandemic in 2020: A modelling study. *Lancet* **2021**, *398*, 522–534. [CrossRef] [PubMed]
4. Ho, L.L.; Gurung, S.; Mirza, I.; Nicolas, H.D.; Steulet, C.; Burman, A.L.; Danovaro-Holliday, M.C.; Sodha, S.V.; Kretsinger, K. Impact of the SARS-CoV-2 pandemic on vaccine-preventable disease campaigns. *Int. J. Infect. Dis.* **2022**, *119*, 201–209. [CrossRef] [PubMed]
5. World Health Organization (WHO); UNICEF. 2021 WHO/UNICEF Estimates of National Immunization Coverage (WUENIC). 2022. Available online: https://www.who.int/teams/immunization-vaccines-and-biologicals/immunization-analysis-and-insights/global-monitoring/immunization-coverage/who-unicef-estimates-of-national-immunization-coverage (accessed on 20 February 2023).
6. Hogan, D.; Gupta, A. Why Reaching Zero-Dose Children Holds the Key to Achieving the Sustainable Development Goals. *Vaccines* **2023**, *11*, 781. [CrossRef] [PubMed]
7. Utazi, C.E.; Pannell, O.; Aheto, J.M.K.; Wigley, A.; Tejedor-Garavito, N.; Wunderlich, J.; Hagedorn, B.; Hogan, D.; Tatem, A.J. Assessing the characteristics of un- and under-vaccinated children in low- and middle-income countries: A multi-level cross-sectional study. *PLOS Glob. Public Health* **2022**, *2*, e0000244. [CrossRef] [PubMed]
8. Wigley, A.; Lorin, J.; Hogan, D.; Utazi, C.E.; Hagedorn, B.; Dansereau, E.; Tatem, A.J.; Tejedor-Garavito, N. Estimates of the number and distribution of zero-dose and under-immunised children across remote-rural, urban, and conflict-affected settings in low and middle income countries. *PLoS Glob. Public Health* **2022**, *2*, e0001126. [CrossRef]
9. Chopra, M.; Bhutta, Z.; Blanc, D.C.; Checchi, F.; Gupta, A.; Lemango, E.T.; Levine, O.S.; Lyimo, D.; Nandy, R.; O'brien, K.L.; et al. Addressing the persistent inequities in immunization coverage. *Bull World Health Organ.* **2020**, *98*, 146–148. [CrossRef] [PubMed]
10. WHO. *Immunization Agenda 2030: A Global Strategy to Leave No One Behind*; World Health Organization: Geneva, Switzerland, 2020; Available online: https://www.who.int/immunization/immunization_agenda_2030/en/ (accessed on 25 June 2021).

11. O'Brien, K.L.; Lemango, E. The big catch-up in immunisation coverage after the COVID-19 pandemic: Progress and challenges to achieving equitable recovery. *Lancet* **2023**, *402*, 510–512. [CrossRef]
12. Shuaib, F.; Garba, A.B.; Meribole, E.; Obasi, S.; Sule, A.; Nnadi, C.; Waziri, N.E.; Bolu, O.; Nguku, P.M.; Ghiselli, M.; et al. Implementing the routine immunisation data module and dashboard of DHIS2 in Nigeria, 2014–2019. *BMJ Glob. Health* **2020**, *5*, e002203. [CrossRef]
13. District Health Information System, Version 2. 2019. Available online: https://www.dhis2.org/ (accessed on 19 March 2023).
14. Sbarra, A.N.; Rolfe, S.; Nguyen, J.Q.; Earl, L.; Galles, N.C.; Marks, A.; Abbas, K.M.; Abbasi-Kangevari, M.; Abbastabar, H.; Abd-Allah, F. Mapping routine measles vaccination in low- and middle-income countries. *Nature* **2021**, *589*, 415–419.
15. Utazi, C.E.; Thorley, J.; Alegana, V.A.; Ferrari, M.J.; Takahashi, S.; Metcalf, C.J.E.; Lessler, J.; Cutts, F.T.; Tatem, A.J. Mapping vaccination coverage to explore the effects of delivery mechanisms and inform vaccination strategies. *Nat. Commun.* **2019**, *10*, 1633. [CrossRef]
16. Utazi, C.E.; Nilsen, K.; Pannell, O.; Dotse-Gborgbortsi, W.; Tatem, A.J. District-level estimation of vaccination coverage: Discrete vs continuous spatial models. *Stat. Med.* **2021**, *40*, 2197–2211. [CrossRef] [PubMed]
17. United Nations (UN). Transforming Our World: The 2030 Agenda for Sustainable Development. UN. 2015. Available online: https://sustainabledevelopment.un.org/post2015/transformingourworld/publication (accessed on 20 August 2023).
18. Gavi The Vaccine Alliance (GAVI). Gavi Strategy 5.0, 2021–2025; GAVI2020, 2020. Available online: https://www.gavi.org/our-alliance/strategy/phase-5-2021-2025 (accessed on 20 June 2023).
19. Nigeria Centre for Disease Control and Prevention (NCDC). An Update of Measles Outbreak in Nigeria. 2023. Available online: https://ncdc.gov.ng/diseases/sitreps (accessed on 20 February 2023).
20. Utazi, C.E.; Aheto, J.M.; Wigley, A.; Tejedor-Garavito, N.; Bonnie, A.; Nnanatu, C.C.; Wagai, J.; Williams, C.; Setayesh, H.; Tatem, A.J.; et al. Mapping the distribution of zero-dose children to assess the performance of vaccine delivery strategies and their relationships with measles incidence in Nigeria. *Vaccine* **2023**, *41*, 170–181. [CrossRef] [PubMed]
21. Baptiste, A.E.J.; Masresha, B.; Wagai, J.; Luce, R.; Oteri, J.; Dieng, B.; Bawa, S.; Ikeonu, O.C.; Chukwuji, M.; Braka, F.; et al. Trends in measles incidence and measles vaccination coverage in Nigeria, 2008–2018. *Vaccine* **2021**, *39*, C89–C95. [CrossRef] [PubMed]
22. Akwataghibe, N.N.; Ogunsola, E.A.; Broerse, J.E.W.; Popoola, O.A.; Agbo, A.I.; Dieleman, M.A. Exploring Factors Influencing Immunization Utilization in Nigeria-A Mixed Methods Study. *Front. Public Health* **2019**, *7*, 392. [CrossRef] [PubMed]
23. Aheto, J.M.K.; Pannell, O.; Dotse-Gborgbortsi, W.; Trimner, M.K.; Tatem, A.J.; Rhoda, D.A.; Cutts, F.T.; Utazi, C.E. Multilevel analysis of predictors of multiple indicators of childhood vaccination in Nigeria. *PLoS ONE* **2022**, *17*, e0269066. [CrossRef] [PubMed]
24. Oku, A.; Oyo-Ita, A.; Glenton, C.; Fretheim, A.; Eteng, G.; Ames, H.; Muloliwa, A.; Kaufman, J.; Hill, S.; Cliff, J.; et al. Factors affecting the implementation of childhood vaccination communication strategies in Nigeria: A qualitative study. *BMC Public Health* **2017**, *17*, 200. [CrossRef] [PubMed]
25. International Vaccine Access Center (IVAC). Landscape Analysis of Routine Immunization in Nigeria. IVAC; 2012. Available online: https://www.jhsph.edu/ivac/wp-content/uploads/2018/05/IVAC-Landscape-Analysis-Routine-Immunization-Nigeria-Brief.pdf (accessed on 10 March 2023).
26. Obanewa, O.A.; Newell, M.L. The role of place of residency in childhood immunisation coverage in Nigeria: Analysis of data from three DHS rounds 2003–2013. *BMC Public Health* **2020**, *20*, 123. [CrossRef]
27. Nigeria Centre for Disease Control (NCDC). First Case of Corona Virus Disease Confirmed in Nigeria. 2020. Available online: https://ncdc.gov.ng/news/227/first-case-of-corona-virus-disease-confirmed-in-nigeria (accessed on 24 March 2023).
28. Presidential Task Force on COVID-19—Nigeria. Presidential Task Force on COVID-19: Mid-Term Report. Nigeria. 2020. Available online: https://statehouse.gov.ng/covid19/2020/10/02/presidential-task-force-on-covid-19-mid-term-report/ (accessed on 30 April 2023).
29. Mathieu, E.; Ritchie, H.; Rodés-Guirao, L.; Appel, C.; Giattino, C.; Hasell, J.; Macdonald, B.; Dattani, S.; Beltekian, D.; Ortiz-Ospina, E.; et al. Coronavirus Pandemic (COVID-19), Vaccinations by Country; Nigeria. Our World in Data. 2020. Available online: https://ourworldindata.org/covid-vaccinations (accessed on 21 February 2023).
30. Essoh, T.A.; Adeyanju, G.C.; Adamu, A.A.; Ahawo, A.K.; Aka, D.; Tall, H.; Aplogan, A.; Wiysonge, C.S. Early Impact of SARS-CoV-2 Pandemic on Immunization Services in Nigeria. *Vaccines* **2022**, *10*, 1107. [CrossRef]
31. Ibrahim, D.; Alyssa, S.; Ismael, H.; Ricardo, I. Analysis of the impact of COVID-19 pandemic and response on routine childhood vaccination coverage and equity in Northern Nigeria: A mixed methods study. *BMJ Open* **2023**, *13*, e076154.
32. Adelekan, B.; Goldson, E.; Abubakar, Z.; Mueller, U.; Alayande, A.; Ojogun, T.; Ntoimo, L.; Williams, B.; Muhammed, I.; Okonofua, F. Effect of COVID-19 pandemic on provision of sexual and reproductive health services in primary health facilities in Nigeria: A cross-sectional study. *Reprod. Health* **2021**, *18*, 166. [CrossRef]
33. National Population Commission (NPC) [Nigeria]; ICF. Nigeria Demographic and Health Survey 2018—Final Report. Abuja, Nigeria, and Rockville, Maryland, USA: NPC and ICF. 2019. Available online: https://dhsprogram.com/publications/publication-fr359-dhs-final-reports.cfm (accessed on 16 March 2021).
34. National Bureau of Statistics (NBS); United Nations Children's Fund (UNICEF). *Multiple Indicator Cluster Survey 2021—Survey Findings Report*; NBS and UNICEF: Abuja, Nigeria, 2022.
35. World Health Organization (WHO). Vaccination Schedule for Nigeria. WHO: 2023. Available online: https://immunizationdata.who.int/pages/schedule-by-country/nga.html?DISEASECODE=&TARGETPOP_GENERAL= (accessed on 19 February 2023).

36. Utazi, C.E.; Wagai, J.; Pannell, O.; Cutts, F.T.; Rhoda, D.A.; Ferrari, M.J.; Dieng, B.; Oteri, J.; Danovaro-Holliday, M.C.; Adeniran, A.; et al. Geospatial variation in measles vaccine coverage through routine and campaign strategies in Nigeria: Analysis of recent household surveys. *Vaccine* **2020**, *38*, 3062–3071. [CrossRef] [PubMed]
37. Utazi, C.E.; Thorley, J.; Alegana, V.A.; Ferrari, M.J.; Takahashi, S.; Metcalf, C.J.E.; Lessler, J.; Tatem, A.J. High resolution age-structured mapping of childhood vaccination coverage in low and middle income countries. *Vaccine* **2018**, *36*, 1583–1591. [CrossRef] [PubMed]
38. WorldPop. Open Spatial Demographic Data and Research. WorldPop. 2021. Available online: https://www.worldpop.org/ (accessed on 20 February 2023).
39. United Nations; Department of Economic and Social Affairs, Population Division. World Population Prospects 2022: Release note. Available online: https://population.un.org/wpp/ (accessed on 19 October 2023).
40. Leckie, G.; Charlton, C. Runmlwin—A Program to Run the MLwiN Multilevel Modelling Software from within Stata. *J. Stat. Softw.* **2013**, *52*, 1–40.
41. Hedeker, D.; Gibbons, R.D. MIXOR: A computer program for mixed-effects ordinal regression analysis. *Comput. Methods Programs Biomed.* **1996**, *49*, 157–176. [CrossRef] [PubMed]
42. Lindgren, F.; Rue, H. Bayesian Spatial Modelling with R-INLA. *J. Stat. Softw.* **2015**, *63*, 25. [CrossRef]
43. Diggle, P.; Ribeiro, P.J.; MyiLibrary. Model-based geostatistics. In *Springer Series in Statistics*; Springer: New York, NY, USA, 2007.
44. Matérn, B. *Spatial Variation*, 2nd ed.; Springer: Berlin, Germany, 1986.
45. Lindgren, F.; Rue, H.; Lindström, J. An explicit link between Gaussian fields and Gaussian Markov random fields: The stochastic partial differential equation approach. *J. R. Stat. Soc. Ser. B* **2011**, *73*, 423–498. [CrossRef]
46. Rue, H.; Martino, S.; Lindgren, F.; Simpson, D.; Riebler, A.; Krainski, E.T. INLA: Functions which allow to perform full Bayesian analysis of latent Gaussian models using Integrated Nested Laplace approximation. R Package Version 0.0-1440400394. 2019. Available online: https://rdrr.io/github/andrewzm/INLA/ (accessed on 11 February 2023).
47. Mosser, J.F.; Gagne-Maynard, W.; Rao, P.C.; Osgood-Zimmerman, A.; Fullman, N.; Graetz, N.; Burstein, R.; Updike, R.L.; Liu, P.Y.; Ray, S.E.; et al. Mapping diphtheria-pertussis-tetanus vaccine coverage in Africa, 2000–2016: A spatial and temporal modelling study. *Lancet* **2019**, *393*, 1843–1855. [CrossRef]
48. Ludlow, L.; Klein, K. Suppressor Variables: The Difference between 'is' Versus 'Acting As'. *J. Stat. Educ.* **2014**, *22*. [CrossRef]
49. Nigeria Centre for Disease Control and Prevention (NCDC). COVID-19 NIGERIA. Nigeria. Available online: https://covid19.ncdc.gov.ng/ (accessed on 20 April 2023).
50. Sato, R. Pattern of vaccination delivery around COVID-19 lockdown in Nigeria. *Hum. Vaccines Immunother.* **2021**, *17*, 2951–2953. [CrossRef]
51. Amouzou, A.; Maïga, A.; Faye, C.M.; Chakwera, S.; Melesse, D.Y.; Mutua, M.K.; Thiam, S.; Abdoulaye, I.B.; Afagbedzi, S.K.; Iknane, A.A.; et al. Health service utilisation during the COVID-19 pandemic in sub-Saharan Africa in 2020: A multicountry empirical assessment with a focus on maternal, newborn and child health services. *BMJ Glob. Health* **2022**, *7*, e008069. [CrossRef]
52. Utazi, C.E.; Aheto, J.M.K.; Chan, H.M.T.; Tatem, A.J.; Sahu, S.K. Conditional probability and ratio-based approaches for mapping the coverage of multi-dose vaccines. *Stat. Med.* **2022**, *41*, 5662–5678. [CrossRef] [PubMed]
53. World Health Organization (WHO). States Adopt Integrated Vaccination Strategy to Reach Unimmunized Children, Nigeria. 2022. Available online: https://www.afro.who.int/countries/nigeria/news/states-adopt-integrated-vaccination-strategy-reach-unimmunized-children (accessed on 19 February 2023).
54. Burgert, C.R.; Colston, J.; Roy, T.; Zachary, B. Geographic displacement procedure and georeferenced data release policy for the Demographic and Health Surveys. In *DHS Spatial Analysis Reports No 7*; ICF International: Calverton, MD, USA, 2013.
55. Leasure, D.R.; Jochem, W.C.; Weber, E.M.; Tatem, A.J. National population mapping from sparse survey data: A hierarchical Bayesian modeling framework to account for uncertainty. *Proc. Natl. Acad. Sci. USA* **2020**, *117*, 24173–24179. [CrossRef] [PubMed]
56. Nilsen, K.; Tejedor-Garavito, N.; Leasure, D.R.; Utazi, C.E.; Ruktanonchai, C.W.; Wigley, A.S.; Dooley, C.A.; Matthews, Z.; Tatem, A.J. A review of geospatial methods for population estimation and their use in constructing reproductive, maternal, newborn, child and adolescent health service indicators. *BMC Health Serv. Res.* **2021**, *21*, 370. [CrossRef] [PubMed]

Disclaimer/Publisher's Note: The statements, opinions and data contained in all publications are solely those of the individual author(s) and contributor(s) and not of MDPI and/or the editor(s). MDPI and/or the editor(s) disclaim responsibility for any injury to people or property resulting from any ideas, methods, instructions or products referred to in the content.

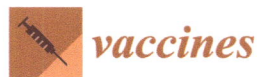

Article

Zero-Dose Childhood Vaccination Status in Rural Democratic Republic of Congo: Quantifying the Relative Impact of Geographic Accessibility and Attitudes toward Vaccination

Branly Kilola Mbunga [1,†], Patrick Y. Liu [2,†], Freddy Bangelesa [1,3], Eric Mafuta [1], Nkamba Mukadi Dalau [1], Landry Egbende [1], Nicole A. Hoff [4], Jean Bosco Kasonga [1], Aimée Lulebo [1], Deogratias Manirakiza [5], Adèle Mudipanu [5], Nono Mvuama [1], Paul Ouma [6], Kerry Wong [6], Paul Lusamba [1] and Roy Burstein [7,*]

1. Kinshasa School of Public Health, University of Kinshasa, Kinshasa H8Q3+2HV, Democratic Republic of the Congo; branly.mbunga@unikin.ac.cd (B.K.M.); ir.fbangelesa@hotmail.fr (F.B.); eric.mafuta@unikin.ac.cd (E.M.); dalau.nkamba@unikin.ac.cd (N.M.D.); landry.egbende@unikin.ac.cd (L.E.); jeanbosco.kasonga@unikin.ac.cd (J.B.K.); aimee.lulebo@ksph-lisanga.org (A.L.); nono.mvuama@unikin.ac.cd (N.M.); paul.lusamba@unikin.ac.cd (P.L.)
2. Health and Life Sciences, Gates Ventures, Seattle, WA 98033, USA; patrick.liu@gatesventures.com
3. Institute of Geography and Geology, University of Würzburg, Am Hubland, 97074 Würzburg, Germany
4. Fielding School of Public Health, University of California, Los Angeles, CA 90095, USA; nhoff84@ucla.edu
5. United Nations Children's Fund (UNICEF) Country Office, Kinshasa M7H9+HQW, Democratic Republic of the Congo; dmanirakiza@unicef.org (D.M.); amudipanu@unicef.org (A.M.)
6. World Health Organization, 1211 Geneva, Switzerland; oumap@who.int (P.O.); wongk@who.int (K.W.)
7. Bill & Melinda Gates Foundation, Seattle, WA 98109, USA
* Correspondence: roy.burstein@gatesfoundation.org
† These authors contributed equally to this work.

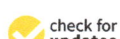

Citation: Mbunga, B.K.; Liu, P.Y.; Bangelesa, F.; Mafuta, E.; Dalau, N.M.; Egbende, L.; Hoff, N.A.; Kasonga, J.B.; Lulebo, A.; Manirakiza, D.; et al. Zero-Dose Childhood Vaccination Status in Rural Democratic Republic of Congo: Quantifying the Relative Impact of Geographic Accessibility and Attitudes toward Vaccination. *Vaccines* **2024**, *12*, 617. https://doi.org/10.3390/vaccines12060617

Academic Editor: Alessandra Casuccio

Received: 2 April 2024
Revised: 24 May 2024
Accepted: 30 May 2024
Published: 4 June 2024

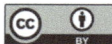

Copyright: © 2024 by the authors. Licensee MDPI, Basel, Switzerland. This article is an open access article distributed under the terms and conditions of the Creative Commons Attribution (CC BY) license (https:// creativecommons.org/licenses/by/ 4.0/).

Abstract: Despite efforts to increase childhood vaccination coverage in the Democratic Republic of the Congo (DRC), approximately 20% of infants have not started their routine immunization schedule (zero-dose). The present study aims to evaluate the relative influence of geospatial access to health facilities and caregiver perceptions of vaccines on the vaccination status of children in rural DRC. Pooled data from two consecutive nationwide immunization surveys conducted in 2022 and 2023 were used. Geographic accessibility was assessed based on travel time from households to their nearest health facility using the AccessMod 5 model. Caregiver attitudes to vaccination were assessed using the survey question "How good do you think vaccines are for your child?" We used logistic regression to assess the relationship between geographic accessibility, caregiver attitudes toward vaccination, and their child's vaccination status. Geographic accessibility to health facilities was high in rural DRC, with 88% of the population living within an hour's walk to a health facility. Responding that vaccines are "Bad, Very Bad, or Don't Know" relative to "Very Good" for children was associated with a many-fold increased odds of a zero-dose status (ORs 69.3 [95%CI: 63.4–75.8]) compared to the odds for those living 60+ min from a health facility, relative to <5 min (1.3 [95%CI: 1.1–1.4]). Similar proportions of the population fell into these two at-risk categories. We did not find evidence of an interaction between caregiver attitude toward vaccination and travel time to care. While geographic access to health facilities is crucial, caregiver demand appears to be a more important driver in improving vaccination rates in rural DRC.

Keywords: zero-dose; children; vaccination; immunization; geographic accessibility; vaccine demand

1. Introduction

Immunization is widely regarded as one of the most important public health interventions for reducing childhood morbidity and mortality. Despite significant progress in global coverage over the past two decades, substantial inequities persist [1–3]. Of the 20.5 million under-immunized (UI) children in 2022, 70% or 14.3 million were considered zero-dose (ZD), operationally defined as children who have not had a single dose of the Pentavalent vaccine [4]. Global efforts, including the Immunization Agenda 2030 (IA2030), have recognized the imperative of reaching zero-dose children as a strategic priority, calling for a 50% reduction in the number of zero-dose children by the year 2030 [5,6]. Beyond the risk of vaccine-preventable diseases, children who are ZD or UI and their families face multiple deprivations related to poverty, gender inequities, and access to other health systems services beyond routine immunization [3,7–9].

The Democratic Republic of the Congo (DRC) persists as one of the most vulnerable countries to vaccine-preventable diseases and has experienced several recent outbreaks, including a measles epidemic in 2019 resulting in more than 300,000 suspected cases and 6000 deaths [10,11]. Prior efforts to understand the drivers of persistently low coverage in DRC identified several system-side challenges, including inequities in service and vaccine availability, variable management and program monitoring, and challenges with health worker motivation [11]. In response, the Ministry of Health developed the Mashako Plan in 2018 with the primary aim of improving coverage interventions focused on improved coordination, service delivery, vaccine availability, real-time service delivery monitoring, and more robust program evaluation. Despite improvements in system targets and increases in vaccination coverage, an estimated 19.1% of children 12–23 months remain ZD (771,000), and 25.5% remain under-immunized (1.03 million) in 2021 [12].

There is a need to move beyond the sole focus on supply-side drivers to more effectively and sustainably overcome the intersecting barriers to vaccination that children who are ZD and UI and their families face [13]. Frameworks like the Behavioral and Social Drivers (BeSD) Framework, UNICEF Journey to Health and Immunization Framework, and Exemplars in Global Health (EGH) Vaccine Delivery Framework identify factors related to vaccine demand, access to services, and supply-side readiness as key drivers of vaccination—and thus barriers to ZD and UI [14–16]. Data across these three domains have been limited to date but are becoming increasingly available to assess their impact on vaccination coverage.

There is a growing body of evidence demonstrating the impact of geospatial access to vaccination services and coverage in sub-Saharan Africa, though this has not yet been characterized in DRC [17–21]. Moreover, recent analyses on self-reported reasons for non-vaccination in DRC identified that 82% of caregivers of children who were ZD expressed no intent to vaccinate their child and that 9.6% experienced barriers related to access to services [22]. While this evidence on intent and access adds nuance to the understanding of drivers of non- and under-vaccination in DRC, this insight is limited when they are evaluated in isolation. A more complete understanding of the drivers of coverage requires analyzing their joint influence related to the individual within the broader health system context [13]. What is the relative impact of geospatial access and caregiver intent on ZD status in DRC, and to what extent do they interact? This understanding is needed to better target and prioritize interventions to overcome barriers to vaccination for children who are ZD.

This current study leverages data from the 2021 and 2022 rounds of the Enquête de Couverture Vaccinale household coverage surveys conducted by the Kinshasa School of Public Health (ECV; vaccine coverage survey; fielded in early 2022 and early 2023, respectively) to assess the relative association between the EGH Vaccine Delivery Framework domains of intent to vaccinate (proxied by caregiver attitudes towards vaccination) and geographic access to services on vaccination status among rural households in DRC [12]. We first linked a constructed geolocated health facility list to estimate travel time from household locations to their closest health facility. We then compared the relative association between the estimated travel time and caregivers' self-reported perceptions of the importance of vaccination on whether their child was ZD, UI, or fully-immunized. Findings from this study may provide important insight relevant to improving targeted programming and policies to address barriers to vaccination in DRC and improve more equitable coverage.

2. Materials and Methods

2.1. Data Source

This is a secondary analysis of pooled data from two consecutive nationwide immunization surveys (Enquête de Couverture Vaccinale (ECV)), conducted in early 2022 and early 2023 and referred to as ECV2021 and ECV2022, respectively. Additional information on sampling protocols for these surveys can be found in the Supplementary Materials and have been described elsewhere [22,23]. Briefly, the ECVs are nationally representative multi-stage cluster cross-sectional randomized surveys, following a modified version of the WHO sampling method for vaccine coverage, targeting a sample of 6–23-month-olds [24]. GPS coordinates were recorded for each household in both study years. Data were pooled across the two surveys for this study.

2.2. Data Preparation

The study sample consisted of children aged 12–23 months and their caregivers. Following the approach used by Gavi, we considered a child to be zero-dose if they did not receive their first dose of the Pentavalent vaccine (DTP-Hib-HepB) by age 12 months [9]. We define under-immunized as receiving the first dose of Pentavalent but not the third or the first dose of the measles-containing vaccine. Given the timing and age cohorts targeted in the two surveys and the randomized sampling, it is extremely unlikely for the same child to appear twice in the two-survey sample.

Our study focused on rural households, defined by the survey's sampling frame. While travel time may be a concern in urban areas, particularly due to traffic congestion, we focused on rural households for this study because our methods for quantifying it do not incorporate traffic and other urban-specific issues and thus would likely underestimate travel time for urban areas relative to rural ones, where travel time is more a function of the distance, ground cover, and road type.

GPS coordinates from the ECV surveys were used to extract travel time to the nearest health facility for each household. Households with missing GPS coordinates or with coordinates not aligned to the AccessMod surface (see below) were dropped. Some households exhibited duplicated GPS coordinates and were consequently excluded from the analysis after being cross-examined against dataset elements, such as health zones, health areas, village names, or household identifiers. This duplication accounted for 12% of the entire dataset. This did not have an appreciable impact on the main results (see sensitivity analysis described in Supplementary Table S3). Further studies are underway to investigate the causes of this duplication and remedy them for future data collection.

Caregiver attitude toward vaccination was reflected using the survey question "How good do you think vaccines are for your child?" (originally surveyed in French as "*Dans quelle mesure pensez-vous que les vaccins sont bons pour votre enfant?*") Responses were grouped as "Very Bad, Bad, Don't Know", "Good", and "Very Good". We combined the "Very bad," "Bad", and "Don't Know" groupings because each had a relatively small sample and each had similar correlations with the outcome. This was one of several questions included in the ECV survey corresponding to well-validated constructs used by the Vaccine Confidence Project and the WHO Behavioral and Social Drivers (BeSD) Tool around vaccine attitudes, including attitudes around vaccine safety, efficacy, peer norms, and more. We selected this single measure to reflect vaccine attitudes because it was highly correlated with the other measures for this sample (Spearman's rank correlation coefficient of 0.53–0.68) and to simplify the interpretation of the primary analysis comparing the effect of vaccine attitudes and geospatial access on vaccination status.

Maternal age, education level of the household head, and birth order were also retained as control variables.

2.3. Quantifying Geographic Accessibility

Health facility locations were derived using a combination of data sources with facility GPS coordinates, including DHIS2 (N = 21,712 facilities, 72% with GPS), monthly Mashako

Plan supervision data (N = 15,565 facilities, 92.5% with GPS) (13), and the ECV facility survey conducted alongside the ECV household survey (N = 2904 facilities, 100% with GPS). We used the DHIS2 as a reference master facility list and supplemented the GPS coordinates in this list with the other two sources based on fuzzy-matching pre-processed facility name strings (e.g., removing non-Latin characters, removing facility type strings) using the Jaro-Winkler metric. An initial threshold score of 0.2 was used to identify potential matches, followed by a manual verification process to identify and reconcile false positive and false negative matches, as well as include facilities not reflected in the DHIS2 list. The final consolidated list used in this study consisted of N = 23,185 facilities with 79% GPS completion.

We estimated travel time using a cost distance algorithm that accounts for variation in travel speeds across differences in land uses, terrain, and barriers to transport, such as forests and water bodies. High-resolution spatial datasets representing these features were used to generate a travel friction surface, which was used to compute accumulated travel time to the nearest health facility in AccessMod version 5 [25]. While AccessMod is capable of producing travel times for both walking and motorized scenarios, we focused on walking time for this analysis for simplicity. Results were similar for both, and motorized results are available in the supplementary information (see Supplementary Table S1).

To derive population coverage statistics, we integrated travel time data with population distribution information from WorldPop [26]. At each gridded location in the country (both urban and rural, in this case), we extracted the population and the travel time from each surface. The population distribution was compared to the population distribution implied by the travel times extracted at the ECV survey locations.

2.4. Statistical Analysis

Descriptive statistics were provided to understand the sample characteristics. We used logistic regression to assess the relationship among geographic accessibility, caregiver attitude toward vaccination, and zero-dose vaccination status. We ran four nested models, successively adding complexity: 1. travel time only; 2. travel time and attitude; 3. travel time and attitude and covariates (maternal age, educational level of the household head, and the child's birth order); and 4. travel time and attitude and covariates with an interaction term between travel time and attitudes. The interaction term tests whether geographic access affects vaccine outcomes differently depending on the level of caregiver attitudes toward vaccination. Travel time was discretized into the following categories: under 5 min, 5–10 min, 10–20 min, 20–40 min, 40–60 min, 60 or more minutes. In addition to the covariates mentioned above, the survey (ECV2021 or ECV2022) was included as a covariate to control for changes in time and due to differences in survey implementation. Ninety-five percent confidence intervals are reported for all statistical tests. All analyses were conducted using R 4.3.1. The code is available at https://github.com/rburstein-IDM/access_attitude (accessed on 30 May 2024).

3. Results

Sample Description

The study sample included 80,313 12–23-month-old children living in rural settings. After removing observations with missing or faulty GPS coordinates (N = 10,828, 13%), we were left with 69,485 observations, 33,489 (48%) from ECV2021 and 35,996 (52%) from ECV2022. Of these 16,157 (23%) were zero-dose, 22,770 (33%) had at least some vaccination, and 30,558 (44%) had completed their vaccination series. Nearly half (47%, or 33,063) of respondents lived within 5 min of a facility, and 88% (N = 61,230) of households were within 60 min. The ECV2022 included a sample of slightly more distant rural households than did the ECV2021 sample. [See Table A1].

Figure A1 compares the population distribution walking time implied by the ECV surveys and WorldPop. Note again that here we included urban, as well as rural, households for a proper comparison. Relative to WorldPop, the ECV sample was nearer to health facilities. The median travel time for the WorldPop population was 6.5 min compared to 3.5 in the full ECV sample, with 70% within 20 min (compared to 82% in ECV), and 88% within 60 min (92% in ECV). Children who live further away from health facilities were more likely to be unvaccinated. Among children who live within 5 min of a health facility, 21% were zero-dose, while 26% of those living more than an hour from a facility were zero-dose (calculated from Table A1). In comparing travel time to the nearest facility and the prevalence of zero-dose, there was a steep increase in zero-dose prevalence within the first 10 min and a gradual increase in prevalence thereafter (Figure A2a). This relationship was similar in both survey rounds, with a slight shift downward in overall zero-dose prevalence in the 2022 survey.

Caregiver attitudes were strongly correlated with non-vaccination. Of the 9% of caregivers (N = 6285) who reported that vaccines are "Bad, Very Bad, or Dont Know", 87% of their children were zero-dose. Only 8.6% of children were zero-dose among caregivers who rated vaccines as "Very Good" for their child. Among caregivers of children who were fully immunized, only 1% reported "Bad" or "Very Bad", while 2% did among under-immunized children and 34% did among zero-dose children. However, within each level of parental attitude, there still appeared to be some effect of travel time (Figure A2b). Figure A2b emphasizes that across every time point in travel time, having a lower attitude status was the more important factor.

The modeled effect of caregiver attitude was much greater than the effect of travel time and was also not impacted much by the addition of the control variables. Unless otherwise noted, reported results are for the fully specified model (Model 3). The odds of being zero-dose for those living over an hour from a health facility relative to those living <5 min from a facility was 1.3 [95%CI: 1.2–1.4] (Table A2). There was a slight decrease from 40–60 min and 60+, but this difference was not significant. The effect of travel time was stable across the models, indicating that there was minimal confounding between the covariates and travel time (Table A2). In contrast, the odds ratio (OR) for "Very bad, bad, don't know" relative to "Very good" was 69.3 [63.4–75.8]. Furthermore, the OR for "Good" in reference to "Very Good" was 2.8 [2.6–2.9]. Covariates, such as maternal age (40+ in reference to <18) and birth order (third or more in reference to first), were in the same order as the geographic access effect (ORs = 1.3 and 1.2 respectively). The effect of education (less than primary in reference to post-secondary) was greater than that of distance (OR: 2.0, 1.8–2.3). We found no significant effect of interaction between travel time and caregiver attitude or on the effect of survey year (see Supplementary Table S2).

4. Discussion

We linked estimates of travel time to the 2021 and 2022 ECV vaccination coverage survey to compare the relative effect of caregiver attitudes towards vaccinations and geographic accessibility to health facilities on child vaccination status. We found that caregiver attitudes toward childhood vaccination, a proxy for intent to vaccinate, is a many-fold stronger predictor of non-vaccination than geographic accessibility. Furthermore, both the ECV and WorldPop indicate that geographic accessibility is high in rural DRC, with 83% of the population living within an hour walk of a health facility.

In recent years, there has been a growing number of geospatial analyses on accessibility to healthcare in low- and middle-income countries [27–29] and the impacts of that on utilization [30–37] and health outcomes [38,39]. At the same time, it has been well understood that demand for services is a critical component of the uptake of health services, including vaccine services [40]. Our study contributes to this body of literature by comparing the relative influence of these two important determinants of utilization jointly. We believe this is the first time this comparison has been performed in DRC.

Our findings add to a growing body of evidence on geographic accessibility and caregiver attitudes to health services in DRC. A previous analysis of the ECV2021 on caregiver-reported reasons for non-vaccination found that 8% of zero-dose caregivers reported distance as a reason for not vaccinating their children, while 64% cited reasons related to people's perceptions and feelings "Confidence in vaccine benefits" [22]. The present study strengthens this finding by confirming it through orthogonally measured variables, rather than self-reported reasons. In a study on antenatal care attendance in two provinces in DRC, Mafuta and Kayembe found that 83.5% of women reported that the distance to reach health facilities was less than 5 km and for 78.4% this distance took them less than an hour [41]. Our study also revealed that vaccine uptake was sensitive to short distances, with a steep increase in zero-dose prevalence from 0–10 min, and that in the model, being 20 min away was similar to being 60+ min away. Karra and colleagues found a similar pattern in their study of child mortality patterns in 21 low and middle-income countries [39].

Reaching zero-dose children is a growing global priority and is a centerpiece of Gavi's 5.0 strategy [42], which is currently disbursing $500M to countries [43] as part of their goal to reduce the global number of zero-dose by 50% by 2030. To achieve this ambitious goal, immunization programs must progress from understanding who is unvaccinated to why caregivers are not taking their children to be vaccinated. This information is critical for making strategic programmatic choices under resource constraints. For example, based on the evidence presented in this paper, an intensive remote rural strategy is likely to reach fewer children than a near-facility demand-generation strategy. Of course, other information, such as cost data, and information about other determinants [44], such as supply chain readiness, and logistical considerations are critical factors as well.

The DRC government committed to strengthening routine immunization services under the Mashako Plan, launched in 2018. However, the plan in its current form does not address demand-related barriers to vaccination and primarily focuses on supply-side improvements, such as increasing the number of immunization sessions, supportive supervision, vaccination stocks, and cold chain improvement [11,45]. To fully address non-vaccination in the country, there will likely need to be an explicit focus on demand generation, for example by mobilizing the network of community health workers (relais communautaire, RECOs in DRC) for educational campaigns.

This paper motivates several areas for future study. First, given the importance of caregiver attitudes toward vaccination, a more thorough investigation of the intent to vaccinate is needed. In addition to caregiver attitudes toward vaccination, components like awareness, knowledge, agency, and community norms interact in complex ways to yield an intent to vaccinate [46,47]. Implementation of the WHO's BeSD questionnaire in future surveys will be a welcome increase in the availability of such data [16]. Further studies should also aim to include a fuller set of determinants across intent to vaccinate, community access, and health facility readiness. For example, future studies may also include measures of health facility readiness to deliver vaccination services (e.g., WHO Service Availability and Readiness Assessment (SARA) immunization indicators) [48] and explore the relative prioritization of child immunization amongst the multiple priorities caregivers have to address possibly through a structural causal modeling framework, similar to work performed by Phillips et al. [44] Even in terms of access, the present analysis is relatively narrowly focused on geographic access, while access is a wider concept that encompasses the convenience and acceptability of services. As such, barriers, including wait times and caregiver costs (both direct and indirect), are not included here but may contribute significantly to the zero-dose status. Furthermore, variation in geographic accessibility due to weather, road conditions, and transportation should be further explored in subsequent studies (see limitations below). Finally, survey sampling in DRC is difficult as there is no recent census to draw on, and this may have impacted ECV sampling. Efforts underway by groups like GRID3 are making alternative geographic data sources available upon which to draw sampling frames for new approaches, such as gridded population survey sampling [49].

This paper has several limitations. First, the households sampled in ECV were nearer to health facilities than the population distribution in WorldPop. While we do not consider this a validation, as WorldPop does not necessarily represent ground truth, it indicates that there is some uncertainty around the true accessibility of the DRC population. The ECV2022 used an updated sampling methodology, segmenting each survey cluster into 16 areas spread across each enumeration unit, and randomly selecting six of them, which likely led to a slightly more remote population being selected (see Figure A1). For this reason, we primarily focus on our results on the modeled impact of distance, rather than reporting it as a representative estimate of distance to care. Second, there may be potential limitations in comparing the relative impact of self-reported attitudes and the objectively measured travel time. For example, while there may exist response bias (e.g., social desirability biases) where individuals do not accurately reflect their true attitudes towards vaccination, the same is not present for measures of travel time to vaccination. However, we note that the construct used to reflect attitudes has been well-validated in other contexts, mitigating some concern for such a bias in this context. Third, and relatedly, since attitudes toward vaccination were measured in the same survey as our outcome and travel time was measured independently, it is likely that travel time is measured with more error. This could lead to attenuation bias in the regression, meaning that the true effect of travel time was likely higher than our estimate. While this should be acknowledged, it is highly unlikely that the attenuation bias rises to the very large magnitude of the difference we observe in the effect of attitude versus access. The approach to estimating travel time may oversimplify the accessibility landscape by not accounting for variations in walking speeds, potential obstacles, or terrain conditions. Additionally, it may not fully capture the nuances of diverse transportation patterns within a population, particularly in areas where alternative modes of transport, such as bicycles or informal public transport, are common. As verification for our approach to estimating travel time, we found that parents who live further away are more likely to cite distance as a reason for non-vaccination (see Supplementary Figure S1). Finally, our operationalization of travel time does not fully account for travel time to all vaccination services. In DRC, some vaccination services are administered via outreach sessions, and we did not have enough information to include those in this analysis. Such strategies are meant to improve equity by reducing the cost for more remote populations to seek care. It is possible that the relatively weak impact of travel time that we observed in our analysis reflects the success of outreach strategies. A more detailed study of the impact of outreach services in DRC is needed.

5. Conclusions

Understanding the relative influence of barriers to vaccination is a critical step in developing effective strategies to reach zero-dose children. In the case of rural areas in DRC, attitudes toward vaccination are much more impactful than geographic accessibility. This evidence suggests that efforts to improve demand and address parental concerns will be a critical component of addressing the large zero-dose problem in DRC.

Supplementary Materials: The following supporting information can be downloaded at: https://www.mdpi.com/article/10.3390/vaccines12060617/s1, Figure S1: The proportion of caregivers who state that distance to care is a factor for non-vaccination increases from 5% next door to over 15% one hour away with distance to the nearest health facility; Table S1: The fully specified model (Model 3) using motorized travel time instead of walking travel time. Results are generally comparable to the walking model; Table S2: Model 4: fully specified model (Model 3), with additional interaction between travel time and parental attitude included. No consistent evidence of interaction was detected; Table S3: Model 3 sensitivity analysis, keeping in all observations with duplicate GPS coordinates. (N= 76,174). Results were nearly identical to the main model; Brief Description of ECV sampling.

Author Contributions: Conceptualization, R.B. and P.Y.L.; statistical analysis, R.B.; geographic analysis (AccessMod), P.O. and K.W.; facility list curation, P.Y.L.; data collection: P.L., F.B., B.K.M., E.M.; interpretation of data, N.A.H.; writing—original draft preparation, B.K.M., F.B., P.Y.L., R.B., L.E.; writing—review and editing, all authors. All authors have read and agreed to the published version of the manuscript.

Funding: The survey that generated the data used in this study was funded by the United Nations Children Emergency Funds (UNICEF) after mobilizing funding from GAVI and BMGF. This particular study was conducted without specific funding.

Institutional Review Board Statement: Ethical approvals were sought for each round of the vaccination coverage survey from the Kinshasa School of Public Health Ethical Committee before data collection (approvals: ESP/CE/175/2021 and ESP/CE/025/2023). Health and politico-administrative authorities at the local level also provided their authorization.

Informed Consent Statement: Oral informed consent was obtained from potential study participants before starting the interview. Potential survey participants were informed about the nature of the survey, including objectives, risks and benefits, the confidentiality of their replies, the contact details of study personnel, and that they were free to participate or not without any negative consequences. Confidentiality was maintained and the dataset was anonymized.

Data Availability Statement: The data underlying this study from the ECV surveys contain sensitive geographic information. Consequently, these datasets are not publicly available to ensure the privacy and confidentiality of the participants involved. Data access can be formally requested by contacting eric.mafuta@unikin.ac.cd. Travel time maps and health facility list will be made available as digital supplements.

Conflicts of Interest: Several authors (R.B., P.Y.L., D.M. and A.M.) work or are contractors at organizations that funded the original collection of the survey data used in this study. This study was conceived and designed by authors without a funding role after data collection was already completed.

Appendix A

Table A1. Sample Characteristics.

	Fully-Immunized		Under-Immunized		Zero-Dose		Total	
	ECV 2021	ECV 2022	ECV 2021	ECV 2022	ECV 2021	ECV 2022	ECV 2021	ECV 2022
	(N = 14,227)	(N = 16,331)	(N = 11,251)	(N = 11,519)	(N = 8011)	(N = 8146)	(N = 33,489)	(N = 35,996)
Travel Time								
<5 min	7913 (55.6%)	7454 (45.6%)	5885 (52.3%)	4944 (42.9%)	3760 (46.9%)	3107 (38.1%)	17,558 (52.4%)	15,505 (43.1%)
5–10 min	2180 (15.3%)	2361 (14.5%)	1872 (16.6%)	1615 (14.0%)	1369 (17.1%)	1144 (14.0%)	5421 (16.2%)	5120 (14.2%)
10–20 min	1456 (10.2%)	1791 (11.0%)	1350 (12.0%)	1386 (12.0%)	990 (12.4%)	986 (12.1%)	3796 (11.3%)	4163 (11.6%)
20–40 min	988 (6.9%)	1524 (9.3%)	881 (7.8%)	1248 (10.8%)	701 (8.8%)	981 (12.0%)	2570 (7.7%)	3753 (10.4%)
40–60 min	463 (3.3%)	875 (5.4%)	392 (3.5%)	667 (5.8%)	391 (4.9%)	556 (6.8%)	1246 (3.7%)	2098 (5.8%)
60+ min	1227 (8.6%)	2326 (14.2%)	871 (7.7%)	1659 (14.4%)	800 (10.0%)	1372 (16.8%)	2898 (8.7%)	5357 (14.9%)
How good are vaccines?								
Very Good	5297 (37.2%)	7156 (43.8%)	2886 (25.7%)	3979 (34.5%)	732 (9.1%)	1096 (13.5%)	8915 (26.6%)	12231 (34.0%)
Good	8840 (62.1%)	9001 (55.1%)	8124 (72.2%)	7236 (62.8%)	4630 (57.8%)	4223 (51.8%)	21594 (64.5%)	20460 (56.8%)
Bad, Very Bad, Don't Know	90 (0.6%)	174 (1.1%)	241 (2.1%)	304 (2.6%)	2649 (33.1%)	2827 (34.7%)	2980 (8.9%)	3305 (9.2%)
Mother's Age								
<18	213 (1.5%)	324 (2.0%)	188 (1.7%)	249 (2.2%)	167 (2.1%)	171 (2.1%)	568 (1.7%)	744 (2.1%)
18–19	698 (4.9%)	1168 (7.2%)	690 (6.1%)	953 (8.3%)	525 (6.6%)	646 (7.9%)	1913 (5.7%)	2767 (7.7%)
20–24	4076 (28.6%)	4961 (30.4%)	3432 (30.5%)	3697 (32.1%)	2472 (30.9%)	2663 (32.7%)	9980 (29.8%)	11321 (31.5%)

Table A1. *Cont.*

	Fully-Immunized		Under-Immunized		Zero-Dose		Total	
	ECV 2021 (N = 14,227)	ECV 2022 (N = 16,331)	ECV 2021 (N = 11,251)	ECV 2022 (N = 11,519)	ECV 2021 (N = 8011)	ECV 2022 (N = 8146)	ECV 2021 (N = 33,489)	ECV 2022 (N = 35,996)
25–29	3522 (24.8%)	3973 (24.3%)	2579 (22.9%)	2564 (22.3%)	1753 (21.9%)	1734 (21.3%)	7854 (23.5%)	8271 (23.0%)
30–39	4826 (33.9%)	4968 (30.4%)	3714 (33.0%)	3358 (29.2%)	2533 (31.6%)	2291 (28.1%)	11073 (33.1%)	10617 (29.5%)
>40	711 (5.0%)	659 (4.0%)	524 (4.7%)	528 (4.6%)	475 (5.9%)	480 (5.9%)	1710 (5.1%)	1667 (4.6%)
Missing	181 (1.3%)	278 (1.7%)	124 (1.1%)	170 (1.5%)	86 (1.1%)	161 (2.0%)	391 (1.2%)	609 (1.7%)
Education Level of HH Head								
Tertiary	869 (6.1%)	1058 (6.5%)	418 (3.7%)	468 (4.1%)	182 (2.3%)	210 (2.6%)	1469 (4.4%)	1736 (4.8%)
Secondary	8295 (58.3%)	9842 (60.3%)	6224 (55.3%)	6511 (56.5%)	4136 (51.6%)	4359 (53.5%)	18655 (55.7%)	20712 (57.5%)
Primary	3776 (26.5%)	4112 (25.2%)	3500 (31.1%)	3312 (28.8%)	2713 (33.9%)	2600 (31.9%)	9989 (29.8%)	10024 (27.8%)
Less than primary	1099 (7.7%)	1063 (6.5%)	970 (8.6%)	1014 (8.8%)	847 (10.6%)	849 (10.4%)	2916 (8.7%)	2926 (8.1%)
Missing	188 (1.3%)	256 (1.6%)	139 (1.2%)	214 (1.9%)	133 (1.7%)	128 (1.6%)	460 (1.4%)	598 (1.7%)
Birth Order								
1	6586 (46.3%)	8298 (50.8%)	5042 (44.8%)	5565 (48.3%)	3757 (46.9%)	4035 (49.5%)	15385 (45.9%)	17898 (49.7%)
2	6498 (45.7%)	6962 (42.6%)	5225 (46.4%)	5017 (43.6%)	3427 (42.8%)	3463 (42.5%)	15150 (45.2%)	15442 (42.9%)
3+	1143 (8.0%)	1071 (6.6%)	983 (8.7%)	937 (8.1%)	826 (10.3%)	648 (8.0%)	2952 (8.8%)	2656 (7.4%)
Missing	0 (0%)	0 (0%)	1 (0.0%)	0 (0%)	1 (0.0%)	0 (0%)	2 (0.0%)	0 (0%)

Table A2. Regression Results.

Variable	Variable Level	Model 3: Fully-Specified (R-Squared = 0.30)			Model 2: Travel Time + Attitudes (R-Squared = 0.29)			Model 1: Travel Time (R-Squared = 0.01)		
		OR	2.5% CI	97.5% CI	OR	2.5% CI	97.5% CI	OR	2.5% CI	97.5% CI
Intercept		0.1	0.0	0.1	0.1	0.1	0.1	0.3	0.3	0.3
Travel time	<5 min (Reference)									
	5–10 min	1.2	1.1	1.3	1.2	1.2	1.3	1.2	1.1	1.3
	10–20 min	1.3	1.2	1.4	1.3	1.2	1.4	1.3	1.2	1.3
	20–40 min	1.4	1.3	1.5	1.5	1.4	1.6	1.4	1.3	1.5
	40–60 min	1.4	1.3	1.6	1.4	1.3	1.6	1.5	1.4	1.6
	60+ min	1.3	1.2	1.4	1.3	1.3	1.4	1.4	1.3	1.4
Attitude	Very Good (Ref.)									
	Good	2.8	2.6	2.9	2.8	2.7	3.0			
	Bad/Very Bad/Don't Know	69.3	63.4	75.8	71.7	65.7	78.3			
Maternal Age	Under-18 (Ref.)									
	18–19	1.0	0.8	1.2						
	20–24	1.0	0.9	1.2						
	25–29	0.9	0.8	1.0						
	30–39	0.9	0.8	1.1						
	40+	1.3	1.1	1.6						

Table A2. Cont.

		Model 3: Fully-Specified (R-Squared = 0.30)	Model 2: Travel Time + Attitudes (R-Squared = 0.29)	Model 1: Travel Time (R-Squared = 0.01)
HH Education	More than secondary (Ref.)			
	Secondary	1.7	1.5	12.0
	Primary	2.0	1.8	2.3
	Less than Primary	2.0	1.8	2.3
Birth Order	First			
	Second	1.0	1.0	1.0
	Third or more	1.2	1.2	1.3
Survey Round	ECV2021 (Ref.)			
	ECV2022	0.9	0.9	1.0

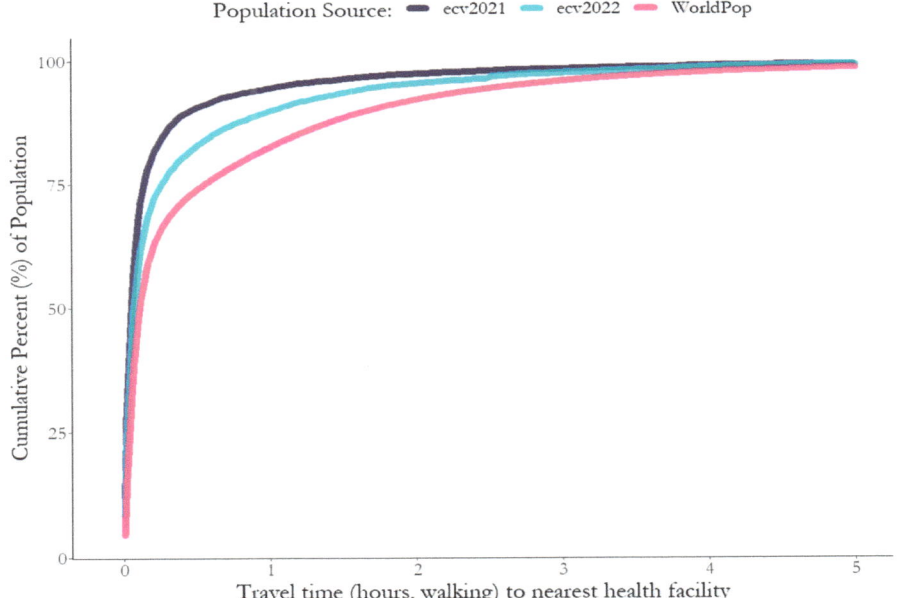

Figure A1. Travel time (walking) in hours to the nearest health facility. ECV2021 and ECV2022 samples were closer to health facilities than the population distribution implied by WorldPop. ECV2022 had a slightly more geographically distant sample, likely due to the addition of segmented sampling in that survey. Median travel time for the WorldPop population was 6.5 min compared to 3.5 in the full ECV sample, with 70% within 20 min (compared to 82% in ECV), and 88% within 60 min (92% in ECV).

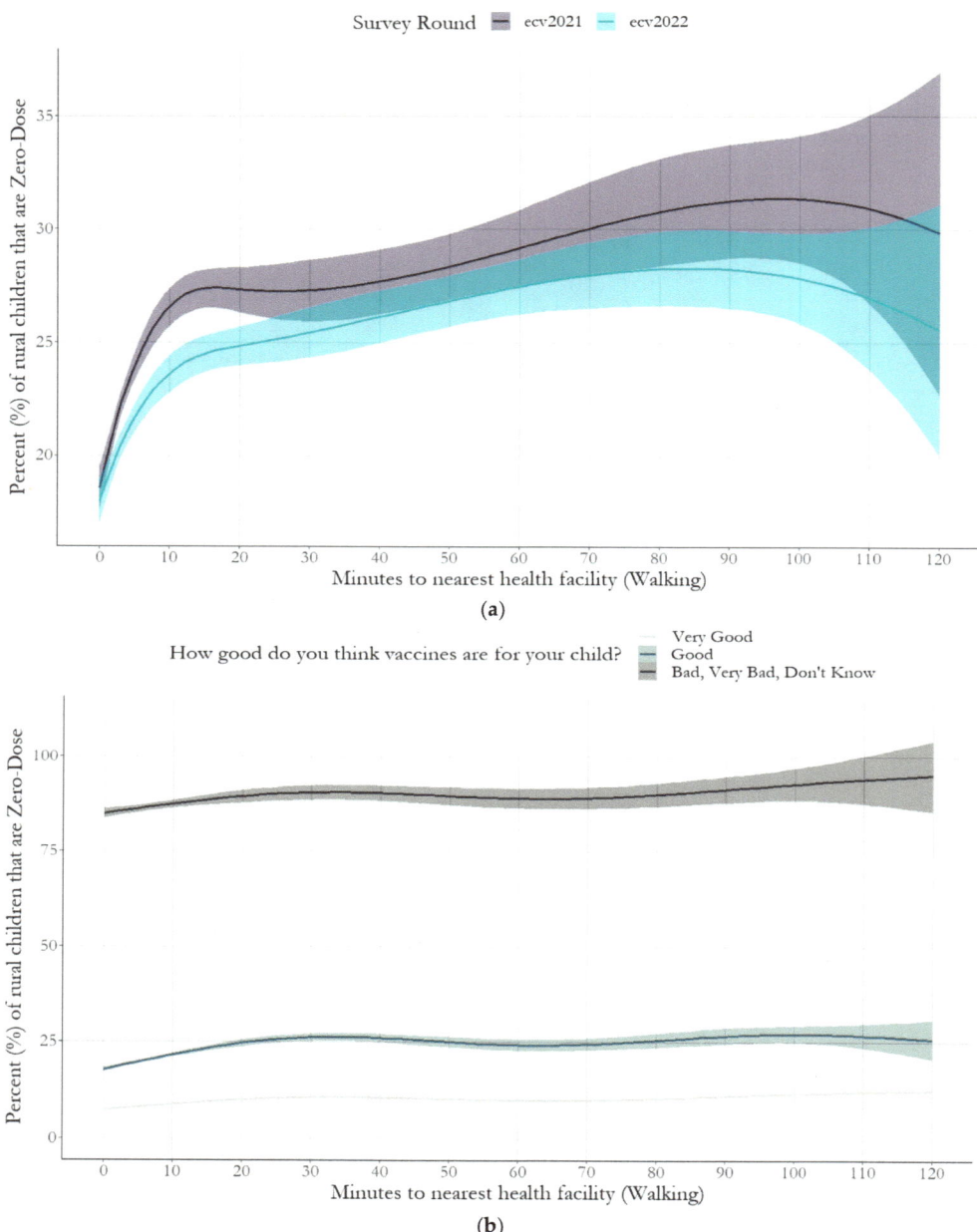

Figure A2. (**a**) Prevalence of zero-dose as a function of travel time (walking) in minutes to the nearest health facility, split by survey round. The lines represent smooths resulting from generalized additive models. (**b**) Prevalence of zero-dose as a function of travel time (walking) in minutes to the nearest health facility, split by parental attitude toward vaccines.

References

1. Lai, X.; Zhang, H.; Pouwels, K.B.; Patenaude, B.; Jit, M.; Fang, H. Estimating global and regional between-country inequality in routine childhood vaccine coverage in 195 countries and territories from 2019 to 2021: A longitudinal study. *EClinicalMedicine* **2023**, *60*, 102042. [CrossRef]
2. Bobo, F.T.; Asante, A.; Woldie, M.; Dawson, A.; Hayen, A. Child vaccination in sub-Saharan Africa: Increasing coverage addresses inequalities. *Vaccine* **2022**, *40*, 141–150. [CrossRef] [PubMed]
3. Hogan, D.; Gupta, A. Why Reaching Zero-Dose Children Holds the Key to Achieving the Sustainable Development Goals. *Vaccines* **2023**, *11*, 781. [CrossRef]
4. World Health Organization. *Immunization Dashboard, Global*; World Health Organization: Geneva, Switzerland, 2022. Available online: https://immunizationdata.who.int/ (accessed on 7 February 2024).
5. World Health Organization. Immunization Agenda 2030: A Global Strategy to Leave No One Behind. 2020. Available online: https://www.who.int/publications/m/item/immunization-agenda-2030-a-global-strategy-to-leave-no-one-behind (accessed on 7 February 2024).
6. Gavi the Vaccine Alliance. The Zero-Dose Child: Explained. 2021. Available online: https://www.gavi.org/vaccineswork/zero-dose-child-explained (accessed on 7 February 2024).
7. Farrenkopf, B.A.; Zhou, X.; Shet, A.; Olayinka, F.; Carr, K.; Patenaude, B.; Chido-Amajuoyi, O.G.; Wonodi, C. Understanding household-level risk factors for zero dose immunization in 82 low- and middle-income countries. *PLoS ONE* **2023**, *18*, e0287459. [CrossRef]
8. Wonodi, C.; Farrenkopf, B.A. Defining the Zero Dose Child: A Comparative Analysis of Two Approaches and Their Impact on Assessing the Zero Dose Burden and Vulnerability Profiles across 82 Low- and Middle-Income Countries. *Vaccines* **2023**, *11*, 1543. [CrossRef]
9. International Vaccines Access Center (IVAC) and Gavi the Vaccine Alliance. Addressing Gender Inequities to Improve Immunization Coverage for Zero-Dose Children. 2022. Available online: https://publichealth.jhu.edu/sites/default/files/2024-02/zero-dosegender-equityadvocacy-briefax.pdf (accessed on 7 February 2024).
10. World Health Organization African Region. Deaths from Democratic Republic of the Congo Measles Outbreak Top 6000. 2024. Available online: https://www.afro.who.int/news/deaths-democratic-republic-congo-measles-outbreak-top-6000 (accessed on 7 February 2024).
11. Lame, P.; Milabyo, A.; Tangney, S.; Mbaka, G.O.; Luhata, C.; Le Gargasson, J.B.; Mputu, C.; Hoff, N.A.; Merritt, S.; Nkamba, D.M.; et al. A Successful National and Multipartner Approach to Increase Immunization Coverage: The Democratic Republic of Congo Mashako Plan 2018–2020. *Glob. Health Sci. Pract.* **2023**, *11*, e2200326. [CrossRef] [PubMed]
12. Kinshasa School of Public Health (KSPH). *Enquête de Couverture Vaccinale (ECV) 2021–2022*; Kinshasa School of Public Health (KSPH): Kinshasa, Democratic Republic of the Congo, 2021.
13. Shearer, J.C.; Nava, O.; Prosser, W.; Nawaz, S.; Mulongo, S.; Mambu, T.; Mafuta, E.; Munguambe, K.; Sigauque, B.; Cherima, Y.J.; et al. Uncovering the Drivers of Childhood Immunization Inequality with Caregivers, Community Members and Health System Stakeholders: Results from a Human-Centered Design Study in DRC, Mozambique and Nigeria. *Vaccines* **2023**, *11*, 689. [CrossRef]
14. World Health Organization. Behavioural and Social Drivers of Vaccination: Tools and Practical Guidance for Achieving High Uptake. 2022. Available online: https://iris.who.int/handle/10665/354459 (accessed on 7 February 2024).
15. Bednarczyk, R.A.; Hester, K.A.; Dixit, S.M.; Ellis, A.S.; Escoffery, C.; Kilembe, W.; Micek, K.; Sakas, Z.M.; Sarr, M.; Freeman, M.C. Exemplars in vaccine delivery protocol: A case-study-based identification and evaluation of critical factors in achieving high and sustained childhood immunisation coverage in selected low-income and lower-middle-income countries. *BMJ Open* **2022**, *12*, e058321. [CrossRef]
16. World Health Organization. *Weekly Epidemiological Record*; World Health Organization: Geneva, Switzerland, 2022.
17. Biset, G.; Woday, A.; Mihret, S.; Tsihay, M. Full immunization coverage and associated factors among children age 12–23 months in Ethiopia: Systematic review and meta-analysis of observational studies. *Hum. Vaccines Immunother.* **2021**, *17*, 2326–2335. [CrossRef] [PubMed]
18. Bangura, J.B.; Xiao, S.; Qiu, D.; Ouyang, F.; Chen, L. Barriers to childhood immunization in sub-Saharan Africa: A systematic review. *BMC Public Health* **2020**, *20*, 1108. [CrossRef]
19. Kiptoo, E.; Esilaba, M.; Kobia, G.; Ngure, R. Factors Influencing Low Immunization Coverage among Children between 12–23 Months in East Pokot, Baringo Country, Kenya. *Int. J. Vaccines Vaccin.* **2015**, *1*, 00012. [CrossRef]
20. Legesse, E.; Dechasa, W. An assessment of child immunization coverage and its determinants in Sinana District, Southeast Ethiopia. *BMC Pediatr.* **2015**, *15*, 31. [CrossRef] [PubMed]
21. Jani, J.V.; De Schacht, C.; Jani, I.V.; Bjune, G. Risk factors for incomplete vaccination and missed opportunity for immunization in rural Mozambique. *BMC Public Health* **2008**, *8*, 161. [CrossRef] [PubMed]
22. Ishoso, D.K.; Mafuta, E.; Danovaro-Holliday, M.C.; Ngandu, C.; Menning, L.; Cikomola, A.M.W.; Lungayo, C.L.; Mukendi, J.C.; Mwamba, D.; Mboussou, F.F.; et al. Reasons for Being "Zero-Dose and Under-Vaccinated" among Children Aged 12–23 Months in the Democratic Republic of the Congo. *Vaccines* **2023**, *11*, 1370. [CrossRef]
23. Ishoso, D.K.; Danovaro-Holliday, M.C.; Cikomola, A.M.W.; Lungayo, C.L.; Mukendi, J.C.; Mwamba, D.; Ngandu, C.; Mafuta, E.; Lusamba Dikassa, P.S.; Lulebo, A.; et al. "Zero Dose" Children in the Democratic Republic of the Congo: How Many and Who Are They? *Vaccines* **2023**, *11*, 900. [CrossRef] [PubMed]

24. World Health Organization. *World Health Organization Vaccination Coverage Cluster Surveys: Reference Manual*; World Health Organization: Geneva, Switzerland, 2018.
25. Ray, N.; Ebener, S. AccessMod 3.0: Computing geographic coverage and accessibility to health care services using anisotropic movement of patients. *Int. J. Health Geogr.* **2008**, *7*, 63. [CrossRef]
26. Lloyd, C.T.; Sorichetta, A.; Tatem, A.J. Data Descriptor: High resolution global gridded data for use in population studies. *Sci. Data* **2017**, *4*, 170001. [CrossRef] [PubMed]
27. Banke-Thomas, A.; Macharia, P.M.; Makanga, P.T.; Beňová, L.; Wong, K.L.; Gwacham-Anisiobi, U.; Wang, J.; Olubodun, T.; Ogunyemi, O.; Afolabi, B.B.; et al. Leveraging big data for improving the estimation of close to reality travel time to obstetric emergency services in urban low- and middle-income settings. *Front. Public Health* **2022**, *10*, 931401. [CrossRef]
28. Bouanchaud, P.; Macharia, P.M.; Demise, E.G.; Nakimuli, D. Comparing modelled with self-reported travel time and the used versus the nearest facility: Modelling geographic accessibility to family planning outlets in Kenya. *BMJ Glob. Health* **2022**, *7*, e008366. [CrossRef]
29. Weiss, D.J.; Nelson, A.; Vargas-Ruiz, C.A.; Gligorić, K.; Bavadekar, S.; Gabrilovich, E.; Bertozzi-Villa, A.; Rozier, J.; Gibson, H.S.; Shekel, T.; et al. Global maps of travel time to healthcare facilities. *Nat. Med.* **2020**, *26*, 1835–1838. [CrossRef]
30. Ogero, M.; Orwa, J.; Odhiambo, R.; Agoi, F.; Lusambili, A.; Obure, J.; Temmerman, M.; Luchters, S.; Ngugi, A. Pentavalent vaccination in Kenya: Coverage and geographical accessibility to health facilities using data from a community demographic and health surveillance system in Kilifi County. *BMC Public Health* **2022**, *22*, 826. [CrossRef]
31. Joseph, N.K.; Macharia, P.M.; Ouma, P.O.; Mumo, J.; Jalang'O, R.; Wagacha, P.W.; Achieng, V.O.; Ndung'U, E.; Okoth, P.; Muniz, M.; et al. Spatial access inequities and childhood immunisation uptake in Kenya. *BMC Public Health* **2020**, *20*, 1407. [CrossRef] [PubMed]
32. Tanou, M.; Kamiya, Y. Assessing the impact of geographical access to health facilities on maternal healthcare utilization: Evidence from the Burkina Faso demographic and health survey 2010. *BMC Public Health* **2019**, *19*, 838. [CrossRef] [PubMed]
33. Wong, K.L.M.; Brady, O.J.; Campbell, O.M.R.; Banke-Thomas, A.; Benova, L. Too poor or too far? Partitioning the variability of hospital-based childbirth by poverty and travel time in Kenya, Malawi, Nigeria and Tanzania. *Int. J. Equity Health* **2020**, *19*, 15. [CrossRef] [PubMed]
34. Masters, S.H.; Burstein, R.; Amofah, G.; Abaogye, P.; Kumar, S.; Hanlon, M. Travel time to maternity care and its effect on utilization in rural Ghana: A multilevel analysis. *Soc. Sci. Med.* **2013**, *93*, 147–154. [CrossRef]
35. Stock, R. Distance and the utilization of health facilities in rural Nigeria☆ rights and content. *Soc. Sci. Med.* **1983**, *17*, 563–570. [CrossRef] [PubMed]
36. Wong, K.L.M.; Benova, L.; Campbell, O.M.R. A look back on how far to walk: Systematic review and meta-analysis of physical access to skilled care for childbirth in Sub-Saharan Africa. *PLoS ONE* **2017**, *12*, e0184432. [CrossRef]
37. Tanser, F.; Gijsbertsen, B.; Herbst, K. Modelling and understanding primary health care accessibility and utilization in rural South Africa: An exploration using a geographical information system. *Soc. Sci. Med.* **2006**, *63*, 691–705. [CrossRef]
38. Moïsi, J.C.; Nokes, D.J.; Gatakaa, H.; Williams, T.N.; Bauni, E.; Levine, O.S.; Scott, J.A.G. Sensibilité de la surveillance hospitalière des maladies graves: Une analyse du système d'information géographique de l'accès aux soins dans le district Kilifi au Kenya. *Bull. World Health Organ.* **2011**, *89*, 102–111. [CrossRef]
39. Karra, M.; Fink, G.; Canning, D. Facility distance and child mortality: A multi-country study of health facility access, service utilization, and child health outcomes. *Int. J. Epidemiol.* **2017**, *46*, 817–826. [CrossRef]
40. Ababu, Y.; Braka, F.; Teka, A.; Getachew, K.; Tadesse, T.; Michael, Y.; Birhanu, Z.; Nsubuga, P.; Assefa, T.; Gallagher, K. Behavioral determinants of immunization service utilization in Ethiopia: A cross-sectional community-based survey. *Pan Afr. Med. J.* **2017**, *27*, 2. [CrossRef] [PubMed]
41. Mafuta, E.M.; Kayembe, K.P. Déterminants de la fréquentation tardive des services de soins prénatals dans les zones de santé de l'Equateur et du Katanga en République Démocratique du Congo Late antenatal care attendance, main determinants, in health zones of Katanga and Equateur. Annales Africaines de Médecine. *Ann. Afr. Med.* **2011**, *4*, 845.
42. Gavi the Vaccine Alliance. Reaching Zero-Dose Children. Available online: https://www.gavi.org/our-alliance/strategy/phase-5-2021-2025/equity-goal/zero-dose-children-missed-communities (accessed on 28 January 2024).
43. Gandhi, G. Charting the evolution of approaches employed by the Global Alliance for Vaccines and Immunizations (GAVI) to address inequities in access to immunization: A systematic qualitative review of GAVI policies, strategies and resource allocation mechanisms through an equity lens (1999–2014). *BMC Public Health* **2015**, *15*, 1198. [CrossRef] [PubMed]
44. Phillips, D.E.; Dieleman, J.L.; Lim, S.S.; Shearer, J. Determinants of effective vaccine coverage in low and middle-income countries: A systematic review and interpretive synthesis. *BMC Health Serv. Res.* **2017**, *17*, 681. [CrossRef] [PubMed]
45. Tangney, S.M. Impact of an Emergency Strategy to Revitalize the Routine Immunization System of the Democratic Republic of the Congo, the "Mashako Plan" Policy. 2023. Available online: https://escholarship.org/uc/item/4b870662 (accessed on 7 February 2024).
46. van Heemskerken, P.G.; Decouttere, C.J.; Broekhuizen, H.; Vandaele, N.J. Understanding the complexity of demand-side determinants on vaccine uptake in sub-Saharan Africa. *Health Policy Plan.* **2022**, *37*, 281–291. [CrossRef] [PubMed]
47. Ajzen, I. The theory of planned behavior. *Organ. Behav. Hum. Decis. Process.* **1991**, *50*, 179–211. [CrossRef]

48. Phillips, D.E.; Dieleman, J.L.; Shearer, J.C.; Lim, S.S. Childhood vaccines in Uganda and Zambia: Determinants and barriers to vaccine coverage. *Vaccine* **2018**, *36*, 4236–4244. [CrossRef] [PubMed]
49. Thomson, D.R.; Rhoda, D.A.; Tatem, A.J.; Castro, M.C. Gridded population survey sampling: A systematic scoping review of the field and strategic research agenda. *Int. J. Health Geogr.* **2020**, *19*, 34. [CrossRef]

Disclaimer/Publisher's Note: The statements, opinions and data contained in all publications are solely those of the individual author(s) and contributor(s) and not of MDPI and/or the editor(s). MDPI and/or the editor(s) disclaim responsibility for any injury to people or property resulting from any ideas, methods, instructions or products referred to in the content.

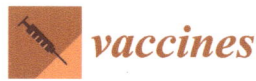 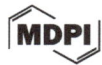

Article

Timeliness of Childhood Vaccinations Following Strengthening of the Second Year of Life (2YL) Immunization Platform and Introduction of Catch-Up Vaccination Policy in Ghana

Pierre Muhoza [1,2,*], Monica P. Shah [1], Kwame Amponsa-Achiano [3], Hongjiang Gao [1], Pamela Quaye [3], William Opare [3], Charlotte Okae [3], Philip-Neri Aboyinga [3], Joseph Kwadwo Larbi Opare [4], Daniel C. Ehlman [1], Melissa T. Wardle [1] and Aaron S. Wallace [1]

1 Global Immunization Division, U.S. Centers for Disease Control and Prevention, Atlanta, GA 30329, USA
2 Epidemic Intelligence Service, U.S. Centers for Disease Control and Prevention, Atlanta, GA 30329, USA
3 Expanded Programme on Immunisation, Disease Control and Prevention Department, Public Health Division, Ghana Health Service, Accra P.O. Box M 44, Ghana
4 Neglected Tropical Diseases Control Programme, Disease Control and Prevention Department, Public Health Division, Ghana Health Service, Accra P.O. Box M 44, Ghana
* Correspondence: pmuhoza@cdc.gov; Tel.: +1-404-698-5942

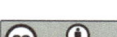

Citation: Muhoza, P.; Shah, M.P.; Amponsa-Achiano, K.; Gao, H.; Quaye, P.; Opare, W.; Okae, C.; Aboyinga, P.-N.; Opare, J.K.L.; Ehlman, D.C.; et al. Timeliness of Childhood Vaccinations Following Strengthening of the Second Year of Life (2YL) Immunization Platform and Introduction of Catch-Up Vaccination Policy in Ghana. *Vaccines* **2024**, *12*, 716. https://doi.org/10.3390/vaccines12070716

Academic Editor: Christian Napoli

Received: 27 April 2024
Revised: 20 June 2024
Accepted: 23 June 2024
Published: 27 June 2024

Copyright: © 2024 by the authors. Licensee MDPI, Basel, Switzerland. This article is an open access article distributed under the terms and conditions of the Creative Commons Attribution (CC BY) license (https://creativecommons.org/licenses/by/4.0/).

Abstract: Strengthening routine immunization systems to successfully deliver childhood vaccines during the second year of life (2YL) is critical for vaccine-preventable disease control. In Ghana, the 18-month visit provides opportunities to deliver the second dose of the measles–rubella vaccine (MR2) and for healthcare workers to assess for and provide children with any missed vaccine doses. In 2016, the Ghana Health Service (GHS) revised its national immunization policies to include guidelines for catch-up vaccinations. This study assessed the change in the timely receipt of vaccinations per Ghana's Expanded Program on Immunizations (EPI) schedule, an important indicator of service quality, following the introduction of the catch-up policy and implementation of a multifaceted intervention package. Vaccination coverage was assessed from household surveys conducted in the Greater Accra, Northern, and Volta regions for 392 and 931 children aged 24–35 months with documented immunization history in 2016 and 2020, respectively. Age at receipt of childhood vaccines was compared to the recommended age, as per the EPI schedule. Cumulative days under-vaccinated during the first 24 months of life for each recommended dose were assessed. Multivariable Cox regression was used to assess the associations between child and caregiver characteristics and time to MR2 vaccination. From 2016 to 2020, the proportion of children receiving all recommended doses on schedule generally improved, the duration of under-vaccination was shortened for most doses, and higher coverage rates were achieved at earlier ages for the MR series. More timely infant doses and caregiver awareness of the 2YL visit were positively associated with MR2 vaccination. Fostering a well-supported cadre of vaccinators, building community demand for 2YL vaccination, sustaining service utilization through strengthened defaulter tracking and caregiver-reminder systems, and creating a favorable policy environment that promotes vaccination over the life course are critical to improving the timeliness of childhood vaccinations.

Keywords: immunization; life course; 2YL; catch-up vaccination; missed opportunities for vaccination (MOV); vaccination timeliness; age appropriate; quality improvement; Ghana; EPI

1. Introduction

Endorsed by the World Health Assembly in 2020, the Immunization Agenda 2030 (IA2030) aims to reduce the morbidity and mortality caused by vaccine-preventable diseases (VPDs) worldwide [1]. The framework calls on countries to strengthen their immunization programs to reach at least 90% vaccination for all vaccines recommended in their national immunization schedule, including coverage with three doses of the diphtheria–tetanus–pertussis vaccine (DTP3) and two doses of the measles-containing vaccine (MCV2). DTP3 coverage by age 12 months indicates routine immunization (RI) program performance. In contrast, timely receipt of MCV2 is essential to prevent the spread of measles and is important for continued progress toward measles elimination goals [2].

In addition to high vaccination coverage, effective VPD control also requires the timely administration of recommended vaccines according to a specified national schedule [3]. Vaccination schedules aim to maximize the benefits of timely protection while minimizing VPD risk or adverse effects following immunization (AEFIs). Thus, schedules consider a range of age-specific factors, including susceptibility to disease and biological response to immunizations. Delayed vaccination increases susceptibility to VPDs, which can lead to increased morbidity and mortality [4–6]. Conversely, vaccine administration before the recommended age may attenuate vaccine effectiveness since maternal antibodies are still present in the child's immune system and may interfere with the immune response to vaccination [7,8]. Thus, vaccination coverage and the timing of vaccination are both important metrics for evaluating the quality and effectiveness of vaccination programs.

The World Health Organization (WHO) recommends countries establish and strengthen a well-child visit in the second year of life (2YL), including vaccination and other services as part of a continuum of care [9]. In addition to providing vaccination opportunities for vaccine doses recommended during the 2YL, such as MCV2, a strengthened 2YL vaccination platform may also provide catch-up vaccination opportunities for children older than one year who are missing vaccine doses recommended during infancy [9].

In 2012, Ghana became the first country in the African region to introduce MCV2, during the 18-month visit, into its RI schedule [10,11]. At the time of MCV2 introduction, Ghana also introduced two infant vaccines, the pneumococcal conjugate vaccine (PCV) and the rotavirus vaccine, to be administered during established visits for pentavalent vaccine [12]. By 2015, coverage with the last doses of the PCV and rotavirus vaccines had reached 88%, levels similar to those of the more established third dose of the pentavalent vaccine, whereas MCV2 (offered as a combined measles–rubella [MR] vaccine since 2013 [13]) coverage lagged at 63%, underscoring challenges with vaccination beyond infancy [14].

From 2015 to 2020, the Ghana Health Service (GHS), in collaboration with the U.S. Centers for Disease Control and Prevention (CDC), designed and implemented interventions to strengthen the 2YL platform and to facilitate the introduction of the meningococcal A conjugate vaccine (Men A) in 2016. During early to mid-2016, the CDC and GHS conducted baseline health facility and household surveys in three underperforming regions of the country to understand the factors associated with poor MCV2 coverage [11]. The baseline assessment highlighted region-level inequities in coverage across various vaccine doses, with several factors contributing to low MCV2 coverage, including a 9-year gap, since the most recent EPI staff training; insufficient supportive supervision and defaulter tracing; weak communication between health care workers (HCWs) and caregivers; and poor HCW practices around documentation of immunization data coupled with inadequate stocks of updated immunization recording and reporting tools [11,15].

To address the gaps highlighted by the baseline assessment, a multifaceted package of 2YL strengthening strategies was designed and implemented in the selected regions. On the service-delivery side, interventions broadly included improving the quality and frequency of EPI training and supportive supervision to improve RI program performance at the district and health-facility levels. HCW capacity-building activities focused on several key areas, including strengthening defaulter tracing, providing catch-up vaccine doses, improving recording and reporting practices of catch-up and 2YL vaccine doses, reinforcing practices related to vaccine vial-opening policies, and enhancing interpersonal communication with caregivers about the importance of 2YL vaccination. Social mobilization and demand-generation activities had a broader scope, primarily centered on increasing vaccine confidence and awareness about the importance of 2YL vaccination among caregivers and their communities. These efforts included several approaches, such as door-to-door interpersonal communication, referring individuals for catch-up vaccinations, disseminating tailored messages for 2YL vaccination through mass-media channels, engaging with local community leaders, and collaborating with daycare proprietors to promote the benefits of immunization.

Additionally, these activities strived to improve screening and referral practices at daycare facilities. In 2016, EPI policies were revised to include guidelines around catch-up vaccination for children under the age of five years with missing vaccine doses. Immunization data-collection tools and databases were also revised to include indicators for 2YL vaccination.

Understanding the impact of the 2YL project activities on the timing of childhood vaccination may provide insights for refining strategies to enhance timely vaccine administration and child survival. In this study, we assessed the change in vaccination timeliness among children aged 24–35 months before and after project implementation from 2016 to 2020 in three regions of Ghana. We also evaluated the extent to which children were under-vaccinated for vaccine doses during the first 24 months of life. This study makes an important contribution to the limited understanding of vaccination timeliness in Ghana, since previous studies had a limited geographic scope, focused solely on infant vaccines, and were conducted prior to the establishment of the 2YL platform [16–19]. Although previous research suggested that delays in infant vaccinations were common in Ghana, similar to other low- and middle-income countries (LMIC), the extent of subnational variation in vaccination timeliness remains to be explored [20].

2. Materials and Methods

2.1. Study Site

The present study includes a subset of data collected as part of the broader 2YL initiative in the Greater Accra Region (GAR), Northern Region (NR), and Volta Region (VR) of Ghana [11]. Although Ghana reorganized its administrative regions in 2018 following a referendum vote to create new regions, this study used the pre-2018 regional boundaries for GAR, NR (now the Northern, North East, and Savannah Regions), and VR (now the Oti and Volta Regions) for both surveys to ensure comparability of findings. According to the 2021 national census, these regions collectively accounted for 37.2% of Ghana's total population of 30.8 million inhabitants [21]. They were selected because they had lower-than-expected MR2 coverage due to various programmatic challenges. GAR is predominantly urban, characterized by higher levels of education, high-income variability, a dense population, and high residential mobility [22]. The population in VR, largely separated from the rest of Ghana by Lake Volta, the country's largest lake, experiences barriers to access to healthcare, including RI services [23]. NR is predominantly rural, and while it is the country's largest region, it has one of the lowest levels of socio-economic and educational attainment in Ghana. Additionally, it is sparsely populated and includes seasonally mobile pastoralist communities with infrequent contact with the health system.

2.2. Sampling and Participant Selection

This study was derived from baseline and endline household surveys conducted in March 2016 and August 2020 to estimate the immunization coverage among children 12–35 months old [11,24]. The details of the baseline and endline household survey design have been previously described elsewhere [11,24]. Briefly, both surveys used a stratified multi-stage cluster sample design. Within each region, enumeration areas (EAs) were selected by probability proportional to size, and, following a listing of all households in selected EAs, a simple random sample was drawn. In households with eligible children in the 12–23 month or 24–35 month age groups, caregivers could respond for up to two children (i.e., one interview per child in each age group). If multiple children were in the 12–23 month or 24–35 month age group, one child was chosen randomly. For the endline survey, children were eligible if they were aged 12–35 months as of March 2020. The selection of the cutoff was intended to minimize potential bias in the analytic sample related to the disruptions in immunization services caused by the COVID-19 pandemic. Trained field staff administered a standardized questionnaire to the selected child's caregiver. The survey questions included demographics and characteristics of the child, caregiver, and household; the caregiver's immunization awareness, knowledge, attitudes, beliefs, and perceptions regarding family, community, and healthcare worker support for immunizations; and the childhood vaccination history assessed by home-based vaccination record (child health record booklet—CHRB) data, health-facility records, or caregiver recall.

The present study reports on data collected from children ages 24 to 35 months with vaccination status and date of vaccination validated using either the child's CHRB or health-facility records.

This project was approved by GHS's Ethics Review Committee and the U.S. Centers for Disease Control and Prevention.

2.3. Definitions and Derived Variables

The age of the vaccination receipt was calculated in days for each recommended dose by subtracting the date of vaccination from the child's date of birth. Vaccination timeliness was assessed by comparing the age of vaccination receipt with the age recommendations listed in Ghana's immunization schedule (Table 1). Based on the age of vaccination receipt, a dose was considered timely if the vaccine was administered within 28 days after the recommended age. Early doses were those received before the earliest nationally accepted valid age. A dose was considered valid if received on or after the minimum recommended age. For multi-dose antigens, validity was determined if they were received on or after the minimum interval (i.e., 4 weeks). For each specific dose, days under-vaccinated were used as a continuous measure to assess the time in days between the end of each recommended age range until either when the child was vaccinated or when 24 months was reached. We considered each recommended age range to begin at the fewest number of days and to end at the greatest number of days possibly composing the given number of months (Table 1).

Table 1. Recommended and minimum ages for Ghana routine childhood immunization schedule.

Vaccine	Recommended Age of Administration	Age in Days When Dose Considered Early	Age in Days after Recommended Age When Under-Vaccination Count Initiated *
BCG	At birth or within 2 weeks of delivery	-	≥21 days
OPV0	At birth or within 2 weeks of delivery	-	≥21 days
OPV1	6 weeks (42 days)	<42 days	≥49 days
PCV1	6 weeks (42 days)	<42 days	≥49 days
Pentavalent 1	6 weeks (42 days)	<42 days	≥49 days
Rotavirus 1	6 weeks (42 days)	<42 days	≥49 days
OPV2	10 weeks (70 days)	<70 days	≥77 days
PCV2	10 weeks (70 days)	<70 days	≥77 days
Pentavalent 2	10 weeks (70 days)	<70 days	≥77 days
Rotavirus 2	10 weeks (70 days)	<70 days	≥77 days
IPV	14 weeks (98 days)	<98 days	≥105 days
OPV3	14 weeks (98 days)	<98 days	≥105 days
PCV3	14 weeks (98 days)	<98 days	≥105 days
Pentavalent 3	14 weeks (98 days)	<98 days	≥105 days
MR1	9 months (273 days)	<273 days	≥303 days
Yellow Fever	9 months (273 days)	<273 days	≥303 days
Men A	18 months (542 days)	<542 days	≥572 days
MR2	18 months (542 days)	<542 days	≥572 days

BCG, bacillus Calmette-Guérin; IPV, inactivated polio vaccine; Men A, meningitis serogroup A conjugate vaccine; MR, measles–rubella vaccine, OPV, oral polio vaccine; Pentavalent vaccine includes diphtheria, pertussis, tetanus, *Haemophilus influenzae* type b, and hepatitis B vaccines; PCV, pneumococcal conjugate vaccine. * Each recommended age range (either week or month of visit) is assumed to end at the greatest number of days that could compose the given number of weeks or months. Since BCG and OPV0 are recommended at birth, they can either be timely or delayed and cannot be administered too early unlike the other tracer vaccines.

2.4. Data and Statistical Analysis

Among children aged 24–35 months with written documentation of their immunization history, we estimated age-specific coverage rates for doses in the MR series calculated as the cumulative percentage of children vaccinated up to that month. Percentage estimates and their 95% confidence intervals (CIs) accounting for survey design and region-specific sampling weights were calculated and displayed graphically. We reported the median number of days for each vaccine dose, with the interquartile range (IQR), during which children were under-vaccinated for the first 24 months of life. Medians and proportions were compared using the Mann–Whitney and chi-square tests, respectively.

To describe factors associated with the timeliness of 2YL vaccination, we conducted an exploratory analysis evaluating the influence of (1) caregiver awareness of the 18-month visit and (2) the number of valid and timely infant doses on time to MR2 vaccination adjusting for key demographic characteristics of the child (age, sex, birth order), mother (age, education, marital status, religion), the household (urban/rural settlement) and year of the survey. Caregiver knowledge of the immunization schedule is an established predictor of childhood vaccination, and improving caregiver awareness of the 2YL visit was a key objective of the intervention package, with elements addressing this issue at the community and health-facility levels. Given that previous studies suggested that delayed vaccinations during infancy may influence the likelihood of completing the immunization schedule recommended during the first year of life [25,26], we extrapolated from those findings to hypothesize timely receipt of infant vaccinations would be associated with timely 2YL vaccine receipt.

Factors associated with time to MR2 vaccination (defined as the number of days between the recommended vaccination age and the date MR2 was given) were examined using univariable and multivariable Cox regression and reported as crude and adjusted hazard ratio (HR and aHR), respectively, where HR < 1 implies delayed vaccination compared with the referent group ("hazard" being the conditional probability of receiving MR2 at time t, given that MR2 has not been received before time t). The hazard ratio compares the average instantaneous risk of vaccination with MR2 over the study period (the hazard) among a randomly chosen pair of children, one from the exposed group and another from the non-exposed group. Children with no MR2 vaccination recorded were right-censored at the age of the interview. We assessed the proportional hazards assumption for each covariate using graphical plots (log-negative log survival plots). The assumption of proportional hazards was violated for the child's age. Thus, we computed age-stratified Cox regression models, allowing the baseline hazards to vary by the child's age. These models were implemented separately for each region, with 'hazard' here on referred to as 'likelihood'.

All analyses were performed using the appropriate clustering and weighting statements to account for the complex survey design described above. Given our analytic sample's inclusion criteria, we used Stata's *subpop* option to conduct analyses using the complete data file to maintain an accurate variance estimation. The Taylor series linearization method was used to calculate the variance of the parameter estimates. Unweighted case frequencies and weighted proportions are reported. All analyses were performed using Stata version 17 [27].

3. Results

3.1. Participant Characteristics

Table 2 describes the characteristics of the surveyed children and their households for each region. A total of 464 and 959 children aged 24–35 months across the three regions were surveyed for the 2016 and 2020 surveys, respectively. The present study included a subset of 392 and 931 children with vaccination records in 2016 and 2020, respectively. A detailed description of the analytic subsets is provided in Supplementary Figure S1. From 2016 to 2020, the vaccination record availability (primarily driven by CHRB availability) increased significantly across all regions (Table 2). In 2016, the vaccination record availability ranged from 76.9% (95% CI: 61.0, 87.7) in GAR to 89.3% (95% CI: 82.8, 93.6) in NR. In 2020, it ranged from 91.4% (95% CI: 86.5, 94.6) in GAR to 99.5% (95% CI: 97.8, 99.9) in VR.

The median age of the children with vaccination records was 29 months (IQR: 27, 33; Table 2). Nearly half of these children were male, with a higher proportion (69.1%) in NR in 2016 compared to 2020. The respondent was primarily the child's mother (94.6% in GAR, 92.6% NR, and 89.9% in VR), and the median maternal age for both survey rounds was 30 years, ranging from 29.5 years in VR in 2016 to 32 in GAR in 2020. While the proportion of children from urban settlements was >92% for GAR in both survey rounds, there was temporal variation in NR (23.8–30.0%) and VR (30.2–26.7%). Most mothers were Christian in GAR and VR ($\geq$88% for both years) and Muslim in NR (49.5% in 2016 and 72.2% in 2020). From 2016 to 2020, caregiver awareness of the need for an 18-month visit before the second birthday increased significantly in NR (19–46.7%) and VR (36.8–57.0%) but decreased in GAR (62.8–58.3%). Timely receipt of infant vaccinations also improved from 2016 to 2020 in NR and VR, but not in GAR, with an increase in the proportion of children who received more than 10 timely infant doses in NR (24.1–30.0%) and VR (49.3–59.6%), but a decrease in GAR (60.1–56.1%). Nonetheless, GAR experienced an improvement in the proportion of children receiving 6–10 timely doses (17.7–24.3%).

3.2. Timing of Vaccinations

Figure 1 illustrates the cumulative percentage of children aged 24–35 months vaccinated with the MR series by region. From 2016 to 2020, the cumulative proportion of children who received MR1 by the recommended age of 9 months increased in GAR (48.2% to 52.5%) and NR (32.6% to 34.7%) but decreased in VR (49.2% to 39.5%). Over the same period, the cumulative proportion of children who received MR2 by the recommended age of 18 months increased in VR (20.5–38.1%) and remained unchanged in GAR (42%) and NR (26.0%).

Figure 1 also highlights the dropout from MR1 to MR2 by region between survey rounds, with a lower coverage of MR2 than MR1 at each survey. In all regions, some children were vaccinated as early as 4 months for MR1 and 10 months for MR2, albeit less frequently in 2020 when compared with 2016. The slopes of the curves around the recommended times of receipt for both doses were steep in 2020 compared to the more gradual slopes observed in 2016, which is indicative of higher coverage levels being achieved more rapidly in 2020 relative to 2016 across all regions. For example, between the ages of 9 and 12 months, MR1 coverage increased from 32.6% to 71.7% in 2016 and from 34.7% to 83.4% in 2020 among children in NR. In this cohort, MR1 coverage reached 83.7% and 92.3% by the end of 2YL during 2016 and 2020, respectively. Similarly, whereas MR2 coverage at 18 months was 26% for both years among children in NR, it increased to 56% in 2016 and to 73.0% in 2020 by 24 months.

In 2016, the recommended minimum coverage of 90% for MR1 was achieved by 11 months in GAR, by 13 months in VR, and not achieved in NR (Figure 1). In 2020, 90% MR1 coverage was achieved by 14 months in both NR and VR and not achieved in GAR. Although the recommended minimum coverage of 90% for MR2 was not achieved in any region by 24 months of age, catch-up vaccination during the 2YL enabled increases in coverage across all regions. VR was closest to achieving the coverage target in 2020, with cumulative MR2 coverage at 24 months reaching 85.8%.

Table 2. Characteristics of children 24–35 months of age in Greater Accra, Northern, and Volta regions, 2016–2020.

	Greater Accra						Northern						Volta					
	2016 N = 100		2020 N = 224				2016 N = 211		2020 N = 535				2016 N = 153		2020 N = 200			
	n	% (95% CIs)	n	% (95% CIs)			n	% (95% CIs)	n	% (95% CIs)			n	% (95% CIs)	n	% (95% CIs)		
Vaccination record availability *																		
Children with vaccination cards	73	76.9 (61.0–87.7)	190	83.1 (75.9–88.5)			189	89.3 (82.8–93.6)	518	96.2 (94.2–97.5)			130	87.5 (80.1–92.3)	193	96.8 (89.2–99.1)		
Children with facility register verification	0	0.0	15	8.3 (4.1–16.0)			0	0.0	10	2.2 (1.2–4.1)			0	0.0	5	2.6 (0.6–11.1)		
Children with either vaccination record	73	76.9 (61.0–87.7)	205	91.4 (86.5–94.6)			189	89.3 (82.8–93.6)	528	98.4 (96.6–99.2)			130	87.5 (80.1–92.3)	198	99.5 (97.8–99.9)		
Child's sex																		
Female	37	45.8 (35.0–57.0)	98	49.8 (41.0–58.6)			75	30.9 (23.2–39.8)	251	47.2 (42.8–51.8)			66	48.9 (40.1–57.7)	105	54.7 (46.5–62.7)		
Male	36	54.2 (43.0–65.0)	107	50.2 (41.4–59.0)			114	69.1 (60.2–76.8)	277	52.8 (48.2–57.2)			64	51.1 (42.3–59.9)	93	45.3 (37.3–53.5)		
Birth order																		
First	26	47.2 (28.4–66.9)	72	38.6 (30.9–46.9)			41	18.9 (13.8–25.2)	108	22.0 (17.9–26.8)			30	22.2 (16.1–29.8)	63	34.8 (27.8–42.7)		
Second	20	18.1 (9.7–31.1)	54	24.6 (18.6–31.7)			39	20.1 (13.5–28.9)	122	23.9 (20.3–27.9)			31	27.0 (20.8–34.3)	36	19.6 (13.6–27.4)		
Third or more	27	34.7 (20.8–51.7)	79	36.8 (30.9–43.2)			109	61.0 (50.4–70.7)	298	54.1 (48.4–59.7)			69	50.8 (43.7–57.9)	99	45.6 (39.9–51.4)		
Maternal age (years)																		
<25	10	13.8 (5.6–30.0)	20	9.0 (5.1–15.5)			37	15.0 (8.6–24.9)	63	12.7 (9.4–16.9)			29	23.3 (16.9–31.1)	44	23.4 (18.6–28.8)		
25–34	33	46.5 (29.4–64.4)	106	50.8 (43.3–58.2)			84	53.7 (38.6–68.2)	137	26.6 (22.2–31.6)			55	40.5 (31.8–50.0)	80	41.2 (33.8–49.0)		
≥35	30	39.7 (24.3–57.5)	79	40.2 (33.8–47.0)			68	31.3 (21.2–43.4)	328	60.7 (54.4–66.6)			46	36.2 (27.8–45.6)	74	35.5 (29.7–41.7)		
Maternal education																		
Never attended school	10	9.6 (4.3–20.1)	15	6.9 (4.1–11.2)			136	74.3 (64.0–82.4)	373	68.1 (60.5–74.8)			40	29.6 (18.8–43.4)	36	17.1 (9.8–28.0)		
Primary	15	30.3 (18.9–44.8)	16	6.6 (4.1–10.4)			14	5.9 (2.9–11.4)	43	8.0 (5.4–11.6)			23	15.5 (10.1–23.0)	34	15.7 (10.5–23.0)		
Secondary or higher	47	60.1 (46.9–72.0)	174	86.5 (80.4–91.0)			39	19.9 (13.9–27.6)	110	24.0 (18.1–31.1)			67	54.9 (40.8–68.3)	127	67.2 (53.2–78.6)		
Maternal marital status																		
Single/Divorced/Separated/Widowed	4	2.8 (1.0–7.9)	27	14.2 (9.1–21.4)			3	1.3 (0.4–4.1)	12	2.8 (1.1–6.6)			6	5.0 (2.1–11.4)	22	9.8 (6.2–15.1)		
Married/Co-habitating	69	97.2 (92.1–99.0)	178	85.8 (78.6–90.9)			186	98.7 (95.9–99.6)	516	97.2 (93.4–98.9)			124	95.0 (88.6–97.9)	176	90.2 (84.9–93.8)		
Maternal religion																		
Christian	64	88.3 (77.6–94.3)	175	88.2 (79.2–93.6)			66	34.9 (23.4–48.4)	125	22.1 (13.6–33.6)			116	88.0 (76.9–94.2)	172	87.8 (79.7–92.9)		
Muslim	7	8.1 (3.1–19.3)	29	11.0 (5.7–20.3)			104	49.5 (32.6–66.5)	359	72.2 (59.2–82.3)			5	4.2 (1.1–14.8)	13	5.6 (2.4–12.7)		
Traditionalist	2	3.6 (0.9–13.4)	0	0.0–4.4			15	13.1 (4.2–33.9)	37	2.5 (1.8–10.1)			9	7.8 (3.4–17.0)	5	2.9 (0.8–7.7)		
None / Do not know	0	0.0–2.6	1	0.7 (0.1–4.8)			4	0.0 (0.8–8.6)	7	1.3 (0.4–4.0)			0	0.7 (0.1–5.2)	8	4.1 (1.8–9.1)		
Settlement type																		
Urban	65	92.2 (71.4–98.2)	183	93.0 (80.6–97.7)			64	23.8 (11.7–42.5)	145	30.0 (16.7–48.0)			45	30.2 (16.0–49.6)	54	26.7 (13.9–45.1)		
Rural	8	7.8 (1.8–28.6)	22	7.0 (2.3–19.4)			125	76.2 (57.5–88.3)	383	70.0 (52.0–83.3)			85	69.8 (50.4–84.0)	144	73.3 (54.9–86.1)		
Caregiver aware of need for 18 mo visit before 2nd birthday																		
No	35	37.2 (23.0–54.0)	94	41.7 (31.4–52.9)			154	81.0 (67.5–89.8)	278	53.3 (43.3–62.9)			78	63.2 (54.8–70.8)	88	43.0 (35.3–50.9)		
Yes	38	62.8 (46.0–77.0)	111	58.3 (47.1–68.6)			35	19.0 (10.2–32.5)	250	46.7 (37.1–56.7)			52	36.8 (29.2–45.2)	110	57.0 (49.1–64.7)		

Table 2. Cont.

	Greater Accra						Northern						Volta			
	2016 N = 100			2020 N = 224			2016 N = 211			2020 N = 535			2016 N = 153		2020 N = 200	
Number of valid timely infant doses [†]																
None timely	3	2.5 (0.8–7.2)		18	11.1 (6.2–18.9)		36	16.2 (9.1–27.1)		82	14.6 (10.5–20.0)		9	6.8 (3.6–12.8)	19	7.5 (3.6–15.1)
1–5 doses	10	19.7 (9.2–37.4)		20	8.6 (5.4–13.4)		61	36.4 (27.6–46.2)		150	27.4 (21.9–33.7)		29	20.6 (14.4–28.6)	34	15.7 (11.6–21.1)
6–10 doses	13	17.7 (9.2–31.2)		46	24.3 (18.1–31.8)		45	23.3 (17.8–30.0)		149	28.0 (23.7–32.7)		29	23.2 (16.4–31.9)	33	17.2 (11.7–24.4)
>10 doses	47	**60.1 (42.2–75.7)**		121	**56.1 (48.6–63.2)**		47	24.1 (14.3–37.6)		147	30.0 (22.7–38.4)		63	49.3 (40.5–58.1)	112	59.6 (49.2–69.1)

* Source vaccination records include child health record books and facility-based registers. Total Ns shown and denominator of proportion includes all sampled children in the region during the specified survey round. Characteristics included in this table are among children with vaccination records. [†] Includes 14 doses total: bacillus Calmette–Guérin (BCG); pentavalent 1, 2, and 3; rotavirus 1, 2, and 2; oral polio vaccine 1, 2, and 3; pneumococcal conjugate vaccine (PCV) 1, 2, and 3; yellow fever, measles–rubella 1. Sample sizes are unweighted, and percentages and 95% CIs are weighted. Bold values denote statistical significance of the design-based chi-square test comparing 2016 to 2020 at the $p < 0.05$ level.

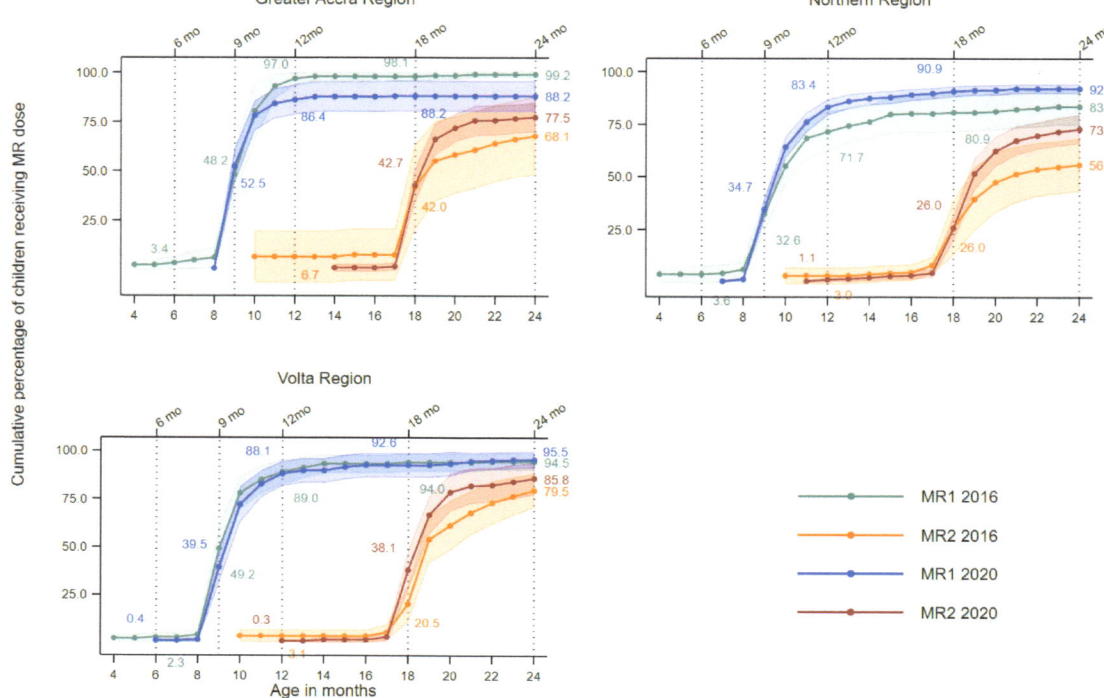

Figure 1. Cumulative vaccination coverage by age in months for the first and second dose of measles–rubella (MR) vaccine among children aged 24–35 months in Greater Accra, Northern, and Volta regions in 2016 and 2020. Values indicate cumulative percentage of children vaccinated by 6, 9, 12, 18, and 24 months of age. Shaded areas represent the 95% confidence intervals for the coverage estimates.

3.3. Duration of Under-Vaccination during the First 24 Months of Life

Across the immunization series, the duration of under-vaccination tended to be longer for most doses in NR compared to other regions for both survey rounds (Table 3). From 2016 to 2020, the median number of days under-vaccinated decreased for most doses across all regions. Nonetheless, the results were mixed in GAR, with the duration of under-vaccination increasing significantly for some doses, including BCG, yellow fever (YF), and the oral poliovirus vaccine (OPV) series. Notably, the median duration of MR2 under-vaccination decreased significantly across all regions, by 68 days in NR and 52 days in both GAR and VR.

Across all regions and for both survey rounds, the duration of under-vaccination generally increased with each subsequent scheduled visit and tended to be similar for scheduled doses during the same visit (Table 3). The exception was the duration of under-vaccination for OPV doses in 2020, which tended to be longer relative to the doses scheduled during the same visit. For instance, the median number of days under-vaccinated with the third dose of OPV in GAR in 2020 was 46 but was only 16 for the third dose of the pentavalent vaccine.

From 2016 to 2020, the proportion of children aged 24–35 months receiving all recommended doses on a timely basis increased in NR (9.9% to 13.6%) and VR (24.6% to 27.3%) but decreased in GAR (33.6% to 30.0%). None of these changes were statistically significant.

Table 3. Days under-vaccinated with various doses of vaccine during the first 24 months among children aged 24–35 months * in Greater Accra, Northern, and Volta Regions, 2016 and 2020.

| | Greater Accra | | | | Northern | | | | Volta | | | |
| | 2016 (N = 71) | | 2020 (N = 205) | | 2016 (N = 189) | | 2020 (N = 528) | | 2016 (N = 128) | | 2020 (N = 198) | |
Vaccine	n	Median (IQR)	n	Median (IQR)	n	Median (IQR)	n	Median (IQR)	n	Median (IQR)	n	Median (IQR)
BCG	62	2 (1, 6)	177	4 (1, 19)	168	22 (8, 65)	506	17 (6, 40)	112	10 (3, 24)	164	7 (2, 51)
OPV1	21	16 (11, 54)	77	29 (11, 90)	124	16 (10, 74)	393	24 (8, 62)	80	14 (7, 25)	113	13 (5, 30)
PCV1	21	18 (11, 96)	56	14 (7, 682)	122	18 (10, 90)	356	16 (6, 34)	83	14 (7, 27)	108	10 (5, 22)
Pentavalent 1	22	16 (11, 96)	57	14 (7, 682)	123	16 (10, 55)	358	17 (6, 34)	81	15 (7, 29)	110	10 (5, 23)
Rota1	20	16 (10, 54)	60	15 (7, 682)	127	17 (10, 77)	357	17 (6, 35)	80	14 (7, 27)	108	10 (5, 22)
OPV2	42	10 (4, 41)	125	29 (7, 75)	159	30 (14, 130)	459	41 (14, 96)	100	18 (8, 37)	138	14 (6, 38)
PCV2	42	19 (4, 41)	104	14 (5, 40)	159	32 (14, 130)	438	23 (9, 48)	99	18 (8, 37)	136	11 (6, 30)
Pentavalent 2	41	10 (4, 41)	105	12 (4, 40)	162	29 (14, 124)	440	24 (9, 49)	101	18 (8, 36)	138	12 (6, 38)
Rota2	42	19 (6, 41)	107	12 (4, 62)	160	33 (14, 146)	439	24 (10, 52)	99	18 (8, 36)	136	12 (6, 30)
OPV3	50	16 (4, 47)	149	46 (12, 169)	173	47 (23, 220)	493	59 (22, 356)	117	21 (9, 47)	161	18 (7, 57)
PCV3	52	17 (4, 46)	128	16 (5, 62)	169	57 (24, 233)	484	33 (14, 65)	116	21 (9, 47)	158	14 (6, 36)
Pentavalent 3	50	18 (4, 47)	130	16 (5, 42)	171	47 (23, 175)	484	33 (14, 67)	118	23 (9, 47)	162	15 (7, 43)
MR1	25	27 (15, 34)	58	54 (12, 428)	99	97 (30, 428)	263	42 (16, 155)	42	47 (13, 121)	87	33 (13, 135)
YF	25	27 (15, 31)	73	58 (12, 428)	99	126 (31, 428)	305	60 (24, 212)	40	47 (13, 122)	90	41 (19, 130)
MR2	44	159 (71, 159)	100	107 (18, 159)	142	159 (61, 159)	335	91 (22, 159)	85	95 (20, 159)	95	43 (17, 159)

* Cumulative days under-vaccinated during the first 24 months of life for a recommended vaccine. Under-vaccination begins after the end of a recommendation period and continues until the child is vaccinated or reaches 24 months of age. Sample includes only children with documented vaccination records. Inactivated polio vaccine and meningitis serogroup A conjugate vaccine were introduced in 2018 and 2016, respectively, and are excluded from this analysis. N represents total number of children under-vaccinated with any dose. Bold values denote statistical significance of the Mann–Whitney Wilcoxon test at the $p < 0.05$ level. BCG, bacillus Calmette–Guérin; MR, measles–rubella vaccine, OPV, oral polio vaccine; Pentavalent vaccine includes diphtheria, pertussis, tetanus, Haemophilus influenzae type b, and hepatitis B vaccines; PCV, pneumococcal conjugate vaccine; Rota, rotavirus vaccine.

3.4. Risk Factors for Time to MR2 Vaccination

In multivariable Cox regression models, several factors were significantly associated with time to MR2 vaccination (Table 4). Across all regions, an increased number of valid, timely vaccine doses during infancy was associated with an increased likelihood of MR2 vaccination. In NR, for example, as compared with children with no timely doses, those receiving 1–5, 6–10, and >10 timely doses, respectively, experienced a 1.9 (95% CI: 1.3, 2.6), 2.1 (95% CI: 1.6, 2.9), and 2.2 (95% CI: 1.6, 3.0) higher likelihood of MR2 vaccination. Caregiver's awareness of the 18-month visit was significantly associated with an increased likelihood of MR2 vaccination in NR (aHR: 1.2, 95% CI: 1.0–1.5) and VR (aHR: 1.5, 95% CI: 1.2–1.8), although the association was not significant in GAR (aHR: 1.2, 95% CI: 0.9–1.6). In GAR and NR, but not VR, children of older mothers had a higher likelihood of MR2 vaccination when compared to those of mothers aged <25 years. Certain factors significantly positively impacted the likelihood of MR2 vaccination in some regions, but not others. These factors included earlier rank in birth order in NR and VR, male sex and rural residence in NR, and Christian religion in GAR and NR.

Table 4. Factors associated with time to vaccination for second dose of measles–rubella (MR2) vaccine among children aged 24–35 months in Greater Accra, Northern, and Volta regions.

	Greater Accra				Northern				Volta			
	Unadjusted		Adjusted		Unadjusted		Adjusted		Unadjusted		Adjusted	
	HR	95% CI	HR	95% CI	HR	95% CI	HR	95% CI	HR	95% CI	HR	95% CI
Child's sex												
Female	REF		REF		REF		REF		REF		REF	
Male	1.1	(0.8–1.4)	1.2	(0.9–1.6)	0.7	(0.6–0.9) **	0.7	(0.6–0.9) **	1.0	(0.9–1.2)	0.9	(0.8–1.2)
Birth order												
First	REF		REF		REF		REF		REF		REF	
Second	0.9	(0.6–1.4)	1.0	(0.7–1.5)	1.0	(0.7–1.5)	1.0	(0.7–1.3)	0.9	(0.6–1.3)	1.0	(0.8–1.4)
Third or more	0.8	(0.5–1.2)	0.8	(0.5–1.1)	1.0	(0.7–1.3)	0.8	(0.6–1.0) *	0.6	(0.5–0.8) *	0.7	(0.6–1.0) *
Maternal education												
Never attended school	REF		REF		REF		REF		REF		REF	
Primary	0.8	(0.4–1.8)	0.8	(0.4–1.6)	1.1	(0.8–1.6)	1.0	(0.7–1.4)	1.1	(0.6–1.8)	0.9	(0.6–1.6)
Secondary or higher	1.0	(0.6–1.7)	1.2	(0.8–1.8)	0.9	(0.7–1.2)	1.0	(0.8–1.3)	1.8	(1.2–2.7)	1.4	(0.9–2.2)
Maternal age (Years)												
<25	REF		REF		REF		REF		REF		REF	
25–34	1.9	(1.1–3.1) *	1.8	(1.0–3.3)	1.2	(0.9–1.6)	1.3	(1.0–1.6)	0.8	(0.5–1.0)	0.9	(0.6–1.3)
≥35	1.8	(1.1–3.0) *	2.1	(1.1–3.9) *	1.3	(1.0–1.7) *	1.5	(1.2–1.9) *	0.8	(0.6–1.1)	1.0	(0.7–1.4)
Maternal marital status												
Single/Divorced/Widowed	REF		REF		REF		REF		REF		REF	
Married/Co-habitating	1.0	(0.6–1.6)	0.8	(0.6–1.2)	1.2	(0.8–2.0)	1.0	(0.6–1.5)	1.2	(0.8–1.7)	1.3	(0.9–1.7)
Maternal religion												
Other	REF		REF		REF		REF		REF		REF	
Christian	1.2	(0.8–2.0)	1.4	(1.0–2.0) *	1.3	(0.9–1.8)	1.4	(1.0–1.9) *	1.6	(1.1–2.5) *	1.4	(0.9–2.1)
Settlement type												
Urban	REF		REF		REF		REF		REF		REF	
Rural	1.1	(0.6–2.1)	1.2	(0.8–1.7)	1.7	(1.3–2.3) **	2.0	(1.4–2.7) ***	1.3	(0.8–2.0)	1.1	(0.8–1.6)
Caregiver aware of need for 18-month visit before second birthday												
No	REF		REF		REF		REF		REF		REF	
Yes	1.8	(1.2–2.7) **	1.2	(0.9–1.6)	1.5	(1.2–2.0) **	1.2	(1.0–1.5) *	1.7	(1.4–2.2) ***	1.5	(1.2–1.8) ***

Table 4. Cont.

	Greater Accra				Northern				Volta			
	Unadjusted		Adjusted		Unadjusted		Adjusted		Unadjusted		Adjusted	
	HR	95% CI	HR	95% CI	HR	95% CI	HR	95% CI	HR	95% CI	HR	95% CI
Number of valid timely doses †												
None timely	REF		REF		REF		REF		REF		REF	
1–5 doses	16.3	(4.3–62.3) ***	20.4	(6.3–65.8) ***	1.9	(1.3–2.6) ***	1.9	(1.3–2.6) ***	4.6	(2.2–9.4) ***	4.2	(2.0–8.9) ***
6–10 doses	25.5	(8.9–72.9) ***	31.3	(12.1–81.2) ***	2.1	(1.6–2.9) ***	2.5	(1.9–3.4) ***	6.4	(3.4–12.1) ***	6.2	(3.1–12.4) ***
>10 doses	31.1	(11.6–83.0) ***	36.4	(14.7–90.0) ***	2.2	(1.6–3.0) ***	3.2	(2.3–4.3) ***	7.1	(3.6–13.8) ***	6.1	(3.0–12.4) ***
Year												
2016	REF		REF		REF		REF		REF		REF	
2020	1.1	(0.7–1.8)	0.8	(0.6–1.2)	1.3	(0.9–1.8)	0.9	(0.7–1.3)	1.0	(0.7–1.3)	0.7	(0.5–1.0) *

† Includes 14 doses total: bacillus Calmette-Guérin (BCG); pentavalent 1, 2, and 3; rotavirus 1, and 2; oral polio vaccine (OPV) 1, 2 and 3; pneumococcal conjugate vaccine (PCV) 1, 2, and 3; yellow fever vaccine, measles–rubella 1. * p-value < 0.05. ** p-value < 0.01. *** p-value < 0.001

4. Discussion

This study highlights improvements in the timely receipt of childhood vaccinations, an important indicator of immunization service quality, following the implementation of an initiative to strengthen the 2YL vaccination platform and introduce catch-up vaccination policies in Ghana. From 2016 to 2020, under-vaccination occurred for fewer doses and shorter duration. The proportion of children vaccinated by the recommended age was higher in 2020 vs. 2016. The improvements were noted for vaccine doses recommended during infancy and those offered during 2YL. Although the improvements varied across doses and regions, the results suggest that, overall, more children were likely protected at earlier ages against VPDs following the implementation of the immunization system strengthening strategies. While the increases in coverage due to catch-up vaccination were marginal in some regions, at the population level, they represent meaningful benefits needed to stop disease transmission. For example, the recent increase in measles cases in Ghana following several years of low disease incidence implies persistent pockets of susceptible hosts sustaining transmission [13,28,29]. In addition to local measles spread, Ghana remains at high risk for case importation given the country's proximity to countries lagging in measles control in an increasingly integrated region [30]. The improvements in vaccination timeliness are, therefore, critical, since immunity gaps resulting from vaccination delays or inadequate immune response to vaccination can be exploited by case importations resulting in disruptive outbreaks.

Vaccination-timing results for the MR series showed improvements in coverage during 2YL, illustrating the importance of strengthening the utilization of the 2YL platform to facilitate catch-up vaccination and, ultimately, sustain progress toward the IA2030 goals. Nonetheless, since the recommended minimum MR2 coverage of 90% was not attained among children aged 24–35 months in any region (consistent with national MR2 coverage of 83% reported in 2021 [31]), further opportunities remain for improvement in coverage. Screening vaccination status at the time of school entry and providing catch-up vaccinations for those with missed doses may be an additional effective strategy to reduce delays and improve coverage among these older cohorts. Ghana has attained high net pre-primary and primary school enrollment rates (~75% and >80%, respectively), particularly among children in urban localities, and has also achieved gender parity in enrollment [32,33]. This means that, for regions like NR, where access to schools has improved [34] and our analysis suggested urban–rural and gender disparities in time to MR2 vaccination, school-based screening and vaccination at school entry could be attractive strategies to provide equitable catch-up vaccination opportunities [35]. Urban–rural disparities in time to MR2 vaccination are especially noteworthy, since they are consistent with previous studies showing lower MR series coverage and higher measles and rubella incidence in Ghanaian urban areas [13,36,37].

Since preventing the administration of invalid vaccine doses is, to a greater degree, the responsibility of healthcare workers, the decrease in the administration of early vaccine doses over the study period points to the relative success of staff training and supervision efforts. According to the Ghana EPI field guide [38], doses administered before the recommended age (age invalid) or not following the minimum spacing intervals (interval invalid) should be readministered to ensure adequate protection. Thus, in addition to potentially reducing vaccine efficacy [39], early vaccination may also inadvertently lead to avoidable increases in programmatic costs and unnecessary risk of AEFIs [40]. Overall, our findings corroborate previous studies showing that age- and interval-invalid vaccine doses are common in African countries [41,42]. Further research is needed to understand better the underlying reasons for invalid dose administration and improve adherence to the EPI schedule.

Because the duration of under-vaccination tended to be similar for doses scheduled during the same visit suggests high levels of receipt of multiple vaccines during the same visit. Leveraging contacts with caregivers of children to provide multiple vaccinations during the same visit, including appropriate catch-up doses, is critical for minimizing missed opportunities for vaccination (MOVs), decreasing the risk of defaulting from the system, and reducing programmatic costs. Further, simultaneous vaccinations, where appropriate, may also reduce caregivers' opportunity costs, such as time away from work, travel time, transportation costs, or the need for childcare while away. Our findings nonetheless point to challenges with the consistent provision of simultaneous vaccinations given that OPV, IPV, and MenA doses tended to have longer delays than the other scheduled doses recommended during the same visit. First, IPV and MenA were, respectively, introduced in Ghana in 2018 and 2016, and it is likely the implementation delays and inefficiencies associated with new vaccine introductions, coupled with a lack of awareness among HCWs and caregivers about the new doses, contributed to the observed vaccination delays. Previous studies evaluating IPV introduction have highlighted that HCWs and caregivers may have concerns about the pain and possible adverse effects of multiple injections, given that the vaccine was scheduled alongside several other more established injectable vaccines [43,44]. While not unique to IPV, such concerns may lead to deliberate delays or refusals [45]. This issue could be addressed by disseminating evidence-based vaccine safety and acceptability communication messages.

Additionally, implementing training and supervision programs focused on improving interpersonal communication between HCWs and caregivers can help address such concerns. Second, due to funding delays, Ghana experienced widespread stockouts for OPV and MenA in 2017 and 2019 [46], respectively, which likely meant many children were left unprotected for long periods. Stockouts adversely impact vaccination timeliness, since HCWs may be reluctant to open multi-dose vials for fewer children [47,48], leading to MOVs and frustration among caregivers who are turned away. This may contribute to hesitation about returning to complete the child's scheduled vaccinations [49]. To increase health-system resiliency when stockouts or other disruptions occur, it is important to have systems in place enabling diligent follow-up and catch-up vaccination for children who have missed vaccines. This requires strengthening of defaulter tracking systems and a focus on strengthening record keeping to identify children with missing doses.

An increasing number of timely doses recommended during infancy was associated with an increased likelihood of MR2 receipt. This is consistent with previous observations that delayed vaccinations are an important predictor of not completing the first-year immunization schedule [25] and that children who complete their infant vaccines by their first year are more likely to receive 2YL vaccines [24]. Overall, the finding suggests that even early deviations from the recommended schedule may have persisting effects that adversely impact the timely receipt of 2YL vaccines, prolonging susceptibility to childhood VPDs. The deviations may reflect barriers to childhood immunization. Still, they may also result from intentional adjustments to the immunization schedule by HCWs to address delayed initiation of a multi-dose series or the re-administration of previous invalid doses while observing dose-spacing requirements. This highlights the importance of supporting HCWs and caregivers to prevent children from falling behind on immunizations and, as appropriate, to utilize 2YL contact points to catch up on missed doses.

Since its establishment in 1979, the Ghanaian EPI schedule has increased in complexity following various vaccine introductions over the years. The increased complexity has implications for vaccination timeliness, since previous studies have suggested assessing the vaccination status and scheduling age-appropriate catch-up regimens for children who have fallen behind on immunizations can be challenging for overburdened HCWs [50–52]. Quality training and supportive supervision, supplemented with simple job aids, may promote improvements in correct screening, recording of tools, and scheduling of doses. Mobile-based immunization decision support systems to automatically construct age-appropriate vaccination schedules for children have also shown promise in LMIC [53] and should be further explored in the Ghana setting. Importantly, field guides should also provide clear instructions and scenarios on what HCWs should do during encounters with children who are behind on immunizations, especially in the absence of written immunization records for the child.

Systematic reviews have shown caregiver reminder/recall systems are effective interventions for improving service utilization and vaccination timeliness [54,55]. These include a wide range of mediums ranging from person-to-person telephone calls, letters, home visits, and text messages to combinations used to remind caregivers that vaccinations are due (reminders) or overdue (recall). Emphasizing the reminder component of these systems would likely be more effective for encouraging timeliness and preventing a build-up of delayed doses, which may be more challenging to address later. Although reminders are effective in increasing vaccination timeliness [56], their impact is less understood in LMIC settings. Nonetheless, a randomized controlled trial in NR evaluating the effect of telephone-call reminders on timely neonatal vaccination showed a 10.5% increase in timely vaccination in the intervention arm compared to the control group [17]. Extending such research to examine the impact of phone-based reminders on vaccination timeliness during 2YL may better inform immunization programming.

In this study, caregiver awareness of the 18-month visit was positively associated with time to MR2 vaccination. The positive association suggests demand generation and social mobilization efforts may be important contributors to improving vaccine timeliness. Our findings suggest that targeted and proactive messaging to communities about the importance and timing of 2YL vaccines should be emphasized to improve vaccination timeliness. In areas like VR and NR, where religious affiliation is an important predictor of 2YL vaccination timeliness, involving local religious leaders and faith-based organizations in raising awareness about 2YL vaccinations and broader vaccine promotion activities may help mitigate community concerns and improve timely vaccine uptake. To incentivize utilization of the 2YL visit, programs may also consider integrated demand-creation strategies that raise awareness of the other preventative health services (e.g., deworming, growth monitoring, and bed net distribution) typically delivered jointly with 2YL immunizations. Lastly, high-quality respectful interpersonal communication skills are essential for HCWs to educate caregivers on the benefits of the 2YL visit and the importance of adherence to the recommended vaccination schedule. Previous research in Ghana and elsewhere has shown that rude HCW behavior, inattention to caregiver questions, and not receiving enough information during healthcare visits are major reasons caregivers do not bring back their children for vaccinations, especially when they fall behind [49,57–60].

5. Strengths and Limitations

The timeliness of childhood vaccinations has seldom been studied in Ghana, and our study is the first to assess the changes following the strengthening of the RI system using data from a household survey specifically designed to assess immunization coverage in the 2YL. We included data from multiple birth cohorts with high levels of vaccination record availability.

Nonetheless, the proportion of children with written documentation of vaccination status was significantly higher in 2020 compared to 2016 across all regions, potentially limiting the interpretation of the pre–post comparisons. CHRB prevalence has markedly improved in Ghana over recent decades [61], and it is possible the health-system improvements achieved by 2020 facilitated increased CHRB availability, such that our 2020 sample of children with CHRBs was more representative of the general population than our 2016 sample, particularly in terms of healthcare access and caregiver motivation to seek timely vaccinations. Given that caregiver awareness of the importance of the CHRB is associated with its retention and improved vaccination uptake [62,63], it is possible that the exclusion of children without vaccination records in our analyses potentially resulted in a sample of those with more knowledgeable and possibly more motivated caregivers in 2016 who were more likely to seek timely vaccinations. Overall, this sampling difference would have the effect of underestimating the true change in timeliness between 2016 and 2020. This is most evident in GAR, where MR1 coverage at 10 months and beyond was higher in 2016 compared with 2020, following significant increases in CHRB prevalence as well as maternal education levels, both of which are known to be correlated with childhood immunization outcomes.

Another limitation of the pre–post study design is the lack of control or comparison regions, which limits direct causal attribution of the observed changes to strengthening the 2YL platform. Thus, we cannot exclude the possibility the observed changes were attributable to contextual changes during the 4-year implementation period. Despite the potential for confounding from other efforts to improve immunization coverage, there were no other interventions in the study regions targeting 2YL vaccination platform strengthening during the study period. Future research should consider including control or comparison areas.

Additionally, the examined factors associated with time to 2YL vaccination were limited to those collected in the two survey rounds. There may be influential factors not captured by this analysis, such as health-system issues related to vaccine supplies or immunization program implementation, contextual barriers such as travel distance and poor infrastructure, and as previously mentioned, caregiver attitudes about vaccinations. Due to the cross-sectional nature of the data, causal inferences cannot be made. The study was designed and powered to make inferences at the regional level, and the results are not intended for national-level inferences. Nevertheless, our exploration of regional variations provides learning opportunities to tailor programs to increase access and utilization of the 2YL immunization services. Lastly, it is impossible to tease apart the relative effects of the different components of the 2YL intervention package. As such, it is unclear how much each component contributed to the observed changes in vaccination timeliness. In the context of limited resources for improving vaccination programs, additional research is needed to determine the relative impact and the cost–benefits of individual strategies and their efficient targeting.

6. Conclusions

While the experience of strengthening the 2YL platform in Ghana was unique, the lessons learned nonetheless provide valuable information for other countries that are considering introducing 2YL vaccines or catch-up vaccination policies into their RI programs, particularly those with regions similar to our study sites. This study has shown substantial improvements in the timeliness of vaccinations in three regions in Ghana following the implementation of a package of interventions to strengthen the 2YL vaccination platform and the revision of the EPI policy to include catch-up vaccination guidelines. The results from this analysis demonstrate that improvements in the timeliness of vaccinations are achievable through comprehensive HCW capacity building, strategic community engagement initiatives, and an enabling policy environment encouraging vaccination during 2YL and beyond. Despite the general successes, regional and urban–rural disparities in vaccination timeliness were noted and will require targeted and multifaceted solutions to address. Additional efforts to not only improve vaccination coverage but to ensure that vaccines are received at their recommended schedule can strengthen the routine immunization platform.

Supplementary Materials: The following supporting information can be downloaded at https://www.mdpi.com/article/10.3390/vaccines12070716/s1: Figure S1: Flowchart of children included in vaccination timeliness analyses in Greater Accra (GAR), Northern (NR), and Volta (VR) regions during 2016 and 2020.

Author Contributions: Conceptualization, P.M., M.T.W., K.A.-A., P.Q., M.P.S., H.G., C.O., P.-N.A., J.K.L.O., W.O. and A.S.W.; methodology, P.M., M.P.S., H.G., D.C.E. and A.S.W.; software, P.M.; validation, H.G. and M.P.S.; formal analysis, P.M. and M.P.S.; investigation, A.S.W.; resources, M.T.W.; writing—original draft preparation, P.M.; writing—review and editing, M.T.W., K.A.-A., P.Q., M.P.S., H.G., C.O., P.-N.A., J.K.L.O., W.O. and A.S.W.; supervision, M.T.W., P.Q., K.A.-A., J.K.L.O., W.O. and A.S.W.; project administration, M.T.W., P.Q., K.A.-A., J.K.L.O., W.O. and A.S.W. All authors have read and agreed to the published version of the manuscript.

Funding: This study was funded by the United States Centers for Disease Control and Prevention.

Institutional Review Board Statement: The protocol was approved by the Ethical Review Board at the Ghana Health Service. The Human Subjects Office at the U.S. Centers for Disease Control and Prevention (CDC) deemed this activity as an assessment of public health practice and determined it as non-research.

Informed Consent Statement: Informed consent was obtained from all persons involved in the household survey.

Data Availability Statement: The datasets used and/or analyzed during the current project may be available upon reasonable request.

Acknowledgments: The efforts of the staff of the Ghana Expanded Program on Immunization and the Centers for Disease and Control, Global Immunization Division, who were involved in the survey-instrument design and data collection are deeply appreciated.

Conflicts of Interest: The authors declare no conflicts of interest. The findings and conclusions in this report are those of the authors and do not necessarily represent the views of the Centers for Disease Control and Prevention.

References

1. World Health Organization. *Immunization Agenda 2030: A Global Strategy to Leave No One Behind*; World Health Organization: Geneva, Switzerland, 2020.
2. Regional Committee for Africa. *Measles Elimination by 2020: A Strategy for the African Region*; World Health Organization, Regional Office for Africa: Brazzaville, Congo, 2011.
3. Dombkowski, K.J.; Lantz, P.M.; Freed, G.L. The need for surveillance of delay in age-appropriate immunization. *Am. J. Prev. Med.* **2002**, *23*, 36–42. [CrossRef] [PubMed]
4. Grant, C.C.; Roberts, M.; Scragg, R.; Stewart, J.; Lennon, D.; Kivell, D.; Ford, R.; Menzies, R. Delayed immunisation and risk of pertussis in infants: Unmatched case-control study. *BMJ* **2003**, *326*, 852. [CrossRef] [PubMed]
5. Kolos, V.; Menzies, R.; McIntyre, P. Higher pertussis hospitalization rates in indigenous Australian infants, and delayed vaccination. *Vaccine* **2007**, *25*, 588–590. [CrossRef] [PubMed]
6. Inskip, H.M.; Hall, A.J.; Chotard, J.; Loik, F.; Whittle, H. Hepatitis B vaccine in the Gambian Expanded Programme on Immunization: Factors influencing antibody response. *Int. J. Epidemiol.* **1991**, *20*, 764–769. [CrossRef] [PubMed]
7. Sato, H.; Albrecht, P.; Reynolds, D.W.; Stagno, S.; Ennis, F.A. Transfer of measles, mumps, and rubella antibodies from mother to infant: Its effect on measles, mumps, and rubella immunization. *Am. J. Dis. Child.* **1979**, *133*, 1240–1243. [CrossRef] [PubMed]
8. Lochlainn, L.M.N.; de Gier, B.; van der Maas, N.; van Binnendijk, R.; Strebel, P.M.; Goodman, T.; de Melker, H.E.; Moss, W.J.; Hahné, S.J.M. Effect of measles vaccination in infants younger than 9 months on the immune response to subsequent measles vaccine doses: A systematic review and meta-analysis. *Lancet Infect. Dis.* **2019**, *19*, 1246–1254. [CrossRef]
9. World Health Organization. *Establishing and Strengthening Immunization in the Second Year of Life: Practices for Vaccination Beyond Infancy*; World Health Organization: Geneva, Switzerland, 2018.
10. Masresha, B.G.; Luce, R.; Okeibunor, J.; Shibeshi, M.E.; Kamadjeu, R.; Fall, A. Introduction of the Second Dose of Measles Containing Vaccine in the Childhood Vaccination Programs Within the WHO Africa Region—Lessons Learnt. *J. Immunol. Sci.* **2018**, 113–121. [CrossRef] [PubMed]
11. Nyaku, M.; Wardle, M.; Eng, J.V.; Ametewee, L.; Bonsu, G.; Opare, J.K.L.; Conklin, L. Immunization delivery in the second year of life in Ghana: The need for a multifaceted approach. *Pan Afr. Med. J.* **2017**, *27* (Suppl. S3), 4. [CrossRef] [PubMed]
12. Le Gargasson, J.-B.; Nyonator, F.K.; Adibo, M.; Gessner, B.D.; Colombini, A. Costs of routine immunization and the introduction of new and underutilized vaccines in Ghana. *Vaccine* **2015**, *33*, A40–A46. [CrossRef]
13. Dongdem, A.Z.; Alhassan, E.; Opare, D.; Boateng, G.; Bonsu, G.; Amponsa-Achiano, K.; Sarkodie, B.; Dzotsi, E.; Adjabeng, M.; Afagbedzi, S.; et al. An 11-year trend of rubella incidence cases reported in the measles case-based surveillance system, Ghana. *Pan Afr. Med. J.* **2021**, *39*, 132. [CrossRef]
14. World Health Organization & UNICEF. Ghana: WHO and UNICEF Estimates of Immunization Coverage: 2021 Revision. 2022. Available online: https://data.unicef.org/wp-content/uploads/cp/immunisation/gha.pdf (accessed on 10 July 2023).
15. Tchoualeu, D.D.; Harvey, B.; Nyaku, M.; Opare, J.; Traicoff, D.; Bonsu, G.; Quaye, P.; Sandhu, H.S. Evaluation of the impact of immunization second year of life training interventions on health care workers in Ghana. *Glob. Health Sci. Pract.* **2021**, *9*, 498–507. [CrossRef] [PubMed]
16. Laryea, D.O.; Abbeyquaye Parbie, E.; Frimpong, E. Timeliness of childhood vaccine uptake among children attending a tertiary health service facility-based immunisation clinic in Ghana. *BMC Public Health* **2014**, *14*, 90. [CrossRef] [PubMed]
17. Levine, G.; Salifu, A.; Mohammed, I.; Fink, G. Mobile nudges and financial incentives to improve coverage of timely neonatal vaccination in rural areas (GEVaP trial): A 3-armed cluster randomized controlled trial in Northern Ghana. *PLoS ONE* **2021**, *16*, e0247485. [CrossRef] [PubMed]

18. Gram, L.; Soremekun, S.; ten Asbroek, A.; Manu, A.; O'Leary, M.; Hill, Z.; Danso, S.; Amenga-Etego, S.; Owusu-Agyei, S.; Kirkwood, B.R. Socio-economic determinants and inequities in coverage and timeliness of early childhood immunisation in rural G hana. *Trop. Med. Int. Health* **2014**, *19*, 802–811. [CrossRef] [PubMed]
19. Akmatov, M.K.; Mikolajczyk, R.T. Timeliness of childhood vaccinations in 31 low and middle-income countries. *J. Epidemiol. Community Health* **2012**, *66*, e14. [CrossRef] [PubMed]
20. Clark, A.; Sanderson, C. Timing of children's vaccinations in 45 low-income and middle-income countries: An analysis of survey data. *Lancet* **2009**, *373*, 1543–1549. [CrossRef] [PubMed]
21. Ghana Statistical Service. Ghana 2021 Population and Housing Census, Volume 1. 2021. Available online: https://census2021.statsghana.gov.gh/gssmain/fileUpload/reportthemelist/PRINT_COPY_VERSION_FOUR%2022ND_SEPT_AT_8_30AM.pdf (accessed on 10 July 2023).
22. Banchani, E.; Tenkorang, E.Y.; Midodzi, W. Examining the effects of individual and neighbourhood socio-economic status/wealth on hypertension among women in the Greater Accra Region of Ghana. *Health Soc. Care Community* **2022**, *30*, 714–725. [CrossRef] [PubMed]
23. Sheff, M.C.; Bawah, A.A.; Asuming, P.O.; Kyei, P.; Kushitor, M.; Phillips, J.F.; Kachur, S.P. Evaluating health service coverage in Ghana's Volta region using a modified Tanahashi model. *Glob. Health Action* **2020**, *13*, 1732664. [CrossRef]
24. Muhoza, P.; Shah, M.P.; Gao, H.; Amponsa-Achiano, K.; Quaye, P.; Opare, W.; Okae, C.; Aboyinga, P.-N.; Opare, K.L.; Wardle, M.T.; et al. Predictors for Uptake of Vaccines Offered during the Second Year of Life: Second Dose of Measles-Containing Vaccine and Meningococcal Serogroup A-Containing Vaccine, Ghana, 2020. *Vaccines* **2023**, *11*, 1515. [CrossRef]
25. Janusz, C.B.; Frye, M.; Mutua, M.K.; Wagner, A.L.; Banerjee, M.; Boulton, M.L. Vaccine Delay and Its Association With Undervaccination in Children in Sub-Saharan Africa. *Am. J. Prev. Med.* **2021**, *60* (Suppl. S1), S53–S64. [CrossRef] [PubMed]
26. Emmanuel, O.W.; Samuel, A.A.; Helen, K.L. Determinants of childhood vaccination completion at a peri-urban hospital in Kenya, December 2013-January 2014: A case control study. *Pan Afr. Med. J.* **2015**, *20*, 277. [CrossRef] [PubMed]
27. StataCorp. *Stata Statistical Software: Release 17*; StataCorp: College Station, TX, USA, 2021.
28. Sheriff, A.A.; Zakariah, A.; Dapaa, S.; Odikro, M.A.; Issahaku, R.G.; Bandoh, D.; Noora, C.L.; Gebru, G.N.; Kenu, E. Ghana's progress towards measles elimination: Surveillance data analysis, Greater Accra Region, 2015–2019. *Front. Trop. Dis.* **2023**, *4*, 1071486. [CrossRef]
29. World Health Organization. Provisional Monthly Measles and Rubella Data: Distribution of Measles Cases by Country and by Month, 2011–2023. 2023. Available online: https://www.who.int/teams/immunization-vaccines-and-biologicals/immunization-analysis-and-insights/surveillance/monitoring/provisional-monthly-measles-and-rubella-data (accessed on 5 January 2024).
30. Wariri, O.; Nkereuwem, E.; Erondu, N.A.; Edem, B.; Nkereuwem, O.O.; Idoko, O.T.; Agogo, E.; Enegela, J.E.; Sesay, T.; Conde, I.S.; et al. A scorecard of progress towards measles elimination in 15 west African countries, 2001–2019: A retrospective, multicountry analysis of national immunisation coverage and surveillance data. *Lancet Glob. Health* **2021**, *9*, e280–e290. [CrossRef] [PubMed]
31. Masresha, B.; Hatcher, C.; Lebo, E.; Tanifum, P.; Bwaka, A.; Minta, A.; Antoni, S.; Grant, G.B.; Perry, R.T.; O'Connor, P. Progress toward measles elimination—African Region, 2017–2021. *Morb. Mortal. Wkly. Rep.* **2023**, *72*, 985. [CrossRef] [PubMed]
32. UNESCO Institute for Statistics. Education and Literacy—Participation in Education 2023. Available online: https://uis.unesco.org/en/country/gh (accessed on 15 August 2023).
33. Education Policy and Data Center (FHI 360). Ghana National Education Profile 2018 Update. 2018. Available online: https://www.epdc.org/sites/default/files/documents/EPDC_NEP_2018_Ghana.pdf (accessed on 5 January 2024).
34. Akyeampong, K.; Djangmah, J.; Oduro, A.; Seidu, A.; Hunt, F. Access to Basic Education in Ghana: The Evidence and the Issues; Country Analytic Report; ERIC: 2007. Available online: https://files.eric.ed.gov/fulltext/ED508809.pdf (accessed on 5 January 2024).
35. Vandelaer, J.; Olaniran, M. Using a school-based approach to deliver immunization—Global update. *Vaccine* **2015**, *33*, 719–725. [CrossRef] [PubMed]
36. Asuman, D.; Ackah, C.G.; Enemark, U. Inequalities in child immunization coverage in Ghana: Evidence from a decomposition analysis. *Health Econ. Rev.* **2018**, *8*, 9. [CrossRef] [PubMed]
37. Moran, E.B.; Wagner, A.L.; Asiedu-Bekoe, F.; Abdul-Karim, A.; Schroeder, L.F.; Boulton, M.L. Socio-economic characteristics associated with the introduction of new vaccines and full childhood vaccination in Ghana, 2014. *Vaccine* **2020**, *38*, 2937–2942. [CrossRef]
38. Ghana Health Service (GHS). *Field Guide for the Ghana Immunization Programme*; Ghana Health Service: Accra, Ghana, 2016.
39. World Health Organization. Measles vaccines: WHO position paper, April 2017—Recommendations. *Vaccine* **2019**, *37*, 219–222. [CrossRef] [PubMed]
40. Feikema, S.M.; Klevens, R.M.; Washington, M.L.; Barker, L. Extraimmunization among US children. *JAMA* **2000**, *283*, 1311–1317. [CrossRef]
41. Akmatov, M.K.; Kimani-Murage, E.; Pessler, F.; Guzman, C.A.; Krause, G.; Kreienbrock, L.; Mikolajczyk, R.T. Evaluation of invalid vaccine doses in 31 countries of the WHO African Region. *Vaccine* **2015**, *33*, 892–901. [CrossRef]
42. Tsega, A.; Hausi, H.; Chriwa, G.; Steinglass, R.; Smith, D.; Valle, M. Vaccination coverage and timely vaccination with valid doses in Malawi. *Vaccine Rep.* **2016**, *6*, 8–12. [CrossRef]

43. Dolan, S.B.; Patel, M.; Hampton, L.M.; Burnett, E.; Ehlman, D.C.; Garon, J.; Cloessner, E.; Chmielewski, E.; Hyde, T.B.; Mantel, C.; et al. Administering multiple injectable vaccines during a single visit—Summary of findings from the accelerated introduction of inactivated polio vaccine globally. *J. Infect. Dis.* **2017**, *216* (Suppl. S1), S152–S160.
44. Preza, I.; Subaiya, S.; Harris, J.B.; Ehlman, D.C.; Wannemuehler, K.; Wallace, A.S.; Huseynov, S.; Hyde, T.B.; Nelaj, E.; Bino, S.; et al. Acceptance of the administration of multiple injectable vaccines in a single immunization visit in Albania. *J. Infect. Dis.* **2017**, *216* (Suppl. S1), S146–S151. [PubMed]
45. Smith, P.J.; Humiston, S.G.; Parnell, T.; Vannice, K.S.; Salmon, D.A. The association between intentional delay of vaccine administration and timely childhood vaccination coverage. *Public Health Rep.* **2010**, *125*, 534–541. [CrossRef] [PubMed]
46. World Health Organization. Joint Reporting form on Immunization for Ghana Vaccine Supply and Logistics. 2022. Available online: https://immunizationdata.who.int/ (accessed on 1 April 2022).
47. Nkwenkeu, S.F.; Jalloh, M.F.; Walldorf, J.A.; Zoma, R.L.; Tarbangdo, F.; Fall, S.; Hien, S.; Combassere, R.; Ky, C.; Kambou, L.; et al. Health workers' perceptions and challenges in implementing meningococcal serogroup a conjugate vaccine in the routine childhood immunization schedule in Burkina Faso. *BMC Public Health* **2020**, *20*, 254.
48. Wallace, A.S.; Krey, K.; Hustedt, J.; Burnett, E.; Choun, N.; Daniels, D.; Watkins, M.L.; Soeung, S.C.; Duncan, R. Assessment of vaccine wastage rates, missed opportunities, and related knowledge, attitudes and practices during introduction of a second dose of measles-containing vaccine into Cambodia's national immunization program. *Vaccine* **2018**, *36*, 4517–4524.
49. Wolff, B.; Aborigo, R.A.; Dalaba, M.; Opare, J.K.; Conklin, L.; Bonsu, G.; Amponsa-Achiano, K. Community Barriers, Enablers, and Normative Embedding of Second Year of Life Vaccination in Ghana: A Qualitative Study. *Glob. Health Sci. Pract.* **2023**, *11*, e2200496. [PubMed]
50. Smalley, H.K.; Keskinocak, P.; Engineer, F.G.; Pickering, L.K. Universal tool for vaccine scheduling: Applications for children and adults. *Interfaces* **2011**, *41*, 436–454.
51. Cohen, N.J.; Lauderdale, D.S.; Shete, P.B.; Seal, J.B.; Daum, R.S. Physician knowledge of catch-up regimens and contraindications for childhood immunizations. *Pediatrics* **2003**, *111*, 925–932. [CrossRef] [PubMed]
52. Engineer, F.G.; Keskinocak, P.; Pickering, L.K. OR practice—Catch-up scheduling for childhood vaccination. *Oper. Res.* **2009**, *57*, 1307–1319. [CrossRef]
53. Siddiqi, D.A.; Ali, R.F.; Shah, M.T.; Dharma, V.K.; Khan, A.A.; Roy, T.; Chandir, S. Evaluation of a Mobile-Based Immunization Decision Support System for Scheduling Age-Appropriate Vaccine Schedules for Children Younger Than 2 Years in Pakistan and Bangladesh: Lessons from a Multisite, Mixed Methods Study. *JMIR Pediatr. Parent.* **2023**, *6*, e40269. [CrossRef] [PubMed Central]
54. Harvey, H.; Reissland, N.; Mason, J. Parental reminder, recall and educational interventions to improve early childhood immunisation uptake: A systematic review and meta-analysis. *Vaccine* **2015**, *33*, 2862–2880. [CrossRef]
55. Oya-Ita, A.; Nwachukwu, C.; Oringanje, C.; Meremikwu, M. Interventions for improving coverage of child immunization in low-income and middle-income countries. *Cochrane Database Syst Rev.* **2009**, *7*. [CrossRef]
56. Yunusa, U.; Garba, S.N.; Umar, A.B.; Idris, S.H.; Bello, U.L.; Abdulrashid, I.; Mohammed, J. Mobile phone reminders for enhancing uptake, completeness and timeliness of routine childhood immunization in low and middle income countries: A systematic review and meta-analysis. *Vaccine* **2021**, *39*, 209–221. [CrossRef] [PubMed]
57. Aksnes, B.N.; Walldorf, J.A.; Nkwenkeu, S.F.; Zoma, R.L.; Mirza, I.; Tarbangdo, F.; Fall, S.; Hien, S.; Ky, C.; Kambou, L.; et al. Vaccination information, motivations, and barriers in the context of meningococcal serogroup A conjugate vaccine introduction: A qualitative assessment among caregivers in Burkina Faso, 2018. *Vaccine* **2021**, *39*, 6370–6377. [CrossRef] [PubMed]
58. Kulkarni, S.; Ishizumi, A.; Eleeza, O.; Patel, P.; Feika, M.; Kamara, S.; Bangura, J.; Jalloh, U.; Koroma, M.; Sankoh, Z.; et al. Using Photovoice Methodology to Uncover Individual-level, Health Systems, and Contextual Barriers to Uptake of Second Dose of Measles Containing Vaccine in Western Area Urban, Sierra Leone, 2020. *Vaccine X* **2023**, *14*, 100338. [CrossRef] [PubMed]
59. Ansong, D.; Tawfik, D.; Williams, E.; Benson, S.; Nyanor, I.; Boakye, I.; Obirikorang, C.; Sallah, L.; Arhin, B.; Boaheng, J.M. Suboptimal vaccination rates in rural Ghana despite positive caregiver attitudes towards vaccination. *J Vaccines Immun.* **2014**, *2*, 7–15.
60. Rahji, F.R.; Ndikom, C.M. Factors influencing compliance with immunization regimen among mothers in Ibadan, Nigeria. *IOSR J. Nurs. Health Sci.* **2013**, *2*, 1–9. [CrossRef]
61. Brown, D.W.; Gacic-Dobo, M. Home-based record prevalence among children aged 12–23 months from 180 demographic and health surveys. *Vaccine* **2015**, *33*, 2584–2593. [CrossRef] [PubMed]
62. Acharya, K.; Lacoul, M.; Bietsch, K. *Factors Affecting Vaccination Coverage and Retention of Vaccination Cards in Nepal*; DHS Further Analysis Report; ICF: Rockville, MD, USA, 2019.
63. Hussain, I.; Khan, A.; Rhoda, D.A.; Ahmed, I.; Umer, M.; Ansari, U.; Shah, M.A.; Yunus, S.; Brustrom, J.; Oelrichs, R.; et al. Routine immunization coverage and immunization card retention in Pakistan: Results from a cross-sectional national survey. *Pediatr. Infect. Dis. J.* **2023**, *42*, 260. [CrossRef]

Disclaimer/Publisher's Note: The statements, opinions and data contained in all publications are solely those of the individual author(s) and contributor(s) and not of MDPI and/or the editor(s). MDPI and/or the editor(s) disclaim responsibility for any injury to people or property resulting from any ideas, methods, instructions or products referred to in the content.

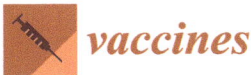

Article

Sociodemographic Trends and Correlation between Parental Hesitancy towards Pediatric COVID-19 Vaccines and Routine Childhood Immunizations in the United States: 2021–2022 National Immunization Survey—Child COVID Module

Olufunto A. Olusanya [1,2,*], Nina B. Masters [1,3], Fan Zhang [4], David E. Sugerman [1,*], Rosalind J. Carter [5], Debora Weiss [6] and James A. Singleton [4]

[1] Division of Viral Diseases, National Center for Immunization and Respiratory Diseases, Centers for Disease Control and Prevention (CDC), Atlanta, GA 30333, USA
[2] Center for Biomedical Informatics, Department of Pediatrics, University of Tennessee Health Science Center, Memphis, TN 38103, USA
[3] Epidemic Intelligence Service, Centers for Disease Control and Prevention (CDC), Atlanta, GA 30333, USA
[4] Immunization Services Division, National Center for Immunization and Respiratory Diseases, Centers for Disease Control and Prevention (CDC), Atlanta, GA 30333, USA; xzs8@cdc.gov (J.A.S.)
[5] Office of the Director, National Center for Immunization and Respiratory Diseases, Centers for Disease Control and Prevention (CDC), Atlanta, GA 30333, USA
[6] Division of Global HIV and TB, Centers for Disease Control and Prevention (CDC), Atlanta, GA 30333, USA
* Correspondence: oolusan1@uthsc.edu (O.A.O.); dsugerman@cdc.gov (D.E.S.)

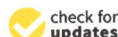

Citation: Olusanya, O.A.; Masters, N.B.; Zhang, F.; Sugerman, D.E.; Carter, R.J.; Weiss, D.; Singleton, J.A. Sociodemographic Trends and Correlation between Parental Hesitancy towards Pediatric COVID-19 Vaccines and Routine Childhood Immunizations in the United States: 2021–2022 National Immunization Survey—Child COVID Module. *Vaccines* 2024, *12*, 495. https://doi.org/10.3390/vaccines12050495

Academic Editor: Pedro Plans-Rubió

Received: 22 March 2024
Revised: 24 April 2024
Accepted: 24 April 2024
Published: 3 May 2024

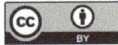

Copyright: © 2024 by the authors. Licensee MDPI, Basel, Switzerland. This article is an open access article distributed under the terms and conditions of the Creative Commons Attribution (CC BY) license (https://creativecommons.org/licenses/by/4.0/).

Abstract: Multiple factors may influence parental vaccine hesitancy towards pediatric COVID-19 vaccines and routine childhood immunizations (RCIs). Using the United States National Immunization Survey—Child COVID Module data collected from parents/guardians of children aged 5–11 years, this cross-sectional study (1) identified the trends and prevalence estimates of parental hesitancy towards pediatric COVID-19 vaccines and RCIs, (2) examined the relationship between hesitancy towards pediatric COVID-19 vaccines and RCIs, and (3) assessed trends in parental hesitancy towards RCIs by sociodemographic characteristics and behavioral and social drivers of COVID-19 vaccination. From November 2021 to July 2022, 54,329 parents or guardians were interviewed. During this 9-month period, the proportion of parents hesitant about pediatric COVID-19 vaccines increased by 15.8 percentage points (24.8% to 40.6%). Additionally, the proportion of parents who reported RCIs hesitancy increased by 4.7 percentage points from November 2021 to May 2022 but returned to baseline by July 2022. Over nine months, parents' concerns about pediatric COVID-19 infections declined; however, parents were increasingly worried about pediatric COVID-19 vaccine safety and overall importance. Furthermore, pediatric COVID-19 vaccine hesitancy was more prevalent among parents of children who were White (43.2%) versus Black (29.3%) or Hispanic (26.9%) and those residing in rural (51.3%) compared to urban (28.9%) areas. In contrast, RCIs hesitancy was higher among parents of children who were Black (32.0%) versus Hispanic (24.5%) or White (23.6%). Pediatric COVID-19 vaccine hesitancy was 2–6 times as prevalent among parents who were RCIs hesitant compared to those who were RCIs non-hesitant. This positive correlation between parental hesitancy towards pediatric COVID-19 vaccines and RCIs was observed for all demographic and psychosocial factors for unadjusted and adjusted prevalence ratios. Parent–provider interactions should increase vaccine confidence, shape social norms, and facilitate behavior change to promote pediatric vaccination rates.

Keywords: COVID-19; immunizations; pediatric COVID-19 vaccines; vaccine hesitancy; vaccine confidence; pandemic; National Immunization Survey—Child COVID Module

1. Introduction

Large-scale childhood vaccination programs are among the most effective and cost-beneficial public health interventions [1]. To offer protection against serious childhood illnesses in the United States (U.S.), the Centers for Disease Control and Prevention's (CDC) Advisory Committee on Immunization Practices (ACIP) recommends the receipt of routine childhood immunizations (RCIs), which are administered based on age [2]. According to the immunization schedule for birth to 6 years, RCIs include vaccines to prevent hepatitis; rotavirus; diphtheria, tetanus, and acellular pertussis (DTaP); *Haemophilus influenzae* type B; pneumococcal conjugate; inactivated polio; influenza; measles, mumps, and rubella (MMR); and varicella [2]. On 29 October 2021, the U.S. Food and Drug Administration (FDA) authorized the Pfizer-BioNTech COVID-19 vaccine for children aged 5–11 years [3], with the first vaccines administered on 2 November 2021. Pediatric COVID-19 vaccines are currently recommended for children aged six months and older [2,4].

Despite the benefits of vaccinations, the COVID-19 pandemic and other factors may have reversed incremental gains in U.S. vaccination rates [5–8] and caused a sustained decline in global immunization coverage [9,10]. The pandemic has caused large-scale disruptions to the delivery and uptake of immunization services [6,11,12] and negatively impacted vaccine equity among susceptible populations and geographical areas [13,14]. Disruptions in child wellness visits and missed vaccinations may have been due to COVID-19 preventive measures, healthcare disparities, long-term school closures, and shortages in testing modalities and treatment therapies [7]. In 2022, vaccination rates for MMR, DTaP, and varicella vaccines among kindergartners were lower in most states in the U.S. compared to the previous school year (i.e., 2019–2020), while the national MMR vaccination rate fell below the Healthy People 2030 target of 95% for kindergartners [15].

Parents' reluctance to accept routine childhood vaccines and adhere to immunization schedules also represents a growing challenge for childhood vaccination programs [5–7,10]. Vaccine hesitancy is a "delay in the acceptance or refusal of safe vaccines despite availability of vaccination services" and is among the top ten global health threats [16,17]. The spike in vaccine hesitancy during the pandemic [18–20] may have been due to the unprecedented speed of development for COVID-19 vaccines, the rapid introduction of these vaccines, and the emergence of new SARS-CoV-2 variants [21–23]. Moreover, COVID-19 vaccine misinformation [8], vaccine mandates, digital hyperconnectivity, and ongoing highly politicized debates surrounding COVID-19 vaccines may have contributed to vaccine hesitancy [23]. Parents' psychosocial factors (e.g., concerns about vaccine safety and effectiveness, mistrust in public health institutions, and belief-based extremism) and access barriers may also be linked to the reluctance to vaccinate children [24].

These complex and dynamic influences (i.e., pandemic disruptions, vaccine hesitancy, the politicization of COVID-19 vaccines, and parental mistrust) could produce unintended consequences that increase parental hesitancy for other childhood vaccines. It is crucial that emerging vaccine concerns within the context of the COVID-19 pandemic are identified and addressed. This cross-sectional study analyzed data from the National Immunization Survey—Child COVID Module (NIS-CCM), which is representative of the U.S. population. Our study had three objectives. We sought to (1) identify the trends and prevalence estimates of parental hesitancy towards pediatric COVID-19 vaccines and RCIs among parents with children aged 5–11 years over 9 months, (2) examine the relationship between parental hesitancy toward pediatric COVID-19 vaccines and hesitancy towards RCIs, and (3) assess the trends in parental hesitancy towards RCIs over the 9-month study period by sociodemographic characteristics and behavioral and social drivers of childhood COVID-19 vaccination.

2. Materials and Methods

2.1. Survey Methods

This cross-sectional study analyzed data from the NIS-CCM, which offers population-based, state, and local area vaccination estimates, using interviews conducted between

November 2021 and July 2022. The NIS-CCM's purpose, beginning in July 2021, is to provide estimates of COVID-19 vaccination coverage, parental intent to vaccinate their children against COVID-19, and behavioral and social indicators related to COVID-19 vaccination in children aged 6 months to 17 years [25–27]. Since November 2021, the NIS-CCM has expanded to include children aged 6 months to 4 years [26]. The NIS-CCM uses a random-digit-dialed sample of cellular numbers belonging to households with children aged 6 months to 17 years. For our study, these analytic data were restricted to households with children aged 5–11 years. The NIS-CCM survey is administered to an adult in a household who is knowledgeable about a child's vaccination history (hereafter referred to as a parent) [28,29]. For households with more than one child, the NIS-CCM randomly selects a child in that household to be the referent. Quarterly telephone samples from 4–5-week periods are compiled into a dataset for timeliness and analytic purposes. The data are then weighted to be representative of children in the U.S. population for analysis. The NIS-CCM is conducted in compliance with applicable federal laws and CDC policies and is determined by CDC to constitute public health surveillance. For our study, pediatric COVID-19 vaccine hesitancy is defined as parental hesitancy towards pediatric COVID-19 vaccines.

2.2. Measures

The NIS-CCM uses the Behavioral and Social Drivers of Vaccination (BeSD) framework to assess socio-behavioral factors influencing pediatric COVID-19 vaccinations [30]. The BeSD proposes four domains that influence the acceptance and uptake of vaccines: (1) what people think and feel about vaccines; (2) social processes and norms that influence vaccinations; (3) environmental context, practical issues, and available resources; and (4) individual motivations (or hesitancy) that shape vaccination behavior. The BeSD domains are presented below with their associated questions.

2.2.1. Outcome Variables
Individual Motivations (or Hesitancy)

Our study outcome measures were (1) parental hesitancy toward pediatric COVID-19 vaccines and (2) parental hesitancy towards routine childhood immunizations (RCIs). For this study, responses to these outcome measures were dichotomized to aid meaningful interpretation.

Pediatric COVID-19 vaccine coverage was determined by asking parents if their children had received at least one dose of a COVID-19 vaccine. Among parents whose eligible children had not yet received any vaccine, parental hesitancy towards the COVID-19 vaccine was assessed with the question, "Once your child is eligible, how likely are you to get [child] a COVID-19 vaccine?" Parents' responses were dichotomized into: "hesitant" (i.e., unvaccinated [child], definitely will not get a vaccine for [child], and probably will not get a vaccine for [child]) and "non-hesitant" (i.e., definitely will get a vaccine for [child] and probably will get a vaccine for [child]). Parents who reported that they were "not sure" about getting the vaccine for [child] or that their child had received "at least one dose of COVID-19 vaccine" were categorized into the "non-hesitant" group. To assess parental hesitancy towards RCIs, parents were asked, "How hesitant about childhood shots would you consider yourself to be?" Parents' responses were dichotomized into two categories for this analysis: "hesitant" (i.e., somewhat hesitant and very hesitant) and "not hesitant" (i.e., not that hesitant and not at all hesitant).

2.2.2. Predictor Variables
What People Think and Feel about Vaccinations

Parents' psychosocial characteristics, including confidence in vaccine safety and benefits, beliefs, perceptions, and regrets, were assessed. Parents' perception of risk for pediatric COVID-19 infections was measured with "How concerned are you about [child's name] getting COVID-19?" Parents' perception of vaccine importance against pediatric COVID-19 infection was measured by asking, "How important do you think getting a COVID-19 vaccine is to protect [child's name] against COVID-19?" Perception of vaccine safety was assessed with the question, "How safe do you think a COVID-19 vaccine is for [child's name]?" Parental regret was measured with, "If I do not get [child's name] a COVID-19 vaccine, I will regret it".

Social Processes and Norms That Influence Vaccinations

This domain measures constructs such as family and social influences, peer norms, and health worker recommendations. Associated questions include, "If you had to guess about how many of your family and friends have gotten a COVID-19 vaccine for their children ages 5–11 years?", "Has a doctor, nurse, or another health professional ever recommended that you get a COVID-19 vaccine for [child's name]?" and "Does [child's name]'s school require a COVID-19 vaccine to attend in-person classes?"

Practical Issues and Available Resources

Practical issues influencing pediatric COVID-19 vaccine uptake, such as knowledge, affordability, ease of access, vaccination availability, etc., were measured with questions such as, "In the past 7 days, how often has [child's name] worn a mask when going into indoor public spaces like schools, stores, etc.?"

Other Sociodemographic Measures

In addition, NIS-CCM collects sociodemographic information such as the child's age, race/ethnicity, relationship of survey respondent to child, mother's educational level, family income, and metropolitan statistical area of residence. Other sociodemographic characteristics assessed include family income and poverty level, number of children under 18 residing in a household, Social Vulnerability Index of county of residence, and Health and Human Services region.

2.3. Statistical Analyses

Our study analyzed parents' or guardians' interview responses from 1 November 2021 through 31 July 2022 [29]. For all analyses, the denominator consisted of all parent survey interviews completed for children aged 5–11 years each month over the course of 9 months. The NIS-CCM accounts for households without cellular phones, as well as variations in sampling, under-representation, and non-response by weighing and adjusting the data [25]. Additionally, survey weights are calibrated to the reported number of children receiving at least one dose of the COVID-19 vaccine by region based on administrative data reported to the CDC by jurisdictions [26].

Descriptive statistics were used to identify trends and estimates for parental hesitancy towards pediatric COVID-19 vaccines and RCIs over the 9-month period. Furthermore, we examined the prevalence and trends of parental perceptions regarding COVID-19 vaccine safety/importance and pediatric COVID-19 infection. We also compared prevalence estimates of demographic and psychosocial characteristics stratified by the study outcome variables (i.e., parental hesitancy towards the pediatric COVID-19 vaccine and parental hesitancy towards RCIs). Nonoverlapping 95% confidence intervals (CI) determined statistically significant estimates between groups.

A logistic regression analysis investigated the relationship between parents' hesitancy towards pediatric COVID-19 vaccines and their hesitancy towards RCI. SUDAAN version 11.0.3 was used to account for the complex survey design. Estimates were quantified as proportions, prevalence ratios (PR), and 95% CIs. During the logistic regression analysis, the PR was calculated as the prevalence of pediatric COVID-19 vaccine hesitancy within the RCIs hesitant group divided by the prevalence of pediatric COVID-19 vaccine hesitancy within the RCIs non-hesitant group of parents across different levels of demographic and psychosocial characteristics. The adjusted PR controlled for socio-demographic variables (child's age and race, mother's educational level, metropolitan statistical area (MSA) status, and poverty status). Results were determined to be statistically significant if the *p*-value was less than 0.05.

We also utilized weighted linear regression models to analyze the temporal trends in parental RCIs hesitancy levels stratified by sociodemographic characteristics and behavioral and social drivers of the child's COVID-19 vaccination. The models examined the linear trends in the prevalence of RCI hesitancy for each subgroup, with the estimated slopes from the regression models representing the average monthly percentage point change in the prevalence of RCIs hesitancy.

3. Results

During the 9-month study period, 54,329 parents or guardians completed the NIS-CCM interviews. The cumulative response rate for the NIS-CCM through July 2022 was 20.4%. The percentage of children who "received at least one dose of the COVID-19 vaccine" increased by 21.6 percentage points (from 11.6% to 33.2%) during this period.

3.1. Prevalence Trend of Parental Hesitancy for COVID-19 Vaccines and RCIs over 9 Months

Parents reported hesitancy towards pediatric COVID-19 vaccines and RCIs for children aged 5–11-years, as shown in Figure 1, depicting the trend over 9 months. The percentage of parents or guardians who expressed pediatric COVID-19 vaccine hesitancy and indicated they would "definitely not get" or "probably not get" their children vaccinated against COVID-19 steadily increased by 15.8 percentage points (24.8% to 40.6%) over the 9 months (Figure 1). Over the initial 7-month period, the percentage of parents or guardians who expressed RCIs hesitancy by stating they were "very hesitant" or "somewhat hesitant" towards administering RCIs to their children rose by 4.7 percentage points (22.2% in November 2021 to 26.9% in May 2022). However, this upward trend declined by 3.6 percentage points (26.0% to 22.4%) from June to July 2022 (Figure 1).

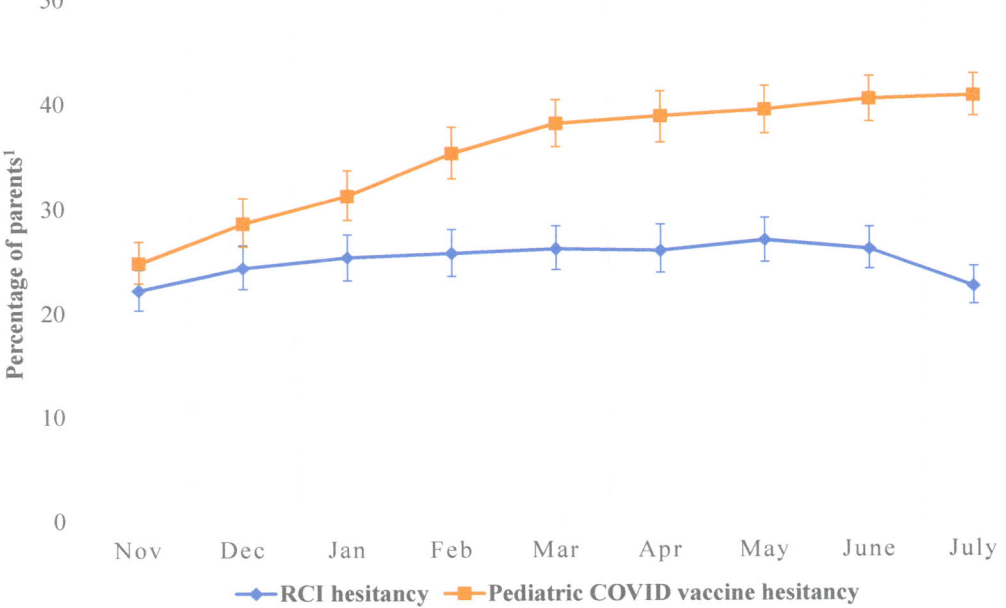

Figure 1. Prevalence of hesitancy towards pediatric COVID-19 vaccines and routine childhood immunizations as reported by parents of children aged 5–11 years, November 2021–July 2022, National

Immunization Survey. Abbreviations: RCIs: Recommended Childhood Immunizations. The denominator of the percentages on the y-axis represents all completed parent interviews for children aged 5–11-years collated monthly between November 2021 and July 2022. (a) *Pediatric COVID-19 vaccine hesitancy* was assessed with, "Once your child is eligible, how likely are you to get a COVID-19 vaccine?" Responses were "definitely not getting vaccine", "probably not getting vaccine", "probably getting vaccine", and "definitely getting vaccine". Responses were dichotomized into two categories: *hesitant* (i.e., unvaccinated [child], definitely not getting vaccine for [child], and probably not getting vaccine for [child]) and *non-hesitant* (i.e., definitely getting vaccine for [child] and probably getting vaccine for [child]). The numerator for *pediatric COVID-19 vaccine hesitancy* in Figure 1 represents parents who reported their children were unvaccinated, probably not getting the vaccine, or definitely not getting the COVID-19 vaccine. (b) *RCIs hesitancy* was assessed with, "How hesitant about childhood shots would you consider yourself to be?" Responses were "not at all hesitant", "not that hesitant", "somewhat hesitant", and "very hesitant". Responses were dichotomized into two categories: *hesitant* (i.e., somewhat hesitant and very hesitant) *and non-hesitant* (i.e., not that hesitant and not at all hesitant). The numerator for *RCIs hesitancy* in Figure 1 represents parents who have reported they were somewhat hesitant or very hesitant towards getting the RCIs for their children. [1] The data obtained from the NIS-CCM are weighted to be representative of children in the US. Accordingly, our results reflect the "percentage of children with a parent who has reported hesitancy either towards pediatric COVID-19 vaccines or RCI". However, to make interpretation easier, we have simplified this as "percentage of parents" on the y-axis.

Throughout the study, parents of children aged 5–11-years expressed fewer concerns about pediatric COVID-19 infections but showed increasing worry about the safety and overall importance of pediatric COVID-19 vaccines (Figure 2).

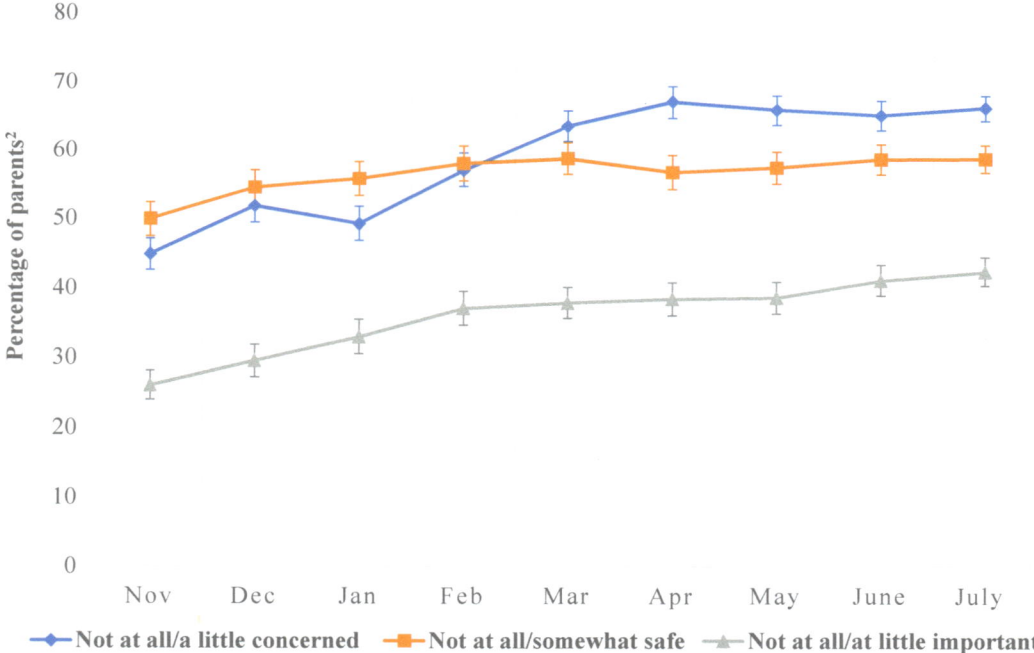

Figure 2. Prevalence of perceptions towards pediatric COVID-19 vaccines as reported by parents of children ages 5–11 years, November 2021–July 2022, National Immunization Survey. The denominator of the percentages on the y-axis represents all completed parent interviews for children aged 5–11-years

collated monthly between November 2021 and July 2022. The numerator represents parents reporting the level of sentiments and perceptions indicated in the graph (e.g., those whose parents reported that COVID-19 vaccines were not at all or somewhat safe, not at all or a little important, etc.). (a) *Not at all concerned/a little*: We assessed parents' *concern for pediatric COVID-19 infections* with, "How concerned are you about your child getting COVID-19?" Responses were not at all concerned, a little concerned, moderately concerned, and very concerned. Responses were dichotomized into two categories: Not at all concerned and a little concerned. (b) *Not at all/somewhat safe*: We assessed parents' *perceptions about COVID-19 vaccine safety* with, "How safe do you think COVID-19 vaccine is for child?" Responses were not at all safe, somewhat safe, very safe, and completely safe. Responses were dichotomized into two categories: Not at all safe and somewhat safe. (c) *Not at all important/a little important*: We assessed parents' *perception of COVID-19 vaccine importance* by asking, "How important do you think getting a COVID-19 vaccine is to protect child against COVID-19?" Responses were not at all important, a little important, somewhat important, and very important. Responses were dichotomized into two categories: Not at all important and a little important. [2] The data obtained from the NIS-CCM are weighted to be representative of children in the US. Accordingly, our results reflect the "percentage of children with a parent who has reported hesitancy either towards pediatric COVID-19 vaccines or RCI". However, to make interpretation easier, we have simplified this as "percentage of parents" on the *y*-axis.

3.2. Prevalence Estimates of Pediatric COVID-19 Vaccine Hesitancy among Socio-Demographic Groups over 9 Months

Pediatric COVID-19 vaccine hesitancy was more prevalent among parents or guardians of children who were White (43.2%) than among Black (29.3%), Hispanic (26.9%), Asian (11.7%), and other/multiple races (35.5%). In addition, mothers with a high school education or equivalent (40.6%) were more hesitant about pediatric COVID-19 vaccines than those with a college degree (28.4%), and parents residing in rural areas (51.3%) were more hesitant than those in urban (28.9%) areas (Table 1).

Parents who were "not at all concerned" or a "little concerned" (48.0%) about pediatric COVID-19 infections were more hesitant towards pediatric COVID-19 vaccines compared to those who were "moderately concerned" or "very concerned" (16.8%). Similarly, the prevalence of COVID-19 vaccine hesitancy was higher among parents who believed that pediatric COVID-19 vaccines were "not at all safe" or "somewhat safe" (55.5%) compared to "very safe" or "completely safe" (5.0%) and among parents who perceived that COVID-19 vaccines were "not at all important" or "a little important" (78.9%) compared with "somewhat important" or "very important" (10.2%). Parents of children aged 5–11 years were more hesitant about pediatric COVID-19 vaccines if they had "none" or "some" family/friends (47.7%) with vaccinated children versus if they had "many" or "almost all" family/friends (7.0%) with vaccinated children. (Table 1).

Table 1. Overall prevalence estimates for pediatric COVID-19 vaccine hesitancy and RCIs hesitancy by demographic indicators and psycho-social characteristics among parents of children aged 5–11 years, United States, November 2021–July 2022, National Immunization Survey—Child COVID Module.

Characteristics	Sample Distribution Weighted % (95% CI)	Pediatric COVID-19 Vaccine Hesitancy [a] Weighted % (95% CI)	RCIs Hesitancy [b] (95% CI)
Child's Age (years)			
5–6 (Referent)	25.3 (24.7–26.0)	36.2 (34.7–37.7)	25.9 (24.5–27.3)
7–9	40.0 (39.2–40.7)	36.0 (34.8–37.2)	24.8 (23.7–25.9)
10–11	34.7 (34.0–35.5)	33.3 (32.0–34.6)	24.4 (23.3–25.7)

Table 1. *Cont.*

Characteristics	Sample Distribution Weighted % (95% CI)	Pediatric COVID-19 Vaccine Hesitancy [a] Weighted % (95% CI)	RCIs Hesitancy [b] (95% CI)
Child's Race/Ethnicity			
Hispanic	27.7 (26.9–28.4)	26.9 (25.3–28.5)	24.5 (23.0–26.0)
White, non-Hispanic (Referent)	48.4 (47.6–49.1)	43.2 (42.1–44.2)	23.6 (22.7–24.5)
Black, non-Hispanic	13.9 (13.3–14.4)	29.3 (27.3–31.4)	32.0 (30.0–34.1)
Asian, non-Hispanic	3.7 (3.4–3.9)	11.7 (9.3–14.6)	18.8 (16.2–21.7)
Multiple races/other, non-Hispanic	6.5 (6.1–6.8)	35.5 (32.9–38.2)	25.8 (23.4–28.4)
Relationship of Respondent to Child			
Mother (Referent)	56.2 (55.5–57.0)	34.6 (33.6–35.7)	24.2 (23.3–25.2)
Father	32.2 (31.5–32.9)	37.9 (36.6–39.2)	27.3 (26.0–28.5)
Other	11.6 (11.1–12.2)	29.4 (27.2–31.7)	21.6 (19.6–23.8)
Mother's Educational Level			
<High school (Referent)	12.0 (11.4–12.6)	31.3 (28.7–34.0)	26.5 (24.0–29.1)
High school or equivalent	22.1 (21.5–22.8)	40.6 (38.9–42.3)	29.4 (27.8–31.0)
Some college/vocational	31.6 (30.9–32.4)	39.9 (38.5–41.3)	27.4 (26.1–28.6)
≥College degree	34.3 (33.6–34.9)	28.4 (27.3–29.5)	19.4 (18.5–20.4)
Urban–Rural Residence (Metropolitan Statistical Area (MSA) Status) [c]			
Urban (MSA, principal city) (Referent)	32.3 (31.6–33.1)	28.9 (27.6–30.2)	24.4 (23.2–25.6)
Suburban (MSA, non-principal city)	54.3 (53.5–55.1)	35.0 (34.0–36.1)	24.1 (23.2–25.1)
Rural (non-MSA)	13.4 (12.9–13.9)	51.3 (49.2–53.3)	30.1 (28.2–32.1)
Poverty Status [d]			
>Poverty, >$75,000/year (Referent)	37.4 (36.7–38.2)	34.3 (33.1–35.5)	21.4 (20.4–22.4)
>Poverty, ≤$75,000/year	25.0 (24.3–25.7)	37.6 (36.0–39.1)	28.6 (27.1–30.1)
Below poverty level	13.8 (13.2–14.4)	33.1 (30.9–35.4)	27.2 (25.1–29.3)
Income not reported	23.8 (23.1–24.5)	34.9 (33.4–36.5)	25.6 (24.2–27.1)
Number of Children Under 18 in Household			
1 child (Referent)	23.5 (22.9–24.1)	31.3 (30.0–32.7)	26.7 (25.4–28.0)
2–3 children	64.4 (63.6–65.1)	34.7 (33.8–35.7)	24.0 (23.2–24.9)
≥4 children	12.1 (11.6–12.7)	44.2 (41.7–46.8)	26.5 (24.3–28.8)
Social Vulnerability Index (SVI) of County of Residence [e]			
Low SVI (Referent)	27.1 (26.5–27.8)	32.9 (31.6–34.3)	21.1 (20.0–22.3)
Moderate SVI	37.2 (36.5–38.0)	35.8 (34.6–37.1)	25.0 (23.8–26.1)
High SVI	35.6 (34.9–36.4)	35.8 (34.4–37.2)	27.2 (25.8–28.5)

Table 1. Cont.

Characteristics	Sample Distribution Weighted % (95% CI)	Pediatric COVID-19 Vaccine Hesitancy [a] Weighted % (95% CI)	RCIs Hesitancy [b] (95% CI)
Health and Human Services (HHS) Region			
Region I: CT, ME, MA, NH, RI, VT (Referent)	3.9 (3.7–4.0)	24.7 (22.7–26.9)	20.9 (19.0–22.9)
Region II: NJ, NY, PR, VI	8.8 (8.4–9.2)	27.1 (24.7–29.7)	24.8 (22.5–27.2)
Region III: DE, DC, MD, PA, VA, WV	8.9 (8.6–9.2)	32.3 (30.5–34.3)	22.9 (21.2–24.6)
Region IV: AL, FL, GA, KY, MS, NC, SC, TN	19.7 (19.1–20.3)	42.3 (40.5–44.1)	28.8 (27.2–30.6)
Region V: IL, IN, MI, MN, OH, WI	15.7 (15.2–16.2)	38.4 (36.4–40.4)	24.7 (23.0–26.5)
Region VI: AR, LA, NM, OK, TX	14.6 (14.1–15.1)	35.5 (33.7–37.4)	25.1 (23.4–26.8)
Region VII: IA, KS, MO, NE	4.5 (4.3–4.7)	42.9 (40.1–45.8)	21.9 (19.6–24.4)
Region VIII: CO, MT, ND, SD, UT, WY	4.0 (3.9–4.2)	37.5 (35.0–40.1)	22.2 (20.0–24.6)
Region IX: AZ, CA, HI, NV, GU	15.6 (14.9–16.2)	27.6 (25.3–30.1)	24.4 (22.2–26.8)
Region X: AK, ID, OR, WA	4.4 (4.1–4.6)	36.4 (33.5–39.4)	24.0 (21.4–26.8)
Concerned about child getting COVID-19 infection? [f]			
Not at all concerned/A little concerned	58.7 (58.0–59.5)	48.0 (47.0–49.0)	26.6 (25.7–27.6)
Moderately concerned/Very concerned (Referent)	41.3 (40.5–42.0)	16.8 (15.8–17.8)	22.6 (21.5–23.7)
I think pediatric COVID-19 vaccine is safe [f]			
Not at all safe/Somewhat safe	56.5 (55.7–57.3)	55.5 (54.3–56.6)	36.4 (35.3–37.5)
Very safe/Completely safe (Referent)	43.5 (42.7–44.3)	5.0 (4.5–5.6)	8.4 (7.7–9.1)
It is important to get pediatric COVID-19 vaccine to protect my child [f]			
Not at all important/A little important	35.9 (35.1–36.6)	78.9 (77.8–80.0)	38.8 (37.5–40.2)
Somewhat important/Very important (Referent)	64.1 (63.4–64.9)	10.2 (9.6–10.9)	16.9 (16.2–17.7)
Family/friends have gotten pediatric COVID-19 vaccine for their children aged 5–11 years [f]			
None/Some	72.0 (71.3–72.7)	46.7 (45.7–47.7)	30.0 (29.1–30.9)
Many/Almost All (Referent)	28.0 (27.3–28.7)	7.0 (6.2–7.9)	12.6 (11.6–13.6)
My health provider has given recommendation to get pediatric COVID-19 vaccine for my child			
Yes	34.4 (33.6–35.1)	21.6 (20.5–22.8)	20.5 (19.4–21.6)
No (Referent)	65.7 (64.9–66.4)	42.9 (41.9–43.9)	27.5 (26.6–28.5)
Child's school requires pediatric COVID-19 vaccine for in-person classes			
Yes	4.5 (4.2–4.8)	6.9 (4.9–9.6)	22.2 (19.2–25.6)
No (Referent)	92.9 (92.5–93.3)	36.9 (36.1–37.7)	25.0 (24.3–25.8)
Not in school, Home schooled	2.6 (2.4–2.9)	47.0 (42.0–52.1)	33.6 (28.8–38.8)

Table 1. Cont.

Characteristics	Sample Distribution Weighted % (95% CI)	Pediatric COVID-19 Vaccine Hesitancy [a] Weighted % (95% CI)	RCIs Hesitancy [b] (95% CI)
Parental regret if pediatric COVID-19 vaccine is not obtained for my child [f]			
Do not agree/Somewhat agree	70.6 (69.9–71.3)	49.2 (48.2–50.2)	31.4 (30.5–32.3)
Strongly agree/Very strongly agree (Referent)	29.4 (28.7–30.1)	3.1 (2.6–3.8)	9.8 (9.0–10.7)
In the last 7 days, my child has worn a mask when going into indoor public spaces [f]			
Never/Rarely/Sometimes	43.8 (43.0–44.5)	51.8 (50.6–52.9)	28.2 (27.2–29.3)
Often/Always (Referent)	56.2 (55.5–57.0)	22.0 (21.0–22.9)	22.4 (21.5–23.4)

Abbreviations: RCIs = Routine Childhood Immunizations; CI = Confidence Interval. The denominator of the percentages represents all completed parent interviews for children aged 5–11-years collated monthly between November 2021–July 2022. [a] Pediatric COVID-19 vaccine hesitancy = unvaccinated (and probably or definitely not getting vaccine). Pediatric COVID-19 vaccine hesitancy was assessed with the following question: "Once your child is eligible, how likely are you to get a COVID-19 vaccine?" Participants' responses were "definitely not getting vaccine", "probably not getting vaccine", "probably getting vaccine", and "definitely getting vaccine". Responses were dichotomized into two categories: pediatric COVID-19 vaccine hesitancy and pediatric COVID-19 vaccine non-hesitancy. [b] RCIs hesitancy = somewhat hesitant or very hesitant to RCIs. RCIs hesitancy was assessed with the following question: "How hesitant about childhood shots would you consider yourself to be?" Response options were "not at all hesitant", "not that hesitant", "somewhat hesitant", and "very hesitant". Participants' responses were dichotomized into RCIs hesitancy and RCIs non-hesitancy. [c] MSA status was determined based on household reported city and county of residence and was grouped into three categories: MSA principal city = urban; MSA non-principal city = suburban; and non-MSA = rural. MSAs and principal cities were as defined by the U.S. Census Bureau at https://www.census.gov/programs-surveys/metro-micro.html, accessed on 23 April 2024. Non-MSA areas include urban populations not located within an MSA and completely rural areas. [d] Income/Poverty level was defined based on total family income in the past calendar year, and the U.S. Census poverty thresholds for that year specified for the applicable family size and the number of children <18 years. Poverty thresholds are available at https://www.census.gov/data/tables/time-series/demo/income-poverty/historical-poverty-thresholds.html, accessed on 23 April 2024. [e] The CDC/ATSDR Social Vulnerability Index was developed using 15 U.S. census variables to help officials identify communities needing support before, during, or after disasters. Categorization of NIS-CCM data into an SVI level was based on the zip code of residence reported by the respondent. Details on the SVI are available at https://www.atsdr.cdc.gov/placeandhealth/svi/index.html, accessed on 23 April 2024. [f] Response options were dichotomized into two categories. Nonoverlapping 95% confidence intervals (CIs) determined statistically significant estimates between groups.

3.3. Prevalence Estimates of RCIs Hesitancy among Socio-Demographic Groups over 9 Months

The prevalence of RCIs hesitancy was higher among parents of children who were Black (32.0%) compared to Hispanic (24.5%), White (23.6%), Asian (18.8%), and other/multiple races (25.8%). Parents residing in rural areas (30.1%) were more hesitant about RCIs than those in urban areas (24.4%). Parents who believed pediatric COVID-19 vaccines were "not at all safe" or "somewhat safe" (36.4%) were more likely to show RCIs hesitancy compared to those who perceived these vaccines as "very safe" or "completely safe" (8.4%). Similarly, those who considered COVID-19 vaccines as "not at all important" or "a little important" (38.8%) were more hesitant about RCIs than those who thought COVID-19 vaccines were "somewhat important" or "very important" (16.9%). Parents with "none/some" family and friends who had vaccinated their children (30.0%) were more hesitant about RCIs than those with "many/almost all" family and friends (12.6%) (Table 1).

3.4. The Relationship between COVID-19 Vaccine Hesitancy and RCIs Hesitancy over 9 Months

Overall, pediatric COVID-19 vaccine hesitancy was approximately 2–6 times as prevalent among parents who were hesitant towards RCIs compared to the RCIs non-hesitant group. This positive correlation was observed across all demographic and psychosocial factors for unadjusted and adjusted prevalence ratios (PRs) (Table 2). For instance, among parents of children who were Asian, pediatric COVID-19 vaccine hesitancy was approximately three times more prevalent among those with RCIs hesitancy compared to those without RCIs hesitancy for unadjusted PR (3.30, CI 2.13–5.10) and adjusted PR (2.97, CI 1.99–4.44) analyses.

Table 2. Overall estimates and prevalence ratios comparing pediatric COVID-19 vaccine hesitancy within the RCIs hesitant group to pediatric COVID-19 vaccine hesitancy within the RCIs non-hesitant group among parents of children ages 5–11 years (logistic regression analysis), November 2021–July 2022, National Immunization Survey—Child COVID Module.

Characteristics	Pediatric COVID-19 Vaccine Hesitancy			
	RCIs Hesitancy Group [a]	RCIs Non-Hesitancy Group [b]	Prevalence Ratio [c]	
	Weighted % (95% CI)	Weighted % (95% CI)	Unadjusted (95% CI)	Adjusted [d] (95% CI)
Child's Age (years)				
5–6	57.0 (53.8–60.1)	28.8 (27.2–30.5)	1.98 (1.83–2.14)	1.88 (1.74–2.04)
7–9	56.4 (53.8–58.9)	29.0 (27.7–30.4)	1.94 (1.82–2.07)	1.89 (1.78–2.02)
10–11	57.1 (54.3–59.9)	25.5 (24.2–26.9)	2.24 (2.08–2.41)	2.17 (2.02–2.33)
Child's Race/Ethnicity				
Hispanic	44.3 (40.7–47.9)	21.2 (19.5–22.9)	2.09 (1.87–2.34)	2.06 (1.84–2.31)
White, non-Hispanic	70.3 (68.3–72.3)	34.5 (33.4–35.7)	2.04 (1.95–2.13)	1.93 (1.84–2.02)
Black, non-Hispanic	46.2 (42.4–50.2)	21.3 (19.1–23.6)	2.18 (1.90–2.49)	2.10 (1.83–2.41)
Asian, non-Hispanic	27.0 (19.6–35.9)	8.2 (6.0–11.2)	3.30 (2.13–5.10)	2.97 (1.99–4.44)
Relationship of Respondent to Child				
Mother	56.0 (53.8–58.1)	27.8 (26.7–28.9)	2.02 (1.91–2.13)	1.95 (1.84–2.06)
Father	60.8 (58.1–63.4)	29.1 (27.6–30.6)	2.09 (1.96–2.24)	2.03 (1.90–2.17)
Other	47.2 (41.8–52.7)	24.4 (22.1–27.0)	1.93 (1.66–2.25)	1.96 (1.70–2.27)
Mother's Educational Level				
<High school	50.0 (44.1–55.2)	25.2 (22.4–28.2)	1.97 (1.68–2.32)	1.81 (1.55–2.11)
High school or equivalent	57.6 (54.4–60.8)	33.5 (31.5–35.4)	1.72 (1.59–1.87)	1.70 (1.57–1.83)
Some college/vocational	59.0 (56.2–61.6)	32.5 (30.9–34.1)	1.81 (1.70–1.94)	1.82 (1.70–1.94)
≥College degree	56.5 (53.7–59.2)	21.5 (20.3–22.6)	2.63 (2.45–2.83)	2.59 (2.41–2.78)
Urban–Rural Residence (Metropolitan Statistical Area (MSA) Status) [e]				
Urban (MSA, principal city)	47.4 (44.4–50.3)	23.0 (21.6–24.4)	2.06 (1.89–2.25)	2.01 (1.84–2.19)
Suburban (MSA, non-principal city)	59.2 (56.9–61.4)	27.2 (26.1–28.4)	2.17 (2.06–2.30)	2.13 (2.02–2.26)
Rural (Non-MSA)	68.3 (64.6–71.9)	43.5 (41.1–45.9)	1.57 (1.46–1.70)	1.55 (1.43–1.67)
Poverty Status [f]				
>Poverty, ≥$75,000/year	61.1 (58.3–63.7)	26.8 (25.5–28.1)	2.28 (2.14–2.43)	2.18 (2.05–2.33)
>Poverty, <$75,000/year	56.4 (53.3–60.0)	30.0 (28.3–31.8)	1.88 (1.73–2.04)	1.87 (1.73–2.02)
Below poverty level	45.3 (40.8–4.98)	28.7 (26.2–31.4)	1.58 (1.38–1.80)	1.48 (1.30–1.69)
Income not reported	58.5 (55.3–61.7)	26.6 (24.9–28.3)	2.20 (2.02–2.40)	2.12 (1.95–2.31)
Number of Children Under 18 in Household				
1 child	50.0 (48.0–53.8)	24.0 (22.7–25.5)	2.12 (1.95–2.30)	2.04 (1.88–2.21)
2–3 children	57.5 (55.4–59.6)	27.4 (26.4–28.4)	2.10 (1.99–2.21)	2.03 (1.93–2.14)
≥4 children	64.5 (59.5–69.2)	37.0 (34.2–40.0)	1.74 (1.56–1.94)	1.70 (1.53–1.89)

Table 2. Cont.

Characteristics	Pediatric COVID-19 Vaccine Hesitancy			
	RCIs Hesitancy Group [a]	RCIs Non-Hesitancy Group [b]	Prevalence Ratio [c]	
	Weighted % (95% CI)	Weighted % (95% CI)	Unadjusted (95% CI)	Adjusted [d] (95% CI)
Social Vulnerability Index (SVI) of County of Residence [g]				
Low SVI	60.2 (57.1–63.2)	25.5 (24.2–27.0)	2.36 (2.19–2.54)	2.27 (2.11–2.45)
Moderate SVI	57.9 (55.2–60.6)	28.4 (27.0–29.8)	2.04 (1.91–2.18)	1.95 (1.82–2.08)
High SVI	53.7 (50.8–56.6)	29.0 (27.4–30.6)	1.86 (1.72–2.00)	1.80 (1.67–1.95)
Human Health Services (HHS) Region				
Region I: CT, ME, MA, NH, RI, VT	51.0 (45.9–56.2)	17.6 (15.6–19.8)	2.90 (2.48–3.40)	2.68 (2.28–3.15)
Region II: NJ, NY, PR, VI	46.4 (41.0–52.0)	20.5 (17.9–23.3)	2.27 (1.90–2.71)	2.16 (1.80–2.58)
Region III: DE, DC, MD, PA, VA, WV	56.5 (52.2–60.7)	25.2 (23.2–27.4)	2.24 (2.00–2.51)	2.16 (1.93–2.42)
Region IV: AL, FL, GA, KY, MS, NC, SC, TN	61.9 (58.3–65.3)	34.3 (32.2–36.4)	1.80 (1.66–1.96)	1.80 (1.66–1.95)
Region V: IL, IN, MI, MN, OH, WI	63.8 (59.7–67.7)	30.1 (27.9–32.3)	2.12 (1.93–2.34)	2.07 (1.88–2.28)
Region VI: AR, LA, NM, OK, TX	53.7 (49.7–57.6)	29.4 (27.4–31.5)	1.83 (1.65–2.02)	1.78 (1.61–1.97)
Region VII: IA, KS, MO, NE	63.4 (57.0–69.3)	36.9 (33.7–40.1)	1.72 (1.51–1.96)	1.67 (1.46–1.91)
Region VIII: CO, MT, ND, SD, UT, WY	69.5 (63.9–74.7)	28.2 (25.6–30.8)	2.47 (2.19–2.79)	2.26 (2.01–2.55)
Region IX: AZ, CA, HI, NV, GU	46.6 (41.2–52.1)	21.3 (18.8–24.0)	2.19 (1.85–2.60)	2.05 (1.73–2.43)
Region X: AK, ID, OR, WA	59.8 (53.3–66.1)	28.6 (25.5–31.9)	2.09 (1.79–2.44)	1.99 (1.71–2.32)
Concerned about child getting COVID-19 infection? [h]				
Not at all concerned/A little concerned	71.8 (69.9–73.5)	39.3 (38.1–40.5)	1.83 (1.76–1.90)	1.78 (1.71–1.85)
Moderately concerned/Very concerned	31.4 (28.9–34.0)	12.3 (11.4–13.3)	2.55 (2.28–2.86)	2.39 (2.13–2.69)
I think pediatric COVID-19 vaccine is safe [h]				
Not at all safe/Somewhat safe	66.8 (64.9–68.7)	48.9 (47.4–50.4)	1.37 (1.31–1.42)	1.35 (1.29–1.40)
Very safe/Completely safe	10.5 (8.0–13.6)	4.5 (3.9–5.0)	2.35 (1.75–3.15)	2.28 (1.70–3.06)
It is important to get pediatric COVID-19 vaccine to protect my child [h]				
Not at all important/A little important	84.9 (83.3–86.5)	75.1 (73.5–76.6)	1.13 (1.10–1.16)	1.13 (1.10–1.16)
Somewhat important/Very important	20.6 (18.6–22.7)	8.1 (7.5–8.7)	2.55 (2.25–2.89)	2.40 (2.11–2.73)
Family/friends have obtained pediatric COVID-19 vaccine for their children aged 5–11 years [h]				
None/Some	63.2 (61.4–65.0)	39.6 (38.4–40.7)	1.60 (1.53–1.66)	1.58 (1.52–1.65)
Many/Almost All	22.1 (18.5–26.2)	4.7 (4.1–5.5)	4.66 (3.71–5.85)	4.49 (3.53–5.71)
My health provider has given recommendation to get pediatric COVID-19 vaccine for my child				
Yes	47.2 (44.1–50.4)	14.8 (13.8–16.0)	3.19 (2.88–3.52)	2.95 (2.66–3.27)
No	60.9 (59.0–62.8)	36.0 (34.8–37.2)	1.69 (1.62–1.77)	1.68 (1.60–1.75)

Table 2. Cont.

Characteristics	Pediatric COVID-19 Vaccine Hesitancy			
	RCIs Hesitancy Group [a]	RCIs Non-Hesitancy Group [b]	Prevalence Ratio [c]	
	Weighted % (95% CI)	Weighted % (95% CI)	Unadjusted (95% CI)	Adjusted [d] (95% CI)
Child's school requires pediatric COVID-19 vaccine for in-person classes.				
Yes	15.8 (9.8–24.5)	4.0 (2.7–7.0)	3.60 (1.87–6.96)	3.28 (1.80–5.99)
No	58.6 (56.9–60.3)	29.5 (28.6–30.4)	1.99 (1.91–2.07)	1.93 (1.85–2.01)
Not in school, Home schooled	73.1 (65.0–79.9)	32.7 (27.3–38.7)	2.23 (1.82–2.74)	2.19 (1.81–2.66)
Parental regret if pediatric COVID-19 vaccine is not obtained for my child [h]				
Do not agree/Somewhat agree	63.1 (61.4–64.8)	42.7 (41.5–43.8)	1.48 (1.42–1.54)	1.48 (1.42–1.53)
Strongly agree/Very strongly agree	13.1 (9.7–17.4)	2.0 (1.6–2.5)	6.56 (4.53–9.50)	5.62 (3.81–8.29)
In the last 7 days, my child has worn a mask when going into indoor public spaces [h]				
Never/Rarely/Sometimes	73.4 (71.4–75.3)	43.0 (41.7–44.3)	1.71 (1.64–1.78)	1.68 (1.61–1.75)
Often/Always	40.4 (38.0–42.8)	16.7 (15.7–17.7)	2.42 (2.23–2.63)	2.29 (2.10–2.49)

Abbreviations: RCIs = Routine Childhood Immunizations; CI = Confidence Interval. Pediatric COVID-19 vaccine hesitancy = unvaccinated [child], definitely not getting vaccine for [child], and probably not getting vaccine for [child]. Pediatric COVID-19 vaccine hesitancy was assessed with, "Once your child is eligible, how likely are you to get a COVID-19 vaccine?" Responses were "definitely not getting vaccine", "probably not getting vaccine", "probably getting vaccine", and "definitely getting vaccine". Participants' responses were dichotomized into two categories: pediatric COVID-19 hesitancy and pediatric COVID-19 non-hesitancy. RCI hesitancy = somewhat hesitant and very hesitant. RCI hesitancy was assessed with, "How hesitant about childhood shots would you consider yourself to be?" Responses were "not at all hesitant", "not that hesitant", "somewhat hesitant", and "very hesitant". Participants' responses were dichotomized into two categories: RCIs hesitancy and RCIs non-hesitancy. [a] RCIs hesitancy group = prevalence estimates of COVID-19 vaccine hesitancy among parents with RCIs hesitancy. [b] RCIs non-hesitancy group (referent group) = prevalence estimates of COVID-19 vaccine hesitancy among parents without RCIs hesitancy. [c] Prevalence ratio = prevalence of COVID-19 vaccine hesitancy among parents with RCIs hesitancy divided by prevalence of COVID-19 vaccine hesitancy among parents without RCIs hesitancy. [d] Adjusted for child age group, child race, relationship of respondent to child, mother's educational level, MSA status, and poverty status. [e] MSA status was determined based on household reported city and county of residence and was grouped into three categories: MSA principal city = urban; MSA non-principal city = suburban; and non-MSA = rural. MSAs and principal cities were as defined by the U.S. Census Bureau at https://www.census.gov/programs-surveys/metro-micro.html, accessed on 23 April 2024. (Non-MSA areas include urban populations not located within an MSA and completely rural areas. [f] Income/Poverty level was defined based on total family income in the past calendar year, and the U.S. Census poverty thresholds for that year specified for the applicable family size and number of children <18 years. Poverty thresholds are available at https://www.census.gov/data/tables/time-series/demo/income-poverty/historical-poverty-thresholds.html, accessed on 23 April 2024. [g] The CDC/ATSDR Social Vulnerability Index was developed using 15 U.S. census variables to help officials identify communities needing support before, during, or after disasters. Categorization of NIS-CCM data into an SVI level was based on the zip code of residence reported by the respondent. Details on the SVI are available at https://www.atsdr.cdc.gov/placeandhealth/svi/index.html, accessed on 23 April 2024. [h] Response options were dichotomized into two categories. Outputs are statistically significant at $p < 0.05$ compared to the referent group. There was consistent statistical association between COVID-19 vaccine and RCIs hesitancy across all demographic and psychosocial factors for both unadjusted and adjusted prevalence ratios.

Notably, parents with *lower* levels of pediatric COVID-19 vaccine hesitancy in both RCIs hesitant and RCIs non-hesitant groups tended to have higher PR (the PR was calculated as the prevalence of pediatric COVID-19 vaccine hesitancy within the RCIs hesitant group divided by the prevalence of pediatric COVID-19 vaccine hesitancy within the RCIs non-hesitant group of parents) estimates (Table 2). For instance, among parents who expressed regret for not having their children vaccinated (unadjusted PR 6.56, CI 4.53–9.50), pediatric COVID-19 vaccine hesitancy rates were relatively low at 13.1% among RCIs hesitant groups and 2.0% among RCIs non-hesitant groups. In comparison, parents with *higher* pediatric COVID-19 vaccine hesitancy levels in both RCIs hesitant and RCIs non-hesitant groups had lower PR estimates. For example, among parents of children residing in rural areas (unadjusted PR 1.57, CI 1.46–1.70), pediatric COVID-19 vaccine hesitancy rates were relatively high at 68.3% and 43.5% for RCIs hesitant and RCIs non-hesitant groups (Table 2). These findings were consistent for both unadjusted and adjusted analyses. Other socio-demographic indicators that indicated low levels of PR estimates but high levels of pediatric COVID-19 vaccine hesitancy included parents of children aged 5–11 years living below the poverty level (adjusted PR 1.48, CI 1.30–1.69) and those who believed that COVID-19 vaccines were unsafe (adjusted PR 1.35, CI 1.29–1.40) and unimportant (adjusted PR 1.13, CI 1.10–1.16).

3.5. Temporal Trends in RCIs Hesitancy by Sociodemographic Characteristics and Behavioral and Social Drivers

Table 3 represents the results of the weighted linear regression models. Over the 9-month period, no linear trends were apparent for RCIs hesitancy for most of the demographic, behavioral, and social characteristics examined. However, parental hesitancy towards RCIs decreased by 1.2 percentage points per month over the 9-month study period among children who never, rarely, or sometimes wore masks in the past 7 days. Also, parental RCIs hesitancy increased by 0.6 percentage points per month over the 9-month study period among children whose parents had received a recommendation for their child's COVID-19 vaccination from a healthcare provider.

Table 3. Trends in parental hesitancy towards routine childhood immunizations by sociodemographic characteristics and behavioral and social drivers of COVID-19 vaccination as reported by parents of children ages 5–11 years (weighted linear regression analysis), November 2021–July 2022, National Immunization Survey—Child COVID Module.

Characteristics	Average Monthly Percentage Point Change in RCIs Hesitancy (95% CI)	p Value
Total	0.1 (−0.4–0.7)	0.60
Child's Age (years)		
5–6	−0.3 (−1.1–0.6)	0.51
7–9	0.4 (−0.2–1.0)	0.19
10–11	0.1 (−0.3–0.5)	0.55
Child's Race/Ethnicity		
Hispanic	0.1 (−0.3–0.5)	0.75
White, non-Hispanic	−0.1 (−0.9–0.8)	0.87
Black, non-Hispanic	0.7 (−0.1–1.4)	0.08
Asian, non-Hispanic	1.1 (−0.3–2.5)	0.10
Other/Multiple	−0.1 (−1.1–0.9)	0.78
Relationship of Respondent to Child		
Mother	0.3 (−0.2–0.8)	0.22
Father	−0.2 (−0.8–0.5)	0.55
Other	0.0 (−1.1–1.2)	0.95
Mother's Educational Level		
<High school	0.7 (−0.3–1.6)	0.13
High school or equivalent	0.3 (−0.6–1.2)	0.43
Some college/vocational	−0.3 (−0.9–0.4)	0.41
≥College degree	0.2 (−0.4–0.7)	0.54

Table 3. Cont.

Characteristics	Average Monthly Percentage Point Change in RCIs Hesitancy (95% CI)	p Value
Urban–Rural Residence (Metropolitan Statistical Area (MSA) Status) [a]		
Urban (MSA, principal city)	0.2 (−0.2–0.6)	0.36
Suburban (MSA, non-principal city)	0.1 (−0.5–0.7)	0.72
Rural (non-MSA)	0.2 (−0.9–1.2)	0.71
Poverty Status [b]		
>Poverty, ≥$75,000/year	0.1 (−0.5–0.6)	0.81
>Poverty, <$75,000/year	−0.2 (−1.1–0.6)	0.55
Below poverty level	0.5 (−0.5–1.4)	0.28
Income not reported	0.4 (−0.2–1.0)	0.18
Number of Children Under 18 in Household		
1 child	−0.1 (−0.8–0.6)	0.71
2–3 children	0.1 (−0.5–0.7)	0.62
≥4 children	0.6 (−0.3–1.6)	0.14
Social Vulnerability Index (SVI) of County of Residence [c]		
Low SVI	−0.1 (−0.9–0.7)	0.80
Moderate SVI	−0.2 (−1.2–0.8)	0.64
High SVI	0.3 (−0.4–0.9)	0.36
Human Health Services (HHS) Region		
Region I: CT, ME, MA, NH, RI, VT	−2.0 (−0.8–0.4)	0.42
Region II: NJ, NY, PR, VI	−0.1 (−0.8–0.5)	0.66
Region III: DE, DC, MD, PA, VA, WV	−0.2 (−1.1–0.6)	0.55
Region IV: AL, FL, GA, KY, MS, NC, SC, TN	0.0 (−0.9–0.8)	0.91
Region V: IL, IN, MI, MN, OH, WI	0.4 (0.0–0.9)	0.06
Region VI: AR, LA, NM, OK, TX	−0.1 (−1.0–0.8)	0.78
Region VII: IA, KS, MO, NE	0.4 (−0.9–1.6)	0.53
Region VIII: CO, MT, ND, SD, UT, WY	0.4 (−0.5–1.4)	0.29
Region IX: AZ, CA, HI, NV, GU	0.5 (−0.6–1.7)	0.28
Region X: AK, ID, OR, WA	0.2 (−1.0–1.3)	0.74
Concerned about child getting COVID-19 infection? [d]		
Not at all concerned/A little concerned	−1.0 (−0.9–0.6)	0.67
Moderately concerned/Very concerned	0.2 (−0.4–0.8)	0.52
I think pediatric COVID-19 vaccine is safe [d]		
Not at all safe/Somewhat safe	−0.2 (−1.1–0.8)	0.66
Very safe/Completely safe	0.3 (−0.1–0.6)	0.16
It is important to get pediatric COVID-19 vaccine to protect my child [d]		
Not at all important/A little important	−0.8 (−2.1–0.5)	0.18
Somewhat important/Very important	0.0 (−0.4–0.4)	0.86

Table 3. Cont.

Characteristics	Average Monthly Percentage Point Change in RCIs Hesitancy (95% CI)	p Value
Family/friends have obtained pediatric COVID-19 vaccine for their children aged 5–11 years [d]		
None/Some	0.2 (−0.7–1.2)	0.58
Many/Almost All	0.5 (0.0–0.9)	0.04 *
My health provider has given recommendation to get pediatric COVID-19 vaccine for my child		
Yes	0.6 (0.1–1.1)	0.02 *
No	0.0 (−0.9–0.9)	0.96
Child's school requires pediatric COVID-19 vaccine for in-person classes.		
Yes	−0.2 (−1.8–1.3)	0.73
No	0.1 (−0.5–0.6)	0.72
Not in school, Home schooled	2.1 (−0.9–5.2)	0.14
Parental regret if pediatric COVID-19 vaccine is not obtained for my child [d]		
Do not agree/Somewhat agree	−0.1 (−0.9–0.7)	0.70
Strongly agree/Very strongly agree	0.1 (−0.3–0.6)	0.44
In the last 7 days, my child has worn a mask when going into indoor public spaces [d]		
Never/Rarely/Sometimes	−1.2 (−1.8–0.5)	0.00 *
Often/Always	0.3 (0.0–0.7)	0.05 *

Abbreviations: CI = Confidence Interval. Pediatric COVID-19 vaccine hesitancy = unvaccinated [child], definitely not getting vaccine for [child], and probably not getting vaccine for [child]. Pediatric COVID-19 vaccine hesitancy was assessed with, "Once your child is eligible, how likely are you to get a COVID-19 vaccine?" Responses were "definitely not getting vaccine", "probably not getting vaccine", "probably getting vaccine", and "definitely getting vaccine". Participants' responses were dichotomized into two categories: pediatric COVID-19 hesitancy and pediatric COVID-19 non-hesitancy. RCIs hesitancy = somewhat hesitant and very hesitant. RCIs hesitancy was assessed with, "How hesitant about childhood shots would you consider yourself to be?" Responses were "not at all hesitant", "not that hesitant", "somewhat hesitant", and "very hesitant". Participants' responses were dichotomized into two categories: RCIs hesitancy and RCIs non-hesitancy. [a] MSA status was determined based on household reported city and county of residence and was grouped into three categories: MSA principal city = urban; MSA non-principal city = suburban; and non-MSA = rural. MSAs and principal cities were as defined by the U.S. Census Bureau at https://www.census.gov/programs-surveys/metro-micro.html, accessed on 23 April 2024. Non-MSA areas include urban populations not located within an MSA and completely rural areas. [b] Income/Poverty level was defined based on total family income in the past calendar year, and the U.S. Census poverty thresholds for that year specified for the applicable family size and number of children <18 years. Poverty thresholds are available at https://www.census.gov/data/tables/time-series/demo/income-poverty/historical-poverty-thresholds.html, accessed on 23 April 2024. [c] The CDC/ATSDR Social Vulnerability Index was developed using 15 U.S. census variables to help officials identify communities needing support before, during, or after disasters. Categorization of NIS-CCM data into an SVI level was based on the zip code of residence reported by the respondent. Details on the SVI are available at https://www.atsdr.cdc.gov/placeandhealth/svi/index.html, accessed on 23 April 2024. [d] Response options were dichotomized into two categories. * Statistically significant at $p < 0.05$ compared to the referent group.

4. Discussion

Our study investigated trends in parental hesitancy towards pediatric COVID-19 vaccines and RCIs over 9 months and examined the relationship between pediatric COVID-19 vaccine hesitancy and RCIs hesitancy. From November 2021 to July 2022, we observed a 15.8 percentage point increase in the proportion of parents who expressed they were "definitely not getting" or "probably not getting" their children vaccinated against COVID-19. This increase in parental hesitancy for pediatric COVID-19 vaccines may be linked to the rapid development and fast-tracked approval process of pediatric COVID-19 vaccines [23].

Moreover, parents' socio-behavioral characteristics, including perceptions that pediatric COVID-19 vaccines were unsafe and unimportant, likely contributed to the increased hesitancy for pediatric COVID-19 vaccines. For instance, some parents' reluctance to vaccinate their children may have been due to rare cases of vaccine-associated adverse events (i.e., myocarditis and pericarditis) following pediatric COVID-19 vaccine administration among adolescents [31]. In addition, some parents believed their children were at a low risk of getting infected, while others reported a lack of family and social support for COVID-19 vaccinations. At the same time, some parents expressed a lack of regret for failing to get their children vaccinated against COVID-19. During the early pandemic, parents' psychosocial characteristics may have been influenced by vaccine misinformation and misconceptions [32]. On the other hand, studies have shown that beliefs in vaccine safety and effectiveness increased vaccine uptake [33]. Our analysis suggests that parents who perceived vaccines as safe, effective, and important and reported positive family/social influences were more likely to accept pediatric COVID-19 vaccines and RCIs. Our research findings align with other observational studies that indicate parents' beliefs, risk perceptions, regret, and personal/family experiences regarding vaccines and infectious diseases significantly influence vaccination behavior [30,34].

Between November 2021 and May 2022, following the introduction of pediatric COVID-19 vaccines, there was a temporary increase in the percentage of parents who expressed they were "very hesitant" or "somewhat hesitant" towards RCIs. This trend plateaued and subsequently declined. Although vaccination is widely recognized as a significant achievement in public health, the recent (i.e., 2020–2022) scientific literature supports this transient upward trend in parental reluctance to consent to some routine childhood vaccines [8,35]. The transient rise in parental hesitancy towards RCIs following the introduction of pediatric COVID-19 vaccines may have been caused by the spike in vaccine misinformation and politicized debates about COVID-19 vaccines [23]. False information that claimed that COVID-19 vaccines could adversely impact female fertility and alter human DNA was widely disseminated but later debunked [36]. Parental hesitancy towards pediatric COVID-19 vaccines, conflicting health information and misinformation, cultural and political factors, and parents' fears/concerns may have influenced this transient rise in parental hesitancy towards RCIs. During this period, no linear trends were evident for RCIs hesitancy for most demographic, behavioral, and social characteristics examined. However, RCIs hesitancy increased among children whose parents had received a recommendation for their child's COVID-19 vaccination from a healthcare provider and decreased among children who never/rarely/sometimes wore masks. It is uncertain why these correlations occurred. However, multiple factors, such as parents' adherence to provider recommendations, school policies on mask usage, and children's compliance with putting on masks, could have influenced these variables. For instance, while some states had policies about mask usage in schools, other states had none in place.

Previous studies have shown that parents' decision-making regarding pediatric uptake for COVID-19 and other childhood vaccines is influenced by socio-demographic indicators [27,37–39]. This scientific evidence is also supported by our study, which found that mothers with a high school education were more likely to be hesitant to vaccinate their children against COVID-19 compared to mothers with a college degree. Parents of children residing in rural areas expressed a higher degree of COVID-19 vaccine hesitancy than parents in urban areas. Furthermore, pediatric COVID-19 vaccine hesitancy was most prevalent among parents of children who were White (43.2%) compared to Black (29.3%) or Hispanic (26.9%). In comparison, RCIs hesitancy was most prevalent among parents of children who were Black (32.0%) compared to Hispanic (24.5%) or White (23.6%). Although RCIs hesitancy was most prevalent among parents of children who were Black, this group was likely more receptive to vaccinating their children against COVID-19 compared to parents of children who were White. This outcome could partly be due to the disproportionately higher COVID-19-related hospitalizations and mortality rates among Black persons during the early stages of the pandemic [40,41]. The African American community has also reported a higher risk perception of COVID-19 infections compared to other racial and ethnic groups [8]. However, historical mistreatment, health disparities [40,42], and the mistrust of healthcare systems may have negatively impacted the uptake of RCIs among African American communities, as shown by their prevalence of RCIs hesitancy, which was higher than the other racial groups in this study.

Additionally, our study found a positive correlation between parental hesitancy towards pediatric COVID-19 vaccines and parental hesitancy towards RCIs across all demographic and psychosocial characteristics examined. This correlation (as depicted by PR estimates) between hesitancy for pediatric COVID-19 vaccines and RCIs tended to be stronger for parent groups with a lower prevalence of COVID-19 vaccine hesitancy among RCIs hesitant and non-hesitant groups, e.g., parents of children who were Asian. On the other hand, the correlation was weaker for groups with a higher prevalence of COVID-19 vaccine hesitancy among RCIs hesitant and non-hesitant groups, e.g., parents of children residing in rural areas. Weaker correlations, a lower PR, and higher COVID-19 vaccine hesitancy may reflect that certain parent groups are more likely to have specific, unique concerns about pediatric COVID-19 vaccines.

This study has several limitations. This cross-sectional study presents a "snapshot" over a 9-month study period of the prevalence of pediatric vaccine hesitancy. Despite this, our findings are consistent with a similar longitudinal study that found a significant increase in the percentage of U.S. parents who believed that childhood vaccines had harmful side effects and may lead to illness or death. Notably, this study was conducted between April 2020 and March 2022, which aligns with our study timeframe (i.e., November 2021–May 2022) [43]. Moreover, our study could not infer cause and effect relationships (i.e., the relative contribution of causality that could indicate that COVID-19 vaccine hesitancy caused RCIs hesitancy). The NIS-CCM relies on parents to report their children's COVID-19 vaccination status) and does not obtain information from health providers to verify children's COVID-19 vaccination coverage. As a result, data may be subject to recall bias and social desirability bias. Additionally, there may be some bias in the data estimates after weighting due to the relatively low response rate (20.4%), which is similar to other NIS surveys. However, survey weights are calibrated based on the COVID-19 vaccine administration data reported to the CDC by jurisdictions, which minimizes potential bias from non-response, incomplete sampling frame (i.e., exclusion of households with no phone service), and misclassification of vaccination coverage estimates due to poor/incomplete parents' recollection. It is important to note that we lacked information on how parents interpreted the RCIs hesitancy question within the context of newly available pediatric COVID-19 vaccines. It is possible that some parents considered the pediatric COVID-19 vaccine as an RCI, which may have contributed to the initial increase in RCIs hesitancy. Also, some parents who were not previously hesitant about RCIs may have reported hesitancy solely due to their concerns about pediatric COVID-19 vaccines. The RCIs hesitancy question was modified in October 2022 to address this issue and expanded into three questions for this age group—hesitancy toward the COVID-19 vaccine, hesitancy toward the influenza vaccine, and hesitancy toward other RCIs. Despite these limitations, this study is of significant public health importance given its assessment of period prevalence, trends, and its depiction of the correlation between parental hesitancy towards COVID-19 vaccines and RCIs using nationally representative data.

Pediatric vaccine hesitancy, along with pandemic disruptions, misinformation, access barriers, politicized debates, and negative perceptions about vaccines, can significantly and adversely impact trusted routine childhood vaccines and new vaccines such as COVID-19 vaccines [23]. Future research is necessary to investigate possible incremental trends in parental hesitancy among different sociodemographic subgroups and examine potentially lower vaccination coverage among children in other age groups, specifically those between 19 and 35 months [44]. Moreover, conducting more in-depth studies to evaluate the impact of introducing new vaccines on parental RCIs hesitancy is essential. As previous pandemics and mass vaccination programs have demonstrated, robust planning and implementation are needed to promote vaccine confidence and ensure public acceptance of vaccines.

Author Contributions: O.A.O.: conceptualization (lead), methodology, resources, writing—original draft preparation (lead), visualization, and writing—review and editing; N.B.M.: conceptualization (lead), methodology, resources, and writing—review and editing; F.Z.: conceptualization, methodology, resources, data curation, formal analysis (lead), and writing—review and editing; D.E.S.: conceptualization, methodology, resources (lead), supervision, and writing—review and editing; R.J.C.: conceptualization, resources, writing—review and editing; D.W.: conceptualization, resources, and writing—review and editing; J.A.S.: conceptualization, methodology, resources, supervision (lead), and writing—review and editing. All authors have read and agreed to the published version of the manuscript.

Funding: This research received no external funding.

Institutional Review Board Statement: This study was conducted in compliance with the applicable federal laws and CDC policies.

Informed Consent Statement: Informed consent was obtained from the person (generally the child's parent or guardian) in the household who was most knowledgeable about the child's vaccination history.

Data Availability Statement: The NIS-CCM data can be accessed at the NCHS Research Data Center following an approval process.

Acknowledgments: We express our gratitude to Yi Mu for their assistance in analyzing and interpreting the NOS-CCM data.

Conflicts of Interest: The authors declare no conflicts of interest.

References

1. Rémy, V.; Zöllner, Y.; Heckmann, U. Vaccination: The cornerstone of an efficient healthcare system. *J. Mark. Access Health Policy* **2015**, *3*, 27041. [CrossRef]
2. Centers for Disease Control and Prevention. Immunization Schedule. 2021. Available online: https://www.cdc.gov/vaccines/schedules/hcp/imz/child-adolescent.html (accessed on 23 April 2024).
3. U.S. Food and Drug Administration. FDA Authorizes Pfizer-BioNTech COVID-19 Vaccine for Emergency Use in Children 5 through 11 Years of Age. Available online: https://www.fda.gov/news-events/press-announcements/fda-authorizes-pfizer-biontech-covid-19-vaccine-emergency-use-children-5-through-11-years-age (accessed on 23 April 2024).
4. Centers for Disease Control and Prevention. Vaccine and Immunizations. 2022. Available online: https://www.cdc.gov/vaccines/index.html (accessed on 23 April 2024).
5. Ackerson, B.K.; Sy, L.S.; Glenn, S.C.; Qian, L.; Park, C.H.; Riewerts, R.J.; Jacobsen, S.J. Pediatric Vaccination During the COVID-19 Pandemic. *Pediatrics* **2021**, *148*, e2020047092. [CrossRef] [PubMed]
6. Bramer, C.A.; Kimmins, L.M.; Swanson, R.; Kuo, J.; Vranesich, P.; Jacques-Carroll, L.A.; Shen, A.K. Decline in child vaccination coverage during the COVID-19 pandemic—Michigan Care Improvement Registry, May 2016–May 2020. *Am. J. Transplant.* **2020**, *20*, 1930. [CrossRef]
7. Santoli, J.M. Effects of the COVID-19 pandemic on routine pediatric vaccine ordering and administration—United States, 2020. *Morb. Mortal. Wkly. Rep.* **2020**, *69*, 591–593. [CrossRef] [PubMed]
8. He, K.; Mack, W.J.; Neely, M.; Lewis, L.; Anand, V. Parental perspectives on immunizations: Impact of the COVID-19 pandemic on childhood vaccine hesitancy. *J. Community Health* **2021**, *23*, 39–52. [CrossRef]
9. World Health Organization. *WHO and UNICEF Warn of a Decline in Vaccinations during COVID-19*; World Health Organization: Geneva, Switzerland, 2020. Available online: https://www.who.int/news/item/15-07-2020-who-and-unicef-warn-of-a-decline-in-vaccinations-during-covid-19 (accessed on 23 April 2024).
10. World Health Organization. *COVID-19 Pandemic Fuels Largest Continued Backslide in Vaccinations in Three Decades*; World Health Organization: Geneva, Switzerland, 2022. Available online: https://www.who.int/news/item/15-07-2022-covid-19-pandemic-fuels-largest-continued-backslide-in-vaccinations-in-three-decades (accessed on 23 April 2024).
11. DeSilva, M.B.; Haapala, J.; Vazquez-Benitez, G.; Daley, M.F.; Nordin, J.D.; Klein, N.P.; Henninger, M.L.; Williams, J.T.B.; Hambidge, S.J.; Jackson, M.L.; et al. Association of the COVID-19 pandemic with routine childhood vaccination rates and proportion up to date with vaccinations across 8 us health systems in the vaccine safety datalink. *JAMA Pediatr.* **2021**, *176*, 68–77. [CrossRef]
12. Murthy, B.P.; Zell, E.; Kirtland, K.; Jones-Jack, N.; Harris, L.; Sprague, C.; Schultz, J.; Le, Q.; Bramer, C.A.; Kuramoto, S.; et al. Impact of the COVID-19 Pandemic on Administration of Selected Routine Childhood and Adolescent Vaccinations—10 US Jurisdictions, March–September 2020. *Morb. Mortal. Wkly. Rep.* **2021**, *70*, 840. [CrossRef] [PubMed]

13. Williams, J.T.; Rice, J.D.; Lou, Y.; Bayliss, E.A.; Federico, S.G.; Hambidge, S.J.; O'Leary, S.T. Parental vaccine hesitancy and vaccination disparities in a safety-net system. *Pediatrics* **2021**, *147*, e2020010710. [CrossRef]
14. Olusanya, O.A.; Bednarczyk, R.A.; Davis, R.L.; Shaban-Nejad, A. Addressing parental vaccine hesitancy and other barriers to childhood/adolescent vaccination uptake during the coronavirus (COVID-19) pandemic. *Front. Immunol.* **2021**, *12*, 663074. [CrossRef]
15. Seither, R. Vaccination Coverage with Selected Vaccines and Exemption Rates Among Children in Kindergarten—United States, 2020–2021 School Year. *Morb. Mortal. Wkly. Rep.* **2022**, *71*, 561–568. [CrossRef]
16. World Health Organization. Vaccine Hesitancy: A Growing Challenge for Immunization Programmes. 2015. Available online: https://www.who.int/news/item/18-08-2015-vaccine-hesitancy-a-growing-challenge-for-immunization-programmes (accessed on 23 April 2024).
17. World Health Organization. Ten Threats to Global Health in 2019. 2022. Available online: https://www.who.int/news-room/spotlight/ten-threats-to-global-health-in-2019 (accessed on 23 April 2024).
18. Agiesta, J. CNN Poll: About a Quarter of Adults Say They Won't Try to Get a COVID-19 Vaccine. CNN Politics. 2021. Available online: https://www.cnn.com/2021/04/29/politics/cnn-poll-covid-vaccines/index.html (accessed on 23 April 2024).
19. Brumfiel, G. 1 in 4 Americans Don't Want a Vaccine, Putting Herd Immunity at Risk. NPR. 2021. Available online: https://www.npr.org/sections/health-shots/2021/04/07/984697573/vaccine-refusal-may-put-herd-immunity-at-risk-researchers-warn (accessed on 16 April 2023).
20. Saad, L.U.S. Readiness to Get COVID-19 Vaccine Steadies at 65%. Gallup. 2021. Available online: https://news.gallup.com/poll/328415/readiness-covid-vaccine-steadies.aspx (accessed on 23 April 2024).
21. Cascini, F.; Pantovic, A.; Al-Ajlouni, Y.; Failla, G.; Ricciardi, W. Attitudes, acceptance and hesitancy among the general population worldwide to receive the COVID-19 vaccines and their contributing factors: A systematic review. *EClinicalMedicine* **2021**, *40*, 101113. [CrossRef] [PubMed]
22. Johnson, N.F.; Velásquez, N.; Restrepo, N.J.; Leahy, R.; Gabriel, N.; El Oud, S.; Zheng, M.; Manrique, P.; Wuchty, S.; Lupu, Y. The online competition between pro-and anti-vaccination views. *Nature* **2020**, *582*, 230–233. [CrossRef] [PubMed]
23. Larson, H.J.; Gakidou, E.; Murray, C.J. The vaccine-hesitant moment. *N. Engl. J. Med.* **2022**, *387*, 58–65. [CrossRef] [PubMed]
24. Al-Amer, R.; Maneze, D.; Everett, B.; Montayre, J.; Villarosa, A.R.; Dwekat, E.; Salamonson, Y. COVID-19 vaccination intention in the first year of the pandemic: A systematic review. *J. Clin. Nurs.* **2022**, *31*, 62–86. [CrossRef] [PubMed]
25. Centers for Disease Control and Prevention. National Immunization Survey. 2018. Available online: https://www.cdc.gov/vaccines/imz-managers/nis/about.html (accessed on 23 April 2024).
26. Centers for Disease Control and Prevention. For Immunization Mangers. 2021. Available online: https://www.cdc.gov/vaccines/imz-managers/coverage/covidvaxview/index.html (accessed on 23 April 2024).
27. Santibanez, T.A.; Lendon, J.P.; Singleton, J.A.; Black, C.L.; Zhou, T.; Kriss, J.L.; Jain, A.; Elam-Evans, L.D.; Masters, N.B.; Peacock, G. Factors Associated with Receipt and Parental Intent for COVID-19 Vaccination of Children Ages 5–11 years. *medRxiv* **2022**. [CrossRef]
28. Centers for Disease Control and Prevention. National Immunization Survey Child COVID Module (NIS-CCM): Vaccination Status and Intent by Demographics I Data I Centers for Disease Control and Prevention (cdc.gov) I Data I Centers for Disease Control and Prevention. 2022. Available online: https://data.cdc.gov/Vaccinations/National-Immunization-Survey-Child-COVID-Module-NI/gr26-95h2/about_data (accessed on 23 April 2024).
29. Vital and Health Statistics: Statistical Methodology of the National Immunization Survey, 2005–2014. December 11. Available online: https://www.cdc.gov/nchs/data/series/sr_01/sr01_061.pdf (accessed on 23 April 2024).
30. Brewer, N.T. What works to increase vaccination uptake. *Acad. Pediatr.* **2021**, *21*, S9–S16. [CrossRef] [PubMed]
31. Centers for Disease Control and Prevention. Vaccines & Immunizations: Clinical Considerations: Myocarditis and Pericarditis after Receipt of COVID-19 Vaccines among Adolescents and Young Adults. 2023. Available online: https://www.cdc.gov/vaccines/covid-19/clinical-considerations/myocarditis.html (accessed on 23 April 2024).
32. Kalichman, S.C.; Eaton, L.A.; Earnshaw, V.A.; Brousseau, N. Faster than warp speed: Early attention to COVID-19 by anti-vaccine groups on Facebook. *J. Public Health* **2022**, *44*, e96–e105. [CrossRef]
33. Wan, X.; Huang, H.; Shang, J.; Xie, Z.; Jia, R.; Lu, G.; Chen, C. Willingness and influential factors of parents of 3–6-year-old children to vaccinate their children with the COVID-19 vaccine in China. *Hum. Vaccines Immunother.* **2021**, *17*, 3969–3974. [CrossRef] [PubMed]
34. Brewer, N.T.; DeFrank, J.T.; Gilkey, M.B. Anticipated regret and health behavior: A meta-analysis. *Health Psychol.* **2016**, *35*, 1264. [CrossRef]
35. Olson, O.; Berry, C.; Kumar, N. Addressing parental vaccine hesitancy towards childhood vaccines in the United States: A systematic literature review of communication interventions and strategies. *Vaccines* **2020**, *8*, 590. [CrossRef]
36. Kassianos, G.; Puig-Barberà, J.; Dinse, H.; Teufel, M.; Türeci, Ö.; Pather, S. Addressing COVID-19 vaccine hesitancy. *Drugs Context* **2022**, *11*, 2021-12-3. [CrossRef] [PubMed]
37. Rhodes, M.E.; Sundstrom, B.; Ritter, E.; McKeever, B.W.; McKeever, R. Preparing for a COVID-19 vaccine: A mixed methods study of vaccine-hesitant parents. *J. Health Commun.* **2020**, *25*, 831–837. [CrossRef] [PubMed]

38. Brownstein, N.C.; Reddy, H.; Whiting, J.; Kasting, M.L.; Head, K.J.; Vadaparampil, S.T.; Giuliano, A.R.; Gwede, C.K.; Meade, C.D.; Christy, S.M. COVID-19 vaccine behaviors and intentions among a national sample of United States adults ages 18–45. *Prev. Med.* **2022**, *160*, 107038. [CrossRef] [PubMed]
39. Cousin, L.; Roberts, S.; Brownstein, N.C.; Whiting, J.; Kasting, M.L.; Head, K.J.; Vadaparampil, S.T.; Giuliano, A.R.; Gwede, C.K.; Meade, C.D.; et al. Factors associated with parental COVID-19 vaccine attitudes and intentions among a national sample of United States adults ages 18–45. *J. Pediatr. Nurs.* **2023**, *69*, 108–115. [CrossRef] [PubMed]
40. Yancy, C.W. COVID-19 and african americans. *JAMA* **2020**, *323*, 1891–1892. [CrossRef] [PubMed]
41. Brakefield, W.S.; Olusanya, O.A.; White, B.; Shaban-Nejad, A. Social Determinants and Indicators of COVID-19 among Marginalized Communities: A Scientific Review and Call to Action for Pandemic Response and Recovery. *Disaster Med. Public Health Prep.* **2022**, *17*, 1–28. [CrossRef] [PubMed]
42. Kolar, S.K.; Wheldon, C.; Hernandez, N.D.; Young, L.; Romero-Daza, N.; Daley, E.M. Human papillomavirus vaccine knowledge and attitudes, preventative health behaviors, and medical mistrust among a racially and ethnically diverse sample of college women. *J. Racial Ethn. Health Disparities* **2015**, *2*, 77–85. [CrossRef]
43. Shah, M.D.; Szilagyi, P.G.; Shetgiri, R.; Delgado, J.R.; Vangala, S.; Thomas, K.; Dudovitz, R.N.; Vizueta, N.; Darling, J.; Kapteyn, A. Trends in Parents' Confidence in Childhood Vaccines During the COVID-19 Pandemic. *Pediatrics* **2022**, *150*, e2022057855. [CrossRef] [PubMed] [PubMed Central]
44. Pingali, C. National Vaccination Coverage Among Adolescents Aged 13–17 Years—National Immunization Survey-Teen, United States, 2021. *Morb. Mortal. Wkly. Rep.* **2022**, *71*, 1101–1108. Available online: https://www.cdc.gov/mmwr/volumes/71/wr/mm7135a1.htm (accessed on 23 April 2024). [CrossRef]

Disclaimer/Publisher's Note: The statements, opinions and data contained in all publications are solely those of the individual author(s) and contributor(s) and not of MDPI and/or the editor(s). MDPI and/or the editor(s) disclaim responsibility for any injury to people or property resulting from any ideas, methods, instructions or products referred to in the content.

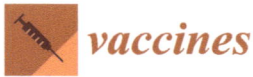

Article

Factors Associated with Uptake of Routine Measles-Containing Vaccine Doses among Young Children, Oromia Regional State, Ethiopia, 2021

Abyot Bekele Woyessa [1,2,*], Monica P. Shah [3], Binyam Moges Azmeraye [4], Jeff Pan [5], Leuel Lisanwork [4], Getnet Yimer [4], Shu-Hua Wang [5], J. Pekka Nuorti [2], Miia Artama [2], Almea M. Matanock [3,6], Qian An [3], Paulos Samuel [1], Bekana Tolera [1], Birhanu Kenate [1], Abebe Bekele [1], Tesfaye Deti [1], Getachew Wako [7], Amsalu Shiferaw [7], Yohannes Lakew Tefera [8], Melkamu Ayalew Kokebie [8], Tatek Bogale Anbessie [9], Habtamu Teklie Wubie [10], Aaron Wallace [3] and Ciara E. Sugerman [3]

1. Oromia Regional Health Bureau, Addis Ababa P.O. Box 24341, Ethiopia; muletagalmesa@gmail.com (T.D.)
2. Health Sciences Unit, Faculty of Social Sciences, Tampere University, 33100 Tampere, Finland
3. Global Immunization Division, Centers for Disease Control and Prevention, Atlanta, GA 30329, USA; hyy9@cdc.gov (M.P.S.); bwf1@cdc.gov (C.E.S.)
4. Global One Health Initiative, Ohio State University, Addis Ababa P.O. Box 1176, Ethiopia
5. College of Medicine, Ohio State University, Columbus, OH 43210, USA
6. Global Immunization Division, CDC-Ethiopia, Addis Ababa P.O. Box 3243, Ethiopia
7. UNICEF, Addis Ababa P.O. Box 1169, Ethiopia
8. Ministry of Health of Ethiopia, Addis Ababa P.O. Box 1234, Ethiopia
9. African Field Epidemiology Network, Addis Ababa P.O. Box 12874, Ethiopia
10. Ethiopian Public Health Institute, Addis Ababa P.O. Box 1242, Ethiopia
* Correspondence: abyot.woyessa@tuni.fi; Tel.: +251-954690454

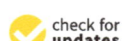

Citation: Woyessa, A.B.; Shah, M.P.; Azmeraye, B.M.; Pan, J.; Lisanwork, L.; Yimer, G.; Wang, S.-H.; Nuorti, J.P.; Artama, M.; Matanock, A.M.; et al. Factors Associated with Uptake of Routine Measles-Containing Vaccine Doses among Young Children, Oromia Regional State, Ethiopia, 2021. Vaccines 2024, 12, 762. https://doi.org/10.3390/vaccines12070762

Academic Editor: Pedro Plans-Rubió

Received: 26 April 2024
Revised: 4 July 2024
Accepted: 10 July 2024
Published: 11 July 2024

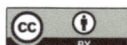

Copyright: © 2024 by the authors. Licensee MDPI, Basel, Switzerland. This article is an open access article distributed under the terms and conditions of the Creative Commons Attribution (CC BY) license (https://creativecommons.org/licenses/by/4.0/).

Abstract: Recommended vaccination at nine months of age with the measles-containing vaccine (MCV1) has been part of Ethiopia's routine immunization program since 1980. A second dose of MCV (MCV2) was introduced in 2019 for children 15 months of age. We examined MCV1 and MCV2 coverage and the factors associated with measles vaccination status. A cross-sectional household survey was conducted among caregivers of children aged 12–35 months in selected districts of Oromia Region. Measles vaccination status was determined using home-based records, when available, or caregivers' recall. We analyzed the association between MCV1 and MCV2 vaccination status and household, caregiver, and child factors using logistic regression. The caregivers of 1172 children aged 12–35 months were interviewed and included in the analysis. MCV1 and MCV2 coverage was 71% and 48%, respectively. The dropout rate (DOR) from the first dose of Pentavalent vaccine to MCV1 was 22% and from MCV1 to MCV2 was 46%. Caregivers were more likely to vaccinate their children with MCV if they gave birth at a health facility, believe that their child had received all recommended vaccines, and know the required number of vaccination visits and doses. MCV2 coverage was low, with a high measles dropout rate (DOR). Caregivers with high awareness of MCV and its schedule were more likely to vaccinate their children. Intensified demand generation, defaulter tracking, and vaccine-stock management should be strengthened to improve MCV uptake.

Keywords: measles; measles-containing vaccine; MCV1; MCV2; second year of life; immunization coverage; dropout rate; barriers; Oromia; Ethiopia

1. Introduction

The Expanded Program on Immunization (EPI) was established by the World Health Organization (WHO) in 1974 to control vaccine-preventable diseases and encourage Member States to establish the EPI in their respective health care delivery system [1,2]. Following the WHO recommendations, Ethiopia established the EPI in 1980, providing selected vaccines, including measles-containing vaccine (MCV), for free to children [3]. Vaccines are provided to children in many modalities, including through campaigns, at health posts, at health facilities, and via mobile health clinics. However, after more than four decades of implementation of the EPI, the coverage of full immunization remains very low in the country [4,5]. It is estimated that the proportion of fully vaccinated children 12-23 months old has increased from 14% in 2000 to 39% in 2016 [6,7], and to 43% in 2019, in Ethiopia [8]; however, this is below the WHO's target goal of 90% coverage for all recommended vaccines by 2030 in every country [9,10]. Despite the availability of effective vaccines, as well as national and substantial government and partner efforts, cases of vaccine-preventable diseases such as measles and polio continue to occur in the country [11]. For instance, between January 2019 and January 2020, an ongoing measles outbreak with a total of 9672 measles cases was reported to the WHO from Ethiopia, of which 5820 (60%) were from Oromia Region, where, nationally, children aged less than five years were the most affected [12]. The mortality rate among children under five years old was 55.2 per 1000 live births in 2019 in Ethiopia [13].

In 2001, Ethiopia adopted the goal of measles elimination for the African Region by the year 2020 and began implementing WHO/UNICEF strategies for accelerating the control of measles. Two of these five key strategies include routine immunization and supplemental immunization. As part of the implementation of the elimination strategies, the WHO recommended all countries to include a second routine dose of MCV (MCV2) in the national vaccination schedules, regardless of the level of MCV1 coverage [14]. In February 2019, the Federal Ministry of Health's EPI introduced MCV2 for children in the second year of life (at 15 months of age) in Ethiopia into the routine immunization schedule to reduce measles morbidity and mortality and accelerate achieving measles elimination goals [15]. While it has been estimated that over 3.3 million children will receive a second dose of this vaccine annually, Ethiopia has experienced low coverage of the measles vaccine, with the most recent data from WHO/UNICEF estimating 56% and 48% coverage in 2022 for the first and second dose of MCV, respectively [16], and a recent mini demographic and health survey (DHS) in Ethiopia similarly estimating coverage at 59% for the first dose of MCV [8]. The drivers of Ethiopia's coverage rates are multiple, however, it has been found that maternal knowledge of immunization and vaccine-preventable diseases is a common factor influencing coverage [17–19].

The introduction of MCV2 offers not only additional protection against measles, but also provides an opportunity to catch children up on the vaccine doses missed in the first year of life and for the integration of other primary healthcare interventions during the second year of life (2YL), such as vitamin A supplementation, nutritional counseling, growth monitoring and promotion, deworming, and pediatric HIV/AIDS care [20].

Oromia Region is the most populous region in Ethiopia and has the third lowest vaccination coverage, thus contributing to a substantial number of unvaccinated children and subsequent measles outbreaks. Per the Ethiopian mini-DHS of 2019, in Oromia Region, routine immunization coverage for MCV1 was 48.7%. Thus, Oromia Region accounts for about half (~600,000) of the unvaccinated children in Ethiopia [21]. Oromia has also been experiencing frequent measles outbreaks; therefore, achieving high coverage of MCV is essential to prevent the spread of outbreaks and achieve the global measles elimination goals. We conducted this survey to examine measles coverage two years after MCV2 introduction and to identify the factors associated with, and barriers to, caretakers vaccinating their age-eligible children with the measles vaccine in select districts of Oromia Region.

2. Materials and Methods

2.1. Study Setting

This study was carried out in Oromia Region, Ethiopia (Figure 1). Oromia Region is the most populated region, with over 40 million people, or 37% of the national population. Routine immunization services in the region are provided in 8622 public health facilities, which includes 108 hospitals, 1399 health centers, and 7115 health posts. In a district, a primary health care unit consists of 4–5 health centers, and each health center has 4–5 satellite health posts.

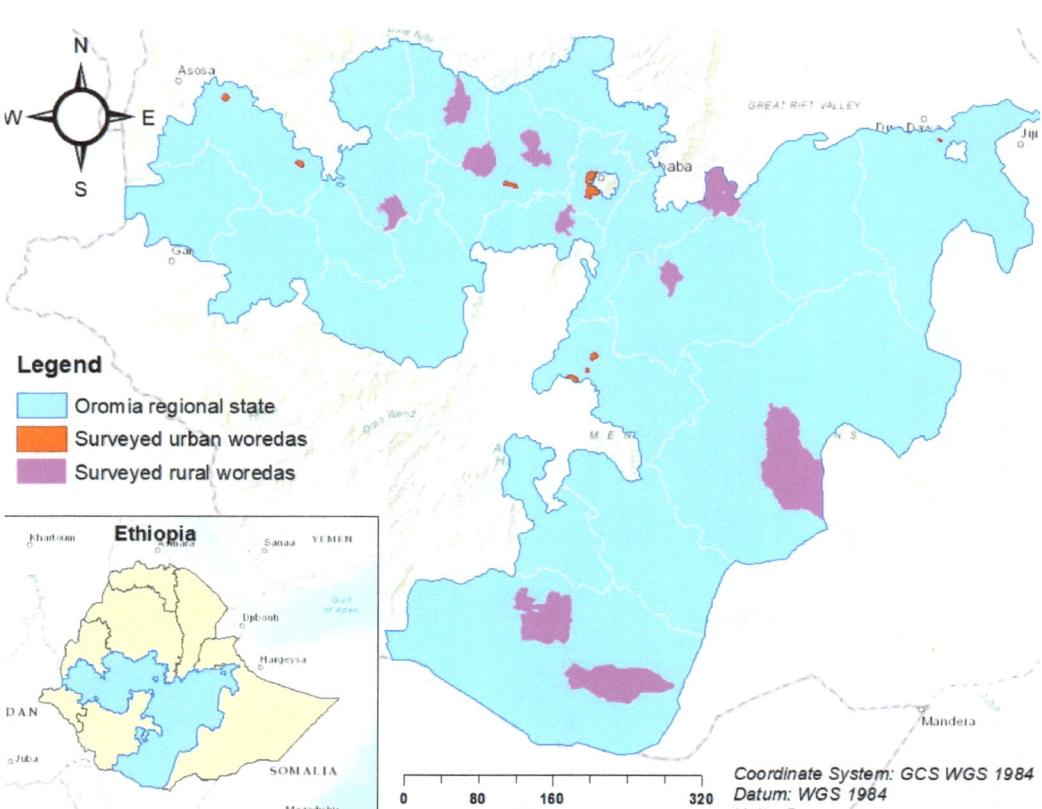

Figure 1. Map showing MCV2 barriers of study surveyed districts (woredas), Oromia region, Ethiopia.

2.2. Study Design

A cross-sectional household survey was conducted among caregivers of children aged 12–35 months from February to March 2021 in randomly selected communities in Oromia Region, Ethiopia.

2.3. Sample Size and Sample Selection

Of the 337 districts across Oromia Region, 18 districts were randomly selected to be included in the survey after an initial stratification by urban/rural settlement and the MCV1 baseline administrative coverage (high: $\geq$80%, low: <80%) and recent measles outbreak status (Figure 2). The sample size for the MCV coverage estimation was calculated using the revised WHO Vaccination Coverage Cluster Survey Reference Manual [22]. We assumed an expected measles coverage rate of 30–70%, precision of $\pm$10, intraclass correlation coefficient (ICC) of 0.333, and 10% non-response rate as the parameters to calculate stratum-specific sample size (SS), with a total of six strata (as indicated in Figure 2).

$$\begin{aligned} SS &= \text{Effective sample size [ESS]} \times (1 + ICC) \times \text{Inflation factor} \\ &= 103 \times (1 + 0.333) \times 100\%/(100\% - 10\%) \\ &= 153 \end{aligned}$$

$$\text{Total sample size (across 6 strata)} = 153 \times 6 = 918$$

To enroll the required sample size, we randomly selected two communities, known as kebeles, the lowest administrative unit in Ethiopia, which made the total selected kebeles 36 in the selected districts. Furthermore, within each selected kebele, we randomly selected one village, known as a Gere or a Gote in rural and urban areas, respectively (Figure 2). Assuming 30 interviews for each selected Gere/Gote (15 caregivers with children aged 12 to 23 months and 15 caregivers with children aged 24 to 35 months), we rounded up the minimum targeted sample size to 1080 (540 caregivers of children aged 12–23 months and 540 caregivers of children aged 24–35 months). To select households, we surveyed the first household at the center of the selected village and moved to the right of where we started until the number of caregivers with eligible children to interview was reached. If there were multiple eligible children in the selected household, the caregiver of the youngest child was surveyed.

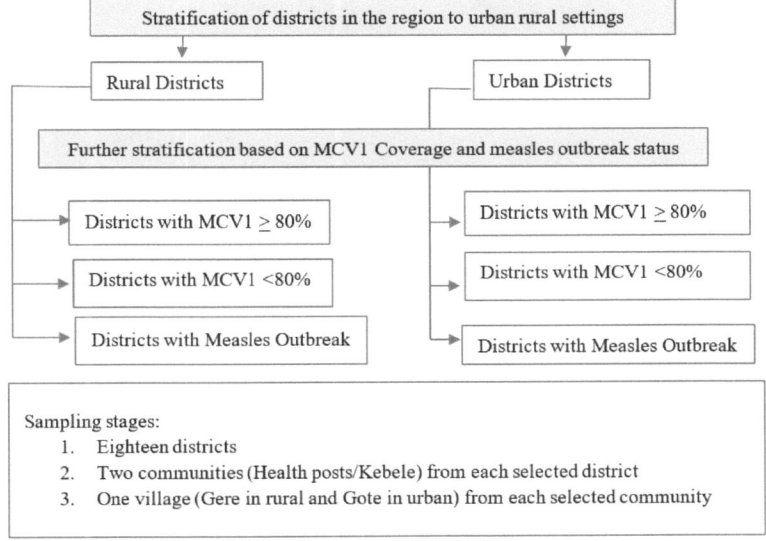

Figure 2. Sample selection flow diagram.

2.4. Data Collection

During the interviews, the caregivers were asked about their demographics and child vaccination status. The household characteristics collected included members involved with vaccine decision making for the child, distance from health facility, residing area, and number of children <5 years of age in the household. The child demographics included age at vaccination, place of birth, sex, and availability of the child's vaccination card. The caregiver demographics included age, education level, religious denomination, marital status, and their awareness, knowledge, attitudes, and practices surrounding vaccination. Child vaccination status for MCV1 and MCV2, the primary outcome of this study, was based on home-based records (HBR, vaccination card), if available, or from the caregivers' recall if absent. Questionnaires were developed and adapted from standardized questionnaires to assess the vaccination status and behavior and social drivers of vaccination. The structured questionnaires were pre-tested prior to data collection and pre-programmed for skip patterns and logic checks using Open Data Kit (ODK) software (https://getodk.org/) and administered on tablets. Experienced data collectors were recruited and trained on the study procedures, data collection tools, and interview techniques for three full days prior to fieldwork. Additionally, one trained supervisor was assigned to each team to ensure the data were collected as per the protocol and to review data quality.

2.5. Data Analysis

Descriptive analyses were stratified by settlement (urban and rural) and age group (12–23 and 24–35 months). The immunization coverage estimates were stratified by settlement and by age group (12–23 and 24–35 months). We calculated the DOR as the difference between the vaccination coverage of the initial and final doses divided by the coverage of the first dose (i.e., Penta1-Penta3 DOR: [Penta1 − Penta3] ÷ Penta1 × 100%), were DORs > 10% reflect underutilization of immunization services.

We performed bivariate regression between the explanatory and outcome variables using logistic regression among children aged 12–23 months for MCV1 and among children aged 18–35 months for MCV2, including children aged 18–23 months here to increase statistical power in the regression. We grouped continuous explanatory variables such as caregiver's age, distance to nearest health facility, and waiting time to better understand their relationship with the outcome variables. All variables with p-value < 0.15 in the bivariate regression analysis were included in the initial multivariate regression model. We used a backward selection approach for model building, and the final model included all variables with p-values < 0.05. Odds ratios (ORs) and 95% confidence intervals (CIs) were reported for all unadjusted and adjusted associations. Adjusted ORs (aOR) with 95% CI and p-values < 0.05 in the multivariate regression analysis were used as the cutoff point to determine the factors associated with MCV1 and MCV2 vaccination uptake. Data were cleaned and analyzed in R.

3. Results

3.1. Household, Caregiver, and Child Characteristics

A total of 1185 caregivers were interviewed across the 18 selected districts and 36 selected kebeles for a 97% response rate. Among those that agreed to participate, 1172 (99%) had a child within the eligible age range for this study (12–23 or 24–35 months) and were included in the analysis. With the exception of the caregivers' educational attainment, the demographic characteristics were similar for both age groups and are described together (12–35 months combined). Nearly all of the caregivers were the child's mother (96%), and many (38%) were the head of the household. The caregivers had a median age of 26 years (interquartile range (IQR), 24–30), were predominantly Christian (70%) or Muslim (27%), and spoke Afan Oromo as their primary language, with differences in spoken language in the rural areas compared to the urban areas (90% overall; 100% rural, 80% urban). Most were married (97%) and in a monogamous marriage (99%). The most frequently reported occupations among the caregivers were housewife (61%), followed by farmer (15%). About one-third of the caregivers had no formal education, and this was higher in the rural areas compared to the urban areas (32% overall; 52% rural, 11% urban). Notably, the proportion without formal education was higher among the caregivers of children aged 24–25 months in the rural areas (57.5%) compared to the caregivers of children aged 12–23 months in the rural areas (46.8%). The median number of children < 59 months of age living in the household was one (IQR, 1–2). The majority of households (94%) were within 1 to 5 km of a health facility (Table 1).

Table 1. Demographic characteristics of households, caregivers, and children surveyed in Oromia Region, Ethiopia.

Characteristic	Total	12–23			24–35		
		All Areas	Rural	Urban	All Areas	Rural	Urban
	N = 1172 n (%)	N = 598 n (%)	N = 299 n (%)	N = 299 n (%)	N = 574 n (%)	N = 287 n (%)	N = 287 n (%)
Relationship to child							
Mother	1124 (95.9)	583 (97.5)	291 (97.3)	292 (97.7)	541 (94.3)	262 (91.3)	279 (97.2)
Father	30 (2.6)	8 (1.3)	4 (1.3)	4 (1.3)	22 (3.8)	19 (6.6)	3 (1.0)
Other relative	18 (1.5)	7 (1.2)	4 (1.3)	3 (1.0)	11 (1.9)	6 (2.1)	5 (1.7)

Table 1. Cont.

Characteristic	Total	12–23			24–35		
		All Areas	Rural	Urban	All Areas	Rural	Urban
	N = 1172 n (%)	N = 598 n (%)	N = 299 n (%)	N = 299 n (%)	N = 574 n (%)	N = 287 n (%)	N = 287 n (%)
Caretaker's age in years, median, IQR	26 (24, 30)	26 (23, 30)	25 (22, 30)	26 (24, 29)	27 (25, 30)	27 (24, 30)	27 (25, 30)
Religion							
Christian	726 (69.5)	373 (69.9)	179 (66.3)	194 (73.5)	353 (69.2)	171 (66.5)	182 (71.9)
Muslim	277 (26.5)	142 (26.6)	75 (27.8)	67 (25.4)	135 (26.5)	70 (27.2)	65 (25.7)
Traditionalist	36 (3.4)	15 (2.8)	12 (4.4)	3 (1.1)	21 (4.1)	15 (5.8)	6 (2.4)
None/Atheist	5 (0.5)	4 (0.7)	4 (1.5)	0 (0.0)	1 (0.2)	1 (0.4)	0 (0.0)
Language							
Afaan Oromo	1054 (89.9)	547 (91.5)	298 (99.7)	249 (83.3)	507 (88.3)	287 (100)	220 (76.7)
Amharic	116 (9.9)	50 (8.4)	1 (0.3)	49 (16.4)	66 (11.5)	0 (0.0)	66 (23.0)
Other	2 (0.2)	1 (0.2)	0 (0.0)	1 (0.3)	1 (0.2)	0 (0.0)	1 (0.3)
Marital status							
Married	1137 (97.0)	583 (97.5)	291 (97.3)	292 (97.7)	554 (96.5)	273 (95.1)	281 (97.9)
Divorced	20 (1.7)	9 (1.5)	3 (1.0)	6 (2.0)	11 (1.9)	6 (2.1)	5 (1.7)
Single	8 (0.7)	3 (0.5)	2 (0.7)	1 (0.3)	5 (0.9)	5 (1.7)	0 (0.0)
Widowed	5 (0.4)	2 (0.3)	2 (0.7)	0 (0.0)	3 (0.5)	2 (0.7)	1 (0.3)
Co-habitation	2 (0.2)	1 (0.2)	1 (0.3)	0 (0.0)	1 (0.2)	1 (0.3)	0 (0.0)
Marriage type							
Monogamous	1145 (99.0)	583 (99.8)	298 (99.7)	285 (100)	562 (98.3)	282 (98.3)	280 (98.2)
Polygamous	11 (1.0)	1 (0.2)	1 (0.3)	0 (0.0)	10 (1.7)	5 (1.7)	5 (1.8)
Caretaker's Occupation							
Housewife	709 (60.5)	375 (62.7)	184 (61.5)	191 (63.9)	334 (58.2)	158 (55.1)	176 (61.3)
Farmer	163 (13.9)	76 (12.7)	72 (24.1)	4 (1.3)	87 (15.2)	78 (27.2)	9 (3.1)
Professional	145 (12.4)	63 (10.5)	10 (3.3)	53 (17.7)	82 (14.3)	30 (10.5)	52 (18.1)
Self-employed	113 (9.6)	55 (9.2)	19 (6.4)	36 (12.0)	58 (10.1)	13 (4.5)	45 (15.7)
Merchant	18 (1.5)	9 (1.5)	6 (2.0)	3 (1.0)	9 (1.6)	7 (2.4)	2 (0.7)
Student	10 (0.9)	8 (1.3)	3 (1.0)	5 (1.7)	2 (0.3)	0 (0.0)	2 (0.7)
Daily laborer	8 (0.7)	6 (1.0)	4 (1.3)	2 (0.7)	2 (0.3)	1 (0.3)	1 (0.3)
Other	6 (0.5)	6 (1.0)	1 (0.3)	5 (1.7)	0 (0.0)	0 (0.0)	0 (0.0)
Highest level of education completed							
No formal education	372 (31.7)	171 (28.6)	140 (46.8)	31 (10.4)	201 (35.0)	165 (57.5)	36 (12.5)
Primary	409 (34.9)	210 (35.1)	115 (38.5)	95 (31.8)	199 (34.7)	83 (28.9)	116 (40.4)
Secondary	222 (18.9)	121 (20.2)	36 (12.0)	85 (28.4)	101 (17.6)	28 (9.8)	73 (25.4)
Tertiary	169 (14.4)	96 (16.1)	8 (2.7)	88 (29.4)	73 (12.7)	11 (3.8)	62 (21.6)
Caretaker is head of household							
Yes	225 (37.6)	89 (29.8)	136 (45.5)		224 (39.0)	84 (29.3)	140 (48.8)
Head of household's occupation							
Farmer	388 (33.2)	192 (32.2)	175 (58.7)	17 (5.7)	196 (34.4)	175 (61.4)	21 (7.4)
Self-employed	380 (32.6)	183 (30.7)	48 (16.1)	135 (45.2)	197 (34.6)	48 (16.8)	149 (52.3)
Professional	296 (25.4)	158 (26.5)	39 (13.1)	119 (39.8)	138 (24.2)	45 (15.8)	93 (32.6)
Other	59 (5.1)	40 (6.7)	27 (9.1)	13 (4.3)	19 (3.3)	10 (3.5)	9 (3.2)
Housewife	44 (3.8)	24 (4.0)	9 (3.0)	15 (5.0)	20 (3.5)	7 (2.5)	13 (4.6)
Number of children under 59 months old living in household, median (IQR)	1 (1, 2)	1 (1, 2)	1 (1, 2)	1 (1, 2)	1 (1, 2)	1 (1, 2)	1 (1, 2)
Distance to nearest health facility							
1 to 5 km	1102 (94.2)	555 (93.1)	266 (89.0)	289 (97.3)	547 (95.3)	271 (94.4)	276 (96.2)
6 to 10 km	32 (2.7)	20 (3.4)	13 (4.3)	7 (2.4)	12 (2.1)	2 (0.7)	10 (3.5)
11 to 15 km	20 (1.7)	14 (2.3)	13 (4.3)	1 (0.3)	6 (1.0)	6 (2.1)	0 (0.0)
15 to 30 km	16 (1.4)	7 (1.2)	7 (2.3)	0 (0.0)	9 (1.6)	8 (2.8)	1 (0.3)
Home-based record (HBR) available							
Yes	674 (57.5)	395 (66.1)	169 (56.5)	226 (75.6)	279 (48.6)	99 (34.5)	180 (62.7)

Table 1. Cont.

Characteristic	Total	12–23			24–35		
		All Areas	Rural	Urban	All Areas	Rural	Urban
	N = 1172 n (%)	N = 598 n (%)	N = 299 n (%)	N = 299 n (%)	N = 574 n (%)	N = 287 n (%)	N = 287 n (%)
		Sex of child					
Male	558 (47.7)	276 (46.2)	130 (43.5)	146 (48.8)	282 (49.2)	127 (44.3)	155 (54.2)
Female	613 (52.3)	322 (53.8)	169 (56.5)	153 (51.2)	291 (50.8)	160 (55.7)	131 (45.8)
		Delivery location					
Home	240 (20.5)	115 (19.2)	97 (32.4)	18 (6.0)	125 (21.8)	108 (37.6)	17 (5.9)
On the way to facility	9 (0.8)	6 (1.0)	5 (1.7)	1 (0.3)	3 (0.5)	2 (0.7)	1 (0.3)
Health facility	922 (78.7)	477 (79.8)	197 (65.9)	280 (93.6)	445 (77.7)	177 (61.7)	268 (93.7)

IQR = interquartile range; km = kilometer.

Nearly half of the children included in the assessment were female (52%). Most of the children were born at a health facility (79%; 94% in urban areas, 64% in rural areas). Over half of the children had HBRs, and HBR retention was higher in the urban areas compared to the rural areas (58%; 46% rural, 70% urban, Table 1).

3.2. Vaccination Coverage

Vaccination coverage for both age groups (12–23 and 24–35 months) exceeded 80% for most antigens and doses and was slightly higher among older (24–35 months) compared to younger (12–23 months) children (Table 2A). However, the coverage of the oral polio vaccine at birth (OPV0), MCV1, and MCV2 was sub-optimal (<80%) (Tables 2A and 3A). Among children 12–23 months of age, OPV0 coverage was 16% and MCV1 coverage was 71%, with higher MCV1 coverage in the urban areas (81%) compared to the rural (61%) areas (Table 2A). The coverage of MCV2 was 48% among children aged 24–35 months, also with higher coverage in the urban areas (53%) compared to rural (42%) settings (Table 3A).

Table 2. Child immunization coverage and indicators based on home-based records (HBR) and caregiver recall among children aged 12–23 months in Oromia Region, Ethiopia, by settlement type.

A: Child Immunization Coverage Based on Home-Based Records (HBR) If Available and Caregiver Recall, N= 598						
Vaccine Dose	All Areas, N = 598		Rural, N = 299		Urban, N = 299	
	n (%)	95% CI	n (%)	95% CI	n (%)	95% CI
BCG	528 (88)	85, 91	258 (86)	82, 90	270 (90)	86, 93
OPV0	96 (16)	13, 19	24 (8.0)	5.3, 12	72 (24)	19, 29
OPV1	544 (91)	88, 93	267 (89)	85, 92	277 (93)	89, 95
OPV2	527 (88)	85, 91	251 (84)	79, 88	276 (92)	89, 95
OPV3	504 (84)	81, 87	236 (79)	74, 83	268 (90)	85, 93
Penta1	544 (91)	88, 93	267 (89)	85, 92	277 (93)	89, 95
Penta2	527 (88)	85, 91	251 (84)	79, 88	276 (92)	89, 95
Penta3	501 (84)	81, 87	233 (78)	73, 82	268 (90)	85, 93
PCV1	545 (91)	88, 93	268 (90)	85, 93	277 (93)	89, 95
PCV2	526 (88)	85, 90	250 (84)	79, 88	276 (92)	89, 95
PCV3	501 (84)	81, 87	233 (78)	73, 82	268 (90)	85, 93
Rota1	545 (91)	88, 93	268 (90)	85, 93	277 (93)	89, 95
Rota2	526 (88)	85, 90	250 (84)	79, 88	276 (92)	89, 95
MCV1	423 (71)	67, 74	182 (61)	55, 66	241 (81)	76, 85
IPV [1]	330 (80)	76, 84	129 (72)	65, 79	201 (86)	81, 90
MCV2 [2]	100 (50)	43, 57	33 (37)	27, 48	67 (61)	51, 70

Table 2. Cont.

B: Child immunization indicators based on home-based records (HBR) only, N = 395						
Vaccine dose	All areas, N = 395		Rural, N = 169		Urban, N = 226	
	n (%)	95% CI	n (%)	95% CI	n (%)	95% CI
Fully immunized for infant vaccines [3]	263 (67)	62, 71	89 (53)	45, 60	174 (77)	71, 82
Penta1 to Penta3 DOR [4]	32 (8.2)	5.7, 11	24 (14)	9.6, 21	8 (3.6)	1.7, 7.1
Penta1 to MCV1 DOR	87 (22)	18, 27	59 (35)	28, 43	28 (12)	8.6, 18

[1] IPV was not consistently assessed through caregiver recall, therefore, these results reflect mainly HBR data (the denominator for IPV was 412 (178 in rural and 234 in urban). [2] MCV2 was not consistently assessed through caregiver recall, therefore, these results reflect mainly HBR data and the coverage estimated among children aged 18–23 months (the denominator for MCV2 was 200 (89 in rural, 111 in urban). [3] Fully immunized children in the first year of life as Ethiopia's EPI criteria is defined as a child receiving 1 dose of BCG, 3 doses of DPT-Hib-HepB (Pentavalent vaccine), 3 doses of OPV, 3 doses of PCV, 2 doses of Rotavirus vaccine, 1 dose of IPV, and 1 dose of measles-containing vaccine. [4] DOR denotes dropout rate, CI: Confidence interval.

Table 3. Child immunization coverage and indicators based on home-based records (HBR) and caregiver recall among children aged 24–35 months in Oromia Region, Ethiopia, by settlement type.

A: Child Immunization Coverage Based on Home-Based Records (HBR) If Available and Caregiver Recall, N = 574						
Vaccine Dose	All areas, N = 574		Rural, N = 287		Urban, N = 287	
	n (%)	95% CI	n (%)	95% CI	n (%)	95% CI
BCG	481 (84)	80, 87	224 (78)	73, 83	257 (90)	85, 93
OPV0	70 (12)	9.7, 15	12 (4.2)	2.3, 7.4	58 (20)	16, 25
OPV1	491 (86)	82, 88	232 (81)	76, 85	259 (90)	86, 93
OPV2	486 (85)	81, 87	224 (78)	73, 83	262 (91)	87, 94
OPV3	462 (80)	77, 84	204 (71)	65, 76	258 (90)	86, 93
Penta1	491 (86)	82, 88	231 (80)	75, 85	260 (91)	86, 94
Penta2	481 (84)	80, 87	219 (76)	71, 81	262 (91)	87, 94
Penta3	462 (80)	77, 84	203 (71)	65, 76	259 (90)	86, 93
PCV1	491 (86)	82, 88	231 (80)	75, 85	260 (91)	86, 94
PCV2	480 (84)	80, 87	220 (77)	71, 81	260 (91)	86, 94
PCV3	459 (80)	76, 83	204 (71)	65, 76	255 (89)	84, 92
Rota1	492 (86)	83, 88	233 (81)	76, 85	259 (90)	86, 93
Rota2	479 (83)	80, 86	219 (76)	71, 81	260 (91)	86, 94
MCV1	425 (74)	70, 78	187 (65)	59, 71	238 (83)	78, 87
IPV [1]	235 (74)	69, 79	76 (59)	50, 68	159 (85)	78, 89
MCV2 [1]	181 (48)	43, 54	65 (42)	34, 50	116 (53)	46, 60

B: Child immunization indicators based on home-based records (HBR) only, N = 279						
Vaccine dose	All areas, N = 279		Rural, N = 99		Urban, N = 180	
	n (%) [2]	95% CI	n (%) [2]	95% CI	n (%) [2]	95% CI
Fully immunized for infant vaccines [2]	183 (66)	60, 71	49 (49)	39, 60	134 (74)	67, 81
Fully immunized for infant vaccines and MCV2 [3]	97 (35)	29, 41	22 (22)	15, 32	75 (42)	34, 49
Penta1 to Penta3 DOR	9 (3.3)	1.6, 6.4	7 (7.2)	3.2, 15	2 (1.1)	0.20, 4.5
Penta1 to MCV1 DOR	40 (15)	11, 19	24 (25)	17, 35	16 (9.0)	5.4, 15
MCV1 to MCV2 DOR	109 (46)	40, 53	36 (49)	37, 60	73 (45)	37, 53

[1] IPV and MCV2 were not consistently assessed through caregiver recall, therefore, these results reflect mainly HBR data (the denominator was 316 for IPV and 371 for MCV2). [2] Fully immunized children in the first year of life as per Ethiopia's EPI criteria, defined as a child who received 1 dose of BCG, 3 doses of DPT-Hib-HepB (Pentavalent vaccine), 3 doses of OPV, 3 doses of PCV, 2 doses of Rotavirus vaccine, 1 dose of IPV, and 1 dose of measles-containing vaccine. [3] Fully immunized children in the second year of life, defined as a child who received 1 dose of BCG, 3 doses of DPT-Hib-HepB (Pentavalent vaccine), 3 doses of OPV, 3 doses of PCV, 2 doses of Rotavirus vaccine, 1 dose of IPV, and 2 doses of measles-containing vaccine. CI: Confidence interval.

Based on HBR, the proportion of children who were fully immunized for all recommended infant EPI vaccines in Ethiopia (one dose of BCG, three doses of Pentavalent vaccine, three doses of OPV, three doses of PCV, two doses of Rotavirus vaccine, one dose of IPV, and one dose of measles vaccine) was 67% (53% rural, 77% urban) among children aged 12–23 months (Table 2B) and 66% (49% rural, 74% urban) among children aged 24–35 months (Table 3B). However, including MCV2 in the fully immunized definition classified 35% of children aged 24–35 months (22% rural, 42% urban) as being fully vaccinated (Table 2B).

The Penta1 to Penta3 DOR was 8% (14% rural, 4% urban) among children aged 12–23 months and 3% (7% rural, 1% urban) among those aged 24–35 months (Table 2B). The Penta1 to MCV1 DOR was 22% (35% rural, 12% urban) among children aged 12–23 months (Table 2B) and 15% (25% rural, 9% urban) among those aged 24–35 months (Table 3B). The DOR between the first and second doses of MCV was much higher, at 46% (49% rural, 45% urban) among children aged 24–35 months (Table 3B).

3.3. Factors Associated with MCV1 Uptake

Based on backwards selection, the final variables in the multivariate model for MCV1 were as follows: caregiver's education, caregiver's age, number of children less than five years old living in the household, caregiver's who believed the child had received all recommended vaccines, and caregiver's who reported being turned away from the health facility due to vaccine stockout. Caregivers with higher levels of education were more likely to vaccinate their children with MCV1, and the strength of this association generally increased with each additional level of educational attainment (aOR 2.6; 95% CI 1.5 to 4.6 for primary, aOR 3.2; 95% CI 1.6 to 6.6 for secondary, and aOR 6.8; 95% CI 2.9 to 17.8 for tertiary education, as compared to no formal education). The caregivers aged 27 to 80 years were more likely to vaccinate their children with MCV1, as compared to the caregivers aged 18 to 26 years (aOR 1.7 95% CI 1.0 to 2.7). The children residing in households with multiple children under the age of five years were less likely to be vaccinated with MCV1 (aOR 0.6, 95% CI 0.4 to 1.0 for two vs.one child under five years and aOR 0.4, 95% CI 0.1 to 1.1 for three or four vs. one child under five years). The caregivers who reported that their child had received all recommended vaccines were more likely to have a child that was vaccinated with MCV1 (aOR 7.8, 95% CI 4.9 to 12.7) compared to caregivers who did not believe that their child was fully immunized. The caregivers who knew the correct number of vaccination visits required to complete vaccination services were more likely to vaccinate their child with MCV1 (aOR 2.44, 95% CI 1.02 to 6.87). The caregivers who reported ever being turned away from a health center due to vaccine stockout were less likely to vaccinate their child with MCV1 (aOR 0.4, 95% CI 0.2 to 0.8) (Table 4).

Table 4. Bivariate and multivariate association between caregiver, household, and child demographic characteristics, caregiver's knowledge, attitude, practice, and awareness factors, and first dose of measles-containing vaccine (MCV1) vaccination status among children aged 12–23 months in Oromia Region, Ethiopia (N = 598).

Characteristic	N	MCV1 = Yes	Bivariate Regression			Multivariate Regression		
			OR	95% CI	p-Value	aOR	95% CI	p-Value
Settlement					<0.001			
Rural	299	182	Ref					
Urban	299	241	2.67	1.85, 3.88				
Caregiver's highest level of education completed					<0.001			<0.001
No formal education	171	88	Ref			Ref		
Primary	210	149	2.30	1.51, 3.53		2.59	1.49, 4.59	
Secondary	121	101	4.76	2.75, 8.56		3.21	1.60, 6.63	
Tertiary	96	85	7.29	3.77, 15.3		6.83	2.89, 17.8	

Table 4. Cont.

Characteristic	N	MCV1 = Yes	Bivariate Regression			Multivariate Regression		
			OR	95% CI	p-Value	aOR	95% CI	p-Value
Caregiver's age in years					0.085			0.039
18 to 26 years	330	225	Ref			Ref		
27 to 80 years	264	197	1.37	0.96, 1.97		1.66	1.03, 2.72	
Number of children under 59 months old living in household					<0.001			0.039
One	383	294	Ref			Ref		
Two	188	116	0.49	0.33, 0.71		0.58	0.35, 0.96	
Three or four	26	12	0.26	0.11, 0.58		0.37	0.12, 1.11	
Sex of child					0.75			
Male	276	197	Ref					
Female	322	226	0.94	0.66, 1.34				
Delivery location					<0.001			
Home	115	55	Ref					
At HF or on the way to HF	483	368	3.99	2.29, 5.33				
Caregiver believes that child has received all recommended vaccines					<0.001			<0.001
No/Do not remember	242	108	Ref			Ref		
Yes	355	315	9.77	6.51, 14.9		7.80	4.88, 12.7	
Number of vaccination visits child needs					<0.001			
0–5 visits	449	307	Ref			Ref		
6 visits (correct as per EPI schedule)	76	70	5.40	2.48, 14.2		2.44	1.02, 6.87	0.045
Named measles as a VPD					0.002			
No	96	55	Ref					
Yes	502	368	2.05	1.30, 3.21				
Heard of immunization against measles					0.003			
No	92	53	Ref					
Yes	506	370	2.00	1.26, 3.16				
Number of doses of measles vaccine that child is supposed to receive					<0.001			
Never heard of measles vaccine or do not know number of doses	347	224	Ref					
Heard of measles vaccine—One dose	92	67	1.47	0.89, 2.48				
Heard of measles vaccine—Two doses	151	126	2.77	1.73, 4.56				
Know of a family or community member who had measles					0.17			
No	428	296	Ref					
Yes	170	127	1.32	0.89, 1.98				
In the household, who makes the decision to immunize the child?					<0.001			
Mother or father only (one parent)	133	73	Ref					
Both father and mother	456	345	2.55	1.71, 3.82				
Ever been sent home from health center due to vaccine stockout?					<0.001			0.005
No	514	381	Ref			Ref		
Yes	80	40	0.35	0.22, 0.56		0.40	0.21, 0.76	

Table 4. Cont.

Characteristic	N	MCV1 = Yes	Bivariate Regression			Multivariate Regression		
			OR	95% CI	p-Value	aOR	95% CI	p-Value
Type of vaccination services available to your child					0.005			
Health facility (fixed)	403	299	Ref					
Outreach site	13	5	0.22	0.06, 0.67				
Both	179	117	0.66	0.45, 0.96				
Frequency of vaccination availability					0.008			
Every month	303	223	Ref					
Every week	171	127	1.04	0.68, 1.60				
Every day	56	51	3.66	1.54, 10.8				
Walking time to vaccination center					0.33			
From 1 to 6 h	39	25	Ref					
30 min to 1 h	85	56	1.08	0.48, 2.38				
30 min or less	461	333	1.46	0.72, 2.85				
How long do you wait at the vaccination center before the child is vaccinated?					0.50			
From 1 to 6 h	129	94	Ref					
30 min to 1 h	145	98	0.78	0.46, 1.30				
30 min or less	311	226	0.99	0.62, 1.56				

N: Total number of surveyed children, MCV: Measles-containing vaccine, OR: Odds ratio, aOR: Adjusted odds ratio, CI: Confidence interval, HF: Health facility, EPI: Expanded program on vaccination, VPD: Vaccine-preventable disease. All independent variables with p-value < 0.15 in the bivariate analysis were added to the initial multivariate regression model.

3.4. Factors Associated with MCV1 Uptake, Stratified by Rural and Urban Settlement

The factors significantly affecting the uptake of MCV1 among children aged 12–23 months differed in rural and urban settings. In the rural areas, only two factors were associated with MCV1 vaccination, as follows: higher levels of educational attainment for the child's caregiver (aOR 2.0, 95% CI 1.1 to 3.8 for primary; aOR 4.4, 95% CI 1.6 to 12.8 for secondary, and aOR 3.7, 95% CI 0.7 to 20.7 for tertiary education levels, as compared to no formal education) and the caregivers' belief that their child had received all recommended vaccines (aOR 13.3, 95% CI 7.5 to 24.5) (Table S1A).

In contrast, in urban settings, several different factors were significantly associated with MCV1 vaccination. The caregivers aged 27 to 80 years were more likely to vaccinate their children with MCV1, as compared to the caregivers aged 18 to 26 years (aOR 2.9, 95% CI 1.3 to 6.9). Children residing in households with multiple children under the age of five years were less likely to be vaccinated with MCV1 (aOR 0.25, 95% CI 0.11 to 0.56 for two vs. one child under five years; and aOR 0.09, 95% CI 0.01 to 0.51 for three or four vs. one child under five years). The caregivers who reported that their child had received all recommended vaccines were more likely to have a child who was vaccinated with MCV1 (aOR 4.55, 95% CI 2.17 to 9.91) compared to the caregivers who did not believe that their child was fully immunized. The caregivers who knew the correct number of vaccinations visits (aOR 4.43, 95% CI 1.26 to 23.1) and named measles as a vaccine-preventable disease (aOR 3.75, 95% CI 1.49 to 9.60) were more likely to have vaccinated their child with MCV1. The caregivers who reported ever being sent home from a health center due to vaccine stockout were less likely to vaccinate their child with MCV1 (aOR 0.33, 95% CI 0.13 to 0.86) (Table S1B).

3.5. Factors Associated with MCV2 Uptake

Children who were delivered at or on the way to a health facility were likely to be vaccinated with MCV2, as compared to children who were delivered at home (aOR 2.37; 95% CI 1.30 to 4.47). Similar to MCV1, the caregivers who reported that their child had received all recommended vaccines were more likely to have a child that was vaccinated with MCV2 (aOR 8.29, 95% CI 4.52 to 16.3) compared to the caregivers who did not believe that their child was fully immunized. The caregivers who knew the recommended number of vaccination visits (aOR 3.12, 95% CI 1.87 to 5.36) and doses of childhood measles vaccine (aOR: 1.62, CI: 1.05 to 2.50) were more likely to vaccinate their children with MCV2 (Table 5).

Table 5. Bivariate and multivariate association between caregiver, household, and child demographic characteristics, caregiver's knowledge, attitude, practice, and awareness factors, and second dose of measles-containing vaccine (MCV2) vaccination status among children aged 18–35 months in Oromia Region, Ethiopia (n = 572).

Characteristic	N	MCV2 = Yes	Bivariate Regression			Multivariate Regression		
			OR	95% CI	p-Value	aOR	95% CI	p-Value
Settlement					<0.001			
Rural	246	96	Ref					
Urban	328	184	1.91	1.36, 2.67				
Caregiver's highest level of education completed					<0.001			
No formal education	155	54	Ref					
Primary	198	93	1.69	1.10, 2.61				
Secondary	119	76	3.31	2.02, 5.48				
Tertiary	102	57	2.37	1.42, 3.97				
Caregiver's age in years					0.20			
18 to 26 years	280	130	Ref					
27 to 80 years	293	149	1.14	0.82, 1.59				
Number of children under 59 months old living in household					0.018			
One	387	196	Ref					
Two	170	80	0.89	0.62, 1.27				
Three or four	14	2	0.16	0.03, 0.61				
Sex of child					0.15			
Male	275	125	Ref					
Female	299	155	1.24	0.89, 1.72				
Delivery location					0.002			0.005
Home	70	20	Ref			Ref		
At HF or on the way to HF	504	260	2.31	1.37, 4.00		2.37	1.30, 4.47	
Caregiver believes that child has received all recommended vaccines					<0.001			<0.001
No/Do not remember	122	16	Ref			Ref		
Yes	451	263	10.2	5.91, 18.7		8.29	4.52, 16.3	
Number of vaccination visits child needs					<0.001			<0.001
0–5	397	174	Ref			Ref		
6 (correct as per EPI schedule)	108	83	3.96	2.47, 6.53		3.12	1.87, 5.36	
Named measles as a VPD					0.051			
No	82	32	Ref					
Yes	492	248	1.60	1.00, 2.60				
Heard of immunization against measles					<0.001			
No	63	15	Ref					
Yes	511	265	3.47	1.94, 6.57				

Table 5. Cont.

Characteristic	N	MCV2 = Yes	Bivariate Regression			Multivariate Regression		
			OR	95% CI	p-Value	aOR	95% CI	p-Value
Number of doses of measles vaccine that child is supposed to receive					<0.001			0.028
Never heard of measles vaccine or do not know number of doses	293	119	Ref			Ref		
Heard of measles vaccine—One dose	77	32	1.03	0.61, 1.70		0.82	0.45, 1.46	
Heard of measles vaccine—Two doses	198	125	2.47	1.71, 3.59		1.62	1.05, 2.50	
Know of a family or community member who had measles					0.33			
No	385	181	Ref					
Yes	189	99	1.19	0.84, 1.69				
In the household, who makes the decision to immunize the child?					<0.001			
Mother or father only (one parent)	121	42	Ref					
Both father and mother	450	235	2.07	1.37, 3.17				
Ever been sent home from health center due to vaccine stockout?					0.22			
No	495	248	Ref					
Yes	73	30	0.74	0.44, 1.20				
Type of vaccination services available to your child					0.82			
Health facility (fixed)	420	206	Ref					
Outreach site	3	2	2.10	0.20, 45.3				
Both	150	71	0.99	0.68, 1.44				
Frequency of vaccination availability					0.46			
Every month	293	142	Ref					
Every week	157	84	1.19	0.81, 1.76				
Every day	71	41	1.34	0.79, 2.26				
Walking time to vaccination center					0.59			
From 1 to 6 h	47	26	Ref					
30 min to 1 h	83	37	0.72	0.35, 1.47				
30 min or less	430	206	0.74	0.40, 1.35				
How long do you wait at the vaccination center before the child is vaccinated?					0.24			
From 1 to 6 h	118	64	Ref					
30 min to 1 h	145	67	0.68	0.41, 1.10				
30 min or less	305	147	0.72	0.47, 1.11				

N: Total number of surveyed children, MCV: Measles-containing vaccine, OR: Odds ratio, aOR: Adjusted odds ratio, CI: Confidence interval, HF: Health facility, EPI: Expanded program on vaccination, VPD: Vaccine-preventable disease. All independent variables with p-value < 0.15 in the bivariate analysis were added to the initial multivariate regression model.

3.6. Factors Associated with MCV2 Uptake, Stratified by Rural and Urban Settlement

Factors statistically associated with the utilization of MCV2 were mostly similar in urban and rural settings. The caregivers who believed that their child had received all recommended vaccines and who knew that six vaccination visits were needed to receive all of the EPI vaccines were more likely to vaccinate their children with MCV2 in both rural and urban settings.

In rural areas only, the caregivers who accessed the nearest health facility within 30 min to 1 hour (aOR 11.3, 95% CI 1.73 to 2.27) and within 30 min or less (aOR 9.1, 95%

CI 1.6 to 1.7) were more likely to vaccinate their children with MCV2, as compared to the caregivers who accessed the health facility within 1–6 h. (Table S2A,B).

4. Discussion

Two years after the introduction of MCV2 in Ethiopia, we found that coverage for both MCV1 and MCV2 in Oromia Region was too low to attain the measles elimination goals. MCV1 coverage in this study was higher compared with previous DHS estimates [7,8], but our study excluded areas inaccessible due to the ongoing conflict where the coverage for routine immunization, including MCV1, could be lower. The MCV2 coverage (48% among children aged 24–35 months), however, was fairly comparable with the findings from other African countries (around 45%) [23]. In addition, the findings from a community-based survey in Tanzania showed slightly lower, but comparable, MCV2 coverage (44%) [24] and lower coverage as compared with the findings in Ghana (67–82%) [25]. MCV2 coverage might be low because it is relatively newly introduced, and often the first vaccine to be introduced in second year of life, as is the case in Ethiopia. In addition, MCV2 was introduced in February 2019, and the COVID-19 pandemic also likely contributed to the lower coverage rate. Similar to MCV1, the coverage for MCV2 was possibly lower than our estimate, as we excluded the inaccessible areas in active conflict. The recent study conducted in March 2022 by Project Hope in remote and underserved communities in Ethiopia also estimated low MCV1 and MCV2 coverage at 66% and 34%, respectively [26].

The coverage for MCV1 and MCV2 was higher in urban areas compared to rural areas, as found in another recent survey [26]. This might be due to the fact that communities in the urban setting have better access to health care services and information. Based on stratified multivariate analyses, households accessing the nearest health facility in less than a 1-hour walk were more likely to vaccinate their children, as compared to households accessing health facilities within a 1–6-h walk in rural areas. This suggested that households situated far from the nearest health facility in the rural area are less likely to vaccinate their children. Establishing locally tailored vaccination sessions, including outreach through discussion with rural communities, could help the communities residing far from the health facility to vaccinate their children.

Although higher levels of educational attainment and awareness of immunizations were associated with MCV1 and MCV2 vaccination, the overall coverage of MCV2 remained low among the study population. The caregivers who believed that their children received all of the recommended doses of the vaccine and those who knew the required number of visits and measles doses were more likely to vaccinate their children. This highlights that adequate knowledge and information about the second dose of the measles vaccine may not be sufficient to increase vaccination uptake. Another study conducted in multiple African countries also reported insufficient sensitization and awareness generation among parents for low MCV2 coverage [27]. The lack of information was also associated with low MCV2 coverage in Kenya [28]. Therefore, building the health workers interpersonal communication skills to provide key immunization messages to all caregivers at each vaccination session is important for increasing the uptake of MCV1 and MCV2. Increasing parental vaccine decision-making power is an essential factor that should be considered when implementing strategies to improve vaccination uptake. As reported in different studies, face-to-face caregiver and health worker interactions are the most recommended strategy to influence parental decisions to vaccinate their children [29]. On the other hand, our study further uncovered the high vaccination dropout rates between Penta1 and MCV1, and MCV1 and MCV2. The dropout rates were relatively high among the rural areas, as compared with urban dwellers. The MCV1 to MCV2 dropout rate was similar to that from a report from Kenya, which was 46.7% [28]. The higher the vaccination dropout rate could be attributed to the absence or inadequate routine immunization defaulter tracking system in the healthcare facilities. Establishing a locally tailored defaulter identification and tracking systems may have a positive effect on the reduction in vaccination dropout rates.

The caregivers who reportedly experienced being sent home from health facilities due to vaccine stockout were less likely to vaccinate their children with MCV1. This is a missed opportunity for vaccination, as the caregivers might come from far away, and may not return for vaccination again. Vaccine stockout was previously documented as being associated with a missed opportunity for vaccination [30]. The monitoring of vaccines and vaccine supply, maintaining the minimum recommended stock level, and the timely submitting of vaccine requests from the health facility level is important to avoid supply constraints in the health facility settings and to reduce missed vaccination opportunities.

Our survey further revealed that the coverage for OPV0 was low, at 16%, while nearly 80% of children were born in health facilities. They had an opportunity to receive OPV0 at birth, as most of them had contact with a health facility and healthcare providers. This indicates a potential missed opportunity for all vaccines, including MCV1 and MCV2, which might be high. Therefore, service integration in healthcare settings, especially at delivery wards, could minimize potential missed opportunities for vaccination. Further research is needed to understand the magnitude of missed opportunities for vaccination and to identify where and why the children visiting the health facilities, including newborns, are missing the vaccine doses for which they are eligible. Plus, the gaps in birth dose coverage should be explored in advance of the introduction of Hepatitis B birth dose in the future.

This study has some limitations. Conflict-affected areas were purposely excluded from the sampling frame, and the findings of this study might not reflect the trends in those areas. Additionally, because of the unavailability of an updated population census, we could not conduct a weighted analysis to account for any sampling error and infer the findings to the general population. We also used the caregiver's recall in the absence of HBR to assess the vaccination status of the children. This might lead to an overestimation or underestimation of vaccination coverage. However, the evidence showed that the concordance between HBR and the caregiver's recall was relatively high in Ethiopia [31]. The discordance between the caregiver's and HBR was reported as minimal for the measles vaccines [32].

5. Conclusions

Two years after MCV2 introduction, coverage remains low, with high measles vaccination dropout rates that illustrate low utilization. The high vaccination dropout rate between MCV1 and MCV2 indicates that the routine immunization defaulter identification, tracking, and follow-up system is weak in healthcare facilities. Caregivers with more awareness of the measles vaccine and its schedule were more likely to vaccinate their children. To improve the uptake of MCV2 in the second year of life and achieve the global measles elimination goals, demand generation, including social mobilization, should be strengthened in the Oromia Region of Ethiopia. In addition, strengthening locally tailored immunization defaulter identification and tracking systems in healthcare facilities is needed to reduce the vaccination dropout rate and increase its utilization. Regular monitoring of vaccines and vaccine supplies and enhancing service integration could have an impact on reducing missed opportunities for vaccination in healthcare settings.

Supplementary Materials: The following supporting information can be downloaded at: https://www.mdpi.com/article/10.3390/vaccines12070762/s1, Table S1. Bivariate and multivariate association between caregiver, household, and child demographic factors and the first dose of measles-containing vaccine (MCV1) vaccination among children aged 12–23 months by settlement in Oromia Region, Ethiopia, N = 598. Table S2. Bivariate and multivariate association between caregiver, household, and child demographic characteristics, caregiver's knowledge, attitude, practice, and awareness factors, and the second dose of measles-containing vaccine (MCV2) vaccination among children aged 18–35 months by settlement in Oromia Region, Ethiopia (N = 572).

Author Contributions: A.B.W., P.S., B.T., B.K., A.B., T.D., G.W., A.S., Y.L.T., M.A.K., H.T.W., A.W. and C.E.S. conceived of and designed the study. A.B.W., B.M.A., L.L., G.Y., S.-H.W., P.S., B.T., B.K., A.B., G.W., A.S., Y.L.T., M.A.K., T.B.A. and C.E.S. facilitated the fieldwork and supervised the data collection. A.B.W., M.P.S., J.P., Q.A., A.M.M., A.W. and C.E.S. guided the analysis. A.B.W., M.P.S., J.P., Q.A., A.M.M., A.W., C.E.S., J.P.N. and M.A. interpreted the results. A.B.W. drafted the manuscript, with input from M.P.S., M.A., J.P.N., A.M.M. and C.E.S. All authors have read and agreed to the published version of the manuscript.

Funding: Funding for this study was provided by Gavi, the Vaccine Alliance via the Ethiopia Targeted Country Assistance, Partner Engagement Framework, through the CDC-Foundation and from the US Centers for Disease Control and Prevention.

Institutional Review Board Statement: This study was conducted according to the guidelines of the Declaration of Helsinki on program assessments. The protocol underwent scientific and ethical review and was granted approval by the Oromia Regional Health Bureau ethical review board and determined as non-research by the U.S. Centers for Disease Control and Prevention. Permission was obtained at each level of the government to conduct the assessment. Approval certificate letter number (BEFO/UBTFU/1-16/875).

Informed Consent Statement: The interviewers read a consent script before the start of the interview for each participant. The participants were given a right to ask questions, decline participation, and withdraw from the interview at any time during the interview process. Verbal consent was obtained from each of the participants before the interview began.

Data Availability Statement: The datasets used to prepare this report are available at the Oromia Regional Health Bureau and can be obtained from the corresponding author upon reasonable request.

Acknowledgments: We would like to thank the Oromia Regional Health Bureau for allowing us to use measles surveillance data for the selection of assessment areas. We also thank Samuel Teshome, and Julianne Gee, CDC, for technical support.

Conflicts of Interest: The authors declare no conflicts of interest.

References

1. Henderson, R.H. The Expanded Programme on Immunization of the World Health Organization. *Rev. Infect. Dis.* **1984**, *6*, S475–S479. [CrossRef] [PubMed]
2. Keja, K.; Chan, C.; Hayden, G.; Henderson, R.H. Expanded Program on Immunization. *World Health Stat. Q.* **1988**, *41*, 59–63. [PubMed]
3. World Health Organization. Measles vaccines: WHO position paper. *Wkly. Epidemiol. Rec.* **2009**, *84*, 349–360.
4. Tamirat, K.S.; Sisay, M.M. Full immunization coverage and its associated factors among children aged 12–23 months in Ethiopia: Further analysis from the 2016 Ethiopia demographic and health survey. *BMC Public Health* **2019**, *19*, 1019. [CrossRef] [PubMed]
5. Federal Democratic Republic of Ethiopia Ministry of Health. *Ethiopia National Expanded Programme on Immunization Comprehensive Multi-Year Plan 2016–2020*; Federal Ministry of Health: Addis Ababa, Ethiopia, 2015.
6. Regassa, N.; Bird, Y.; Moraros, J. Preference in the use of full childhood immunizations in Ethiopia: The role of maternal health services. *Patient Prefer Adherence* **2019**, *13*, 91–99. [PubMed]
7. Central Statistical Agency (CSA) Ethiopia and ICF. *Demographic and Health Survey 2016*; CSA and ICF: Addis Ababa, Ethiopia; Rockville, MD, USA, 2016.
8. Ethiopian Public Health Institute [Ethiopia] and ICF. *Mini Demographic and Health Survey 2019: Key Indicators*; EPHI and ICF: Addis Ababa, Ethiopia; Rockville, MD, USA, 2019.
9. World Health Organization. *EB154/9 Immunization Agenda 2030 Progress towards Global Immunization Goals and Implementation of the Immunization Agenda 2030*; World Health Organization: Geneva, Switzerland, 2023; pp. 1–10.
10. World Health Organization. *Global Vaccine Action Plan: Monitoring, Evaluation and Accountability. Secretariat Annual Report 2020*; World Health Organization: Geneva, Switzerland, 2020.
11. Wondwossen, L.; Gallagher, K.; Braka, F.; Karengera, T. Advances in the control of vaccine preventable diseases in Ethiopia. *Pan Afr. Med. J.* **2017**, *27*, 1. [CrossRef] [PubMed]
12. World Health Organization (WHO) Regional Office for Africa. Weekly Bulletin on Outbreaks and Other Emergencies. 2020, Week 4: 1–17. Available online: https://apps.who.int/iris/bitstream/handle/10665/330642/OEW04-2026012020.pdf (accessed on 12 October 2020).
13. UN Inter-Agency Group for Child Mortality Estimation. Under-Five Mortality Rate in Ethiopia. 2019. Available online: https://childmortality.org/all-cause-mortality/data?refArea=ETH (accessed on 10 December 2020).
14. World Health Organization (WHO). Measles vaccines: WHO position paper—April 2017. *Wkly Epidemiol. Rec.* **2017**, *92*, 205–227.

15. World Health Organization (WHO). *Ethiopia Launches Measles Vaccine Second Dose (MCV2) Introduction: Over 3.3 Million Children will Receive the Vaccine Annually*; World Health Organization: Addis Ababa, Ethiopia, 2019; Available online: https://www.afro.who.int/news/ethiopia-launches-measles-vaccine-second-dose-mcv2-introduction-over-33-million-children-will (accessed on 12 October 2020).
16. WHO/UNICEF. Estimates of National Immunization Coverage, 2022 Revision. 2022. Available online: https://worldhealthorg.shinyapps.io/wuenic-trends-2023/ (accessed on 12 October 2020).
17. Lakew, Y.; Bekele, A.; Biadgilign, S. Factors influencing full immunization coverage among 12–23 months of age children in Ethiopia: Evidence from the national demographic and health survey in 2011. *BMC Public Health* **2015**, *15*, 728. [CrossRef]
18. Biellik, R.J.; Davis, R. The new World Health Organization recommendation on the 2-dose measles vaccine schedule and the way forward in African Region. *Pan Afr. Med. J.* **2017**, *27*, 14. [CrossRef] [PubMed]
19. Legesse, E.; Dechasa, W. An assessment of child immunization coverage and its determinants in Sinana District, Southeast Ethiopia. *BMC Pediatr.* **2015**, *15*, 31. [CrossRef]
20. World Health Organization. *A Guide to Introducing a Second Dose of Measles Vaccine into Routine Immunization Schedules. WHO Guidelines*; WHO: Geneva, Switzerland, 2013; p. 11.
21. Global Vaccine Alliance. *Gavi Ethiopia Joint Appraisal Report, 2019*; Gavi, the Vaccine Alliance: Geneva, Switzerland, 2019.
22. World Health Organization. *Vaccination Coverage Cluster Surveys: Reference Manaul*; WHO/IVB: Geneva, Swizerland, 2018.
23. Chilot, D.; Belay, D.G.; Shitu, K.; Gela, Y.Y.; Getnet, M.; Mulat, B.; Muluneh, A.G.; Merid, M.W.; Bitew, D.A.; Alem, A.Z. Measles second dose vaccine utilization and associated factors among children aged 24–35 months in Sub-Saharan Africa, a multi-level analysis from recent DHS surveys. *BMC Public Health* **2022**, *22*, 2070. [CrossRef]
24. Magodi, R.; Mmbaga, E.J.; Massaga, J.; Lyimo, D.; Mphuru, A.; Abade, A. Factors associated with non-uptake of measles-rubella vaccine second dose among children under five years in Mtwara district council, Tanzania, 2017. *Pan Afr. Med. J.* **2019**, *33*, 67. [CrossRef] [PubMed]
25. Muhoza, P.; Shah, M.P.; Gao, H.; Amponsa-Achiano, K.; Quaye, P.; Opare, W.; Okae, C.; Aboyinga, P.-N.; Opare, K.L.; Wardle, M.T.; et al. Predictors for Uptake of Vaccines Offered during the Second Year of Life: Second Dose of Measles-Containing Vaccine and Meningococcal Serogroup A-Containing Vaccine, Ghana, 2020. *Vaccines* **2023**, *11*, 1515. [CrossRef] [PubMed]
26. Project HOPE M of H (Ethiopia) and AHA. *Reaching Zero-Dose and Under-Immunized Children in Remote and Underserved Settings of Ethiopia: Evaluation Zero Tolerance for Zero*; Project HOPE: Addis Ababa, Ethiopia, 2022.
27. Masresha, B.G.; Luce, R.; Okeibunor, J.; Shibeshi, M.E.; Kamadjeu, R.; Fall, A. Introduction of The Second Dose of Measles Containing Vaccine in the Childhood Vaccination Programs within the WHO Africa Region-Lessons Learnt. *J. Immunol. Sci.* **2018**, *2*, 113–121. [CrossRef]
28. Ogutu, J.O.; Francis, G.M.; Kamau, D.M.; Owiny, M.O.; Oyugi, E.O.; Ettyang, G.K. Factors Associated with Low Coverage of the Second Dose of Measles Containing Vaccine among Children Aged 19–59 Months, Alego-Usonga Sub-County, Kenya, 2020. *J. Interv. Epidemiol. Public Health* **2023**, *6*, 1. [CrossRef]
29. Ekezie, W.; Awwad, S.; Krauchenberg, A.; Karara, N.; Dembiński, Ł.; Grossman, Z.; del Torso, S.; Dornbusch, H.J.; Neves, A.; Copley, S.; et al. Access to Vaccination among Disadvantaged, Isolated and Difficult-to-Reach Communities in the WHO European Region: A Systematic Review. *Vaccines* **2022**, *10*, 1038. [CrossRef] [PubMed]
30. Garib, Z.; Vargas, A.L.; Trumbo, S.P.; Anthony, K.; Diaz-Ortega, J.L.; Bravo-Alcántara, P.; Leal, I.; Danovaro-Holliday, M.C.; Velandia-González, M. Missed Opportunities for Vaccination in the Dominican Republic: Results of an Operational Investigation. *BioMed Res. Int.* **2016**, *2016*, 4721836. [CrossRef] [PubMed]
31. Porth, J.M.; Wagner, A.L.; Tefera, Y.A.; Boulton, M.L. Childhood immunization in Ethiopia: Accuracy of maternal recall compared to vaccination cards. *Vaccines* **2019**, *7*, 48. [CrossRef] [PubMed]
32. Mansour, Z.; Brandt, L.; Said, R.; Fahmy, K.; Riedner, G.; Danovaro-Holliday, M.C. Home-based records' quality and validity of caregivers' recall of children's vaccination in Lebanon. *Vaccine* **2019**, *37*, 4177–4183. [CrossRef] [PubMed]

Disclaimer/Publisher's Note: The statements, opinions and data contained in all publications are solely those of the individual author(s) and contributor(s) and not of MDPI and/or the editor(s). MDPI and/or the editor(s) disclaim responsibility for any injury to people or property resulting from any ideas, methods, instructions or products referred to in the content.

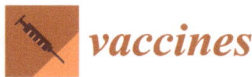

Article

Enhancing COVID-19 Vaccine Uptake among Tribal Communities: A Case Study on Program Implementation Experiences from Jharkhand and Chhattisgarh States, India

Ankita Meghani [1,*], Manjula Sharma [2,†], Tanya Singh [2], Sourav Ghosh Dastidar [2], Veena Dhawan [3], Natasha Kanagat [4], Anil Gupta [2], Anumegha Bhatnagar [2], Kapil Singh [5], Jessica C. Shearer [1] and Gopal Krishna Soni [2]

[1] PATH, Seattle, WA 98102, USA; jshearer@path.org
[2] John Snow India Pvt. Ltd., Delhi 110070, India; manjula.sharma1972@gmail.com (M.S.); tanya.25@gmail.com (T.S.); gdsourav@gmail.com (S.G.D.); gupta.dranil@gmail.com (A.G.); anumegha_bhatnagar@in.jsi.com (A.B.); sonigk70@gmail.com (G.K.S.)
[3] Ministry of Health & Family Welfare, Government of India, New Delhi 110011, India; veena.dhawan@gov.in
[4] John Snow Inc., Arlington, VA 22202, USA; natasha_kanagat@jsi.com
[5] World Health Organization, New Delhi 110011, India; singhkap@who.int
* Correspondence: ameghani@path.org
† Deceased.

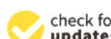

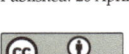 

Citation: Meghani, A.; Sharma, M.; Singh, T.; Dastidar, S.G.; Dhawan, V.; Kanagat, N.; Gupta, A.; Bhatnagar, A.; Singh, K.; Shearer, J.C.; et al. Enhancing COVID-19 Vaccine Uptake among Tribal Communities: A Case Study on Program Implementation Experiences from Jharkhand and Chhattisgarh States, India. *Vaccines* **2024**, *12*, 463. https://doi.org/10.3390/vaccines12050463

Academic Editor: Alessandra Casuccio

Received: 26 February 2024
Revised: 13 April 2024
Accepted: 19 April 2024
Published: 26 April 2024

Copyright: © 2024 by the authors. Licensee MDPI, Basel, Switzerland. This article is an open access article distributed under the terms and conditions of the Creative Commons Attribution (CC BY) license (https:// creativecommons.org/licenses/by/ 4.0/).

Abstract: Tribal populations in India have health care challenges marked by limited access due to geographical distance, historical isolation, cultural differences, and low social stratification, and that result in weaker health indicators compared to the general population. During the pandemic, Tribal districts consistently reported lower COVID-19 vaccination coverage than non-Tribal districts. We assessed the MOMENTUM Routine Immunization Transformation and Equity (the project) strategy, which aimed to increase access to and uptake of COVID-19 vaccines among Tribal populations in Chhattisgarh and Jharkhand using the reach, effectiveness, adoption, implementation, and maintenance framework. We designed a qualitative explanatory case study and conducted 90 focus group discussions and in-depth interviews with Tribal populations, community-based nongovernmental organizations that worked with district health authorities to implement the interventions, and other stakeholders such as government and community groups. The active involvement of community leaders, targeted counseling, community gatherings, and door-to-door visits appeared to increase vaccine awareness and assuage concerns about its safety and efficacy. Key adaptations such as conducting evening vaccine awareness activities, holding vaccine sessions at flexible times and sites, and modifying messaging for booster doses appeared to encourage vaccine uptake among Tribal populations. While we used project resources to mitigate financial and supply constraints where they arose, sustaining long-term uptake of project interventions appears dependent on continued funding and ongoing political support.

Keywords: tribal populations; COVID-19 vaccination; India; implementation science; case study; community-based strategies

1. Introduction

Tribal populations make up roughly 8% (104 million people) of the Indian population and comprise 700 scheduled tribes [1,2]. Tribal populations in India are heterogeneous, distinct in language, culture, and belief systems. Nearly 90% of all Tribal populations live in rural areas, often in dense forests which make it hard to access and deliver health services [1]. About 45% of all scheduled tribes, which have been acknowledged as among the most disadvantaged socio-economic groups in India, fall below the poverty line and have literacy rates that are persistently lower than the national average [1]. Furthermore, several studies on Tribal populations' health care preferences have highlighted their lack of trust in medical treatments or prevention measures and their preference for traditional medicines, practices, [3] and healers [4,5]. Socioeconomic differences, inadequate access to health care, geographic remoteness, cultural practices, and unique perspectives on health contribute to disparities in health outcomes among Tribal populations, compared to the general population [3].

Furthermore, connection with one's community appears to be central to Tribal populations. This connection fosters the strong sense of belonging that has been observed among tribal and indigenous populations living in India [6], Australia [7], and the United States [8]. Consequently, tribal populations often prefer to seek care from traditional providers within their community, as noted also in Bangladesh [9]. Strategies that employ individuals within Tribal communities to deliver health services, and leverage the social capital of key opinion leaders, such as village leaders and community health workers from those communities, have been shown to bridge gaps with the local health system in India [10]. Broader community participation has also been considered to be critical for expanding access to services [6]. Despite these distinct characteristics and preferences, India's health system has taken a uniform approach to Tribal and non-Tribal population health, with inconsistent attention paid to the differences in economic and educational attainment, language, geographic access to health professionals, and cultural beliefs that shape care-seeking behaviors [6]. A 2021 UNICEF study from India citing 2015–2016 NFHS-4 data noted that only 56% of Tribal children were fully vaccinated (compared to 62% nationally) [11]. Tribal populations also have disproportionately higher rates of diseases such as malaria, leprosy, and tuberculosis, and higher rates of malnutrition than the non-Tribal population [3]. The under-five mortality rate among scheduled tribes is 50 per 1000 live births; the national average is 42 per 1000 live births [12].

Tribal populations' health challenges were exacerbated during the pandemic. India introduced COVID-19 vaccines in January 2021 [13], and in the early stages of the vaccination campaigns that year, the national government initially reported that 72% of Tribal districts were surpassing the national average in terms of vaccination coverage [14]. However, coverage disparities quickly emerged between Tribal- and non-Tribal-majority districts. The lowest coverage was observed in Tribal districts in the Northeast, followed by those in Jharkhand and Chhattisgarh [15]. In October 2021, 63% of districts with Scheduled Tribe populations exceeding 20% were falling behind the national average of 53% of people having received at least the first dose of the vaccine [14,16]. Lower vaccination coverage among Tribal populations was attributed to lack of awareness [15] and misinformation about COVID-19 [17]; overburdened community health workers having to travel longer distances to reach Tribal populations [18]; and fluctuations in vaccine supply [15].

MOMENTUM Routine Immunization Transformation and Equity (the project) began working across 18 states in India to catalyze the government's efforts to increase COVID-19 vaccine coverage among priority populations. Increasing vaccine uptake among Tribal populations was a key focus for the project in Chhattisgarh and Jharkhand, where roughly one-third and one-quarter of the population, respectively, identify as scheduled tribes [19]. In collaboration with the state government, the project partnered with two community-based nongovernmental organizations (CBOs)—Samarthan in Chhattisgarh and the Indian Society of Agri-Business Professionals in Jharkhand—to increase awareness and vaccination uptake among Tribal populations, beginning in January 2022.

The project entered the two states after the initial COVID-19 vaccination rollout by the government, and at a time when resources from the COVID-19 program were diminishing and significant human resource capacity gaps were emerging. The project was positioned to address these gaps by creating awareness and demand among Tribal populations who remained unvaccinated, in collaboration with the CBOs and the government.

Based on a series of formative discussions with Tribal community members, community health workers, and government staff, the project began uncovering the multiple reasons why some Tribal populations remained unvaccinated. Some strongly believed that COVID-19 was not a major concern, as they had not witnessed significant illness in their communities. This led to a strong sense of complacency in Tribal communities, particularly among elderly members, who felt that death was imminent and therefore did not seek vaccination. Younger Tribal members were concerned about potential side effects from vaccination, particularly infertility. Even among those who were vaccinated, there seemed to lack a clear understanding of the benefits of vaccination. However, social factors, such as the influence of family members, did motivate some individuals to receive the vaccine. There were instances where unvaccinated elders, despite their own complacency, encouraged their family members to get vaccinated to prevent illness. Tribal populations also reported trusting those within their community, such as their community health workers and village leaders, for advice on health issues such as vaccination. Receiving the COVID-19 vaccination certificate, which at the time was a requirement for travel and work, was also seen as an important motivator.

Taking account of these factors, the project implemented four key interventions to increase vaccine uptake among Tribal populations across both states (Table 1). These interventions focused on: (i) developing strong partnerships with government and frontline community health workers to identify the unvaccinated and arrange vaccination sessions; (ii) collaborating with trusted community members from the Tribal community to expand outreach within the Tribal community; (iii) conducting interpersonal outreach and awareness campaigns by hiring Tribal community members who speak the local language and can build trust with unvaccinated Tribal members; and, more broadly, (iv) leveraging community events to raise awareness and encourage vaccine uptake using existing forums.

Table 1. Key interventions to increase vaccine uptake implemented during the project period in Chhattisgarh and Jharkhand.

Strategy	Intervention	Frequency
Partner with district government and frontline community health workers to identify Tribal populations that need vaccination	District- and block-level CBO staff collaborated with district immunization officers and other government officials to identify individuals, including those from Tribal populations, who were due for COVID-19 vaccines. This initial step informed the development of microplans, which were essential for conducting door-to-door vaccination.	Initially, interactions were frequent (weekly/twice a week) to establish relationships, but later occurred fortnightly.
Collaborate with and integrate trusted community members into project activities	CBOs partnered with village heads to serve as community coordinators, who, in turn, made announcements about government- and project-sponsored vaccine awareness activities and vaccination sessions.	Initially, interactions were frequent (weekly/twice a week) to establish relationships, but later occurred fortnightly.
	CBOs trained community volunteers, sometimes referred to as vaccine ambassadors, to provide accurate information about the COVID-19 vaccine. These individuals were selected for their leadership qualities and ability to engage the community. Some volunteers were paid by the CBOs.	Training sessions were conducted when beginning the position, and refresher training sessions were held monthly.
	CBOs collaborated with local groups like *yuva mitan* clubs (youth groups) and women's self-help groups (SHGs) to expand their outreach within the Tribal community.	Weekly

Table 1. Cont.

Strategy	Intervention	Frequency
Implement interpersonal communication activities to allay vaccination concerns	Vaccine ambassadors conducted door-to-door visits, often in collaboration with community health workers, to create general awareness about the vaccine and mobilize community members to attend vaccination camps. Often, they also accompanied community members to the vaccination site.	Biweekly
	Ratri chaupals (evening community gatherings) were held to actively listen to Tribal populations' concerns about vaccination and answer their questions. Implemented exclusively in the state of Chhattisgarh.	Weekly
Use government health- and non-health-sector platforms to increase awareness about the COVID-19 vaccines	At government events such as *Apki Yojana Apki Sarkar Apke Dwar* ("The Government is in Service to You"), the project set up vaccination stalls alongside government program booths and instructed staff at those booths to check vaccination status and refer people who were un- or under-vaccinated to the vaccination stall.	Project teams participated twice during these government events.
	Additionally, the project set up vaccination stalls at cultural and religious events like Durga Puja, Chhath Puja, local community gatherings, sports matches, and weekly markets to promote vaccination and vaccinate a broader audience, including Tribal populations.	Participation at cultural and religious events happened annually. Participation in community gatherings occurred on an ad hoc basis as these events arose.

Note: The interventions were implemented in both states unless otherwise stated.

In this paper, we applied the reach, effectiveness, adoption, implementation, and maintenance (RE-AIM) framework to assess the success of the project's interventions for increasing vaccine uptake among Tribal populations [20]. We conclude by reflecting on how these insights might inform the design and implementation of interventions for other health programs for Tribal populations.

Overview of Conceptual Framework

Applying the RE-AIM framework was relevant in our case study, where interventions are complex and may enable a deeper understanding of various outcomes, including unintended benefits and consequences. This approach not only enhanced our understanding of the project interventions' effectiveness, but also of the mechanisms behind the outcomes, accounting for external factors influencing implementation, adoption, long-term sustainability, and potential scale [21].

Table 2 provides the definitions of the RE-AIM framework dimensions examined in our study. We adapted these definitions to align with our study context. For the implementation dimension, instead of primarily assessing fidelity to a rigid intervention design, we modified the definition to recognize and capture adaptations made to the interventions for the unique Tribal sub-contexts in which the project was implemented.

Table 2. Description of the RE-AIM Framework.

Dimension	Definition
Reach	Whether, how, and why the interventions reached the Tribal populations
Effectiveness	Whether the interventions improved access to, demand for, and uptake of COVID-19 vaccines
Adoption	Whether, why, and how project staff and other stakeholders, such as the community-based CBOs and government, agreed to initiate/support the implementation of the interventions
Implementation	Whether, why, and how the interventions were delivered as intended, including adaptations made based on need and the evolving context
Maintenance	The sustainability of the interventions in the setting

Source: [20].

2. Materials and Methods

A. Study Design

We designed a qualitative, retrospective, and explanatory case study guided by the RE-AIM framework to assess the success of the project strategies. Because the project strategies collectively aimed to increase COVID-19 vaccination uptake among Tribal populations in both states, our evaluation centers on the project strategies as a unified case, rather than separately assessing each intervention. This approach also acknowledges the interdependence of these project strategies. Therefore, the case is the implementation of project strategies, and the unit of analysis is the community covered by the project. A case study approach was considered appropriate because it can help to answer not just what happened, but why and how it happened within the complex and evolving contexts where the case was unfolding [22].

This case study conducted qualitative in-depth interviews (IDIs) or focus group discussions (FGDs) with three key respondent groups: (1) Tribal populations that interacted with the project's activities; (2) CBOs that designed and implemented project interventions; and (3) key community-, district-, and state-level stakeholders who supported the implementation of project interventions. The interview and discussion guides were informed by the RE-AIM framework.

B. Study Context

Data collection took place in two districts each in Jharkhand and Chhattisgarh. District selection was determined based on two criteria: (1) whether the district was an M-RITE project district; and (2) whether it had a significant Tribal population, so that we could glean insights into how the project strategies were working. According to these criteria, data collection was conducted in Giridih and West Singhbhum in Jharkhand, and Gariabandh and Kanker districts in Chhattisgarh.

In Chhattisgarh, the project implementation in both districts began in October 2021, and implementation concluded in January 2023 in Kanker, and June 2023 in Gariabandh. Project implementation in both districts of Jharkhand started in March 2022 and ran until January 2023 in Giridih, and June 2023 in West Singhbhum.

Based on the most recent district-level census data available on Tribal populations [2], West Singhbhum and Giridih in Jharkhand, respectively, have Tribal populations of 1,011,296 and 238,188. Kanker and Gariabandh districts have populations of 414,770 and 173,977, respectively. The Tribal communities in Jharkhand and Chhattisgarh are linguistically diverse and live in densely forested areas. Some rely on foraging in the forests for sustenance, while others engage in various occupations such as agricultural labor, iron smelting, rope making, and household industries [23]. Each Tribal community is tightly knit, and their village and community leaders can have a significant influence on their decision-making. In this context, CBOs became instrumental project partners; they came with a deep understanding of the local context and used their existing infrastructure and community networks to develop and implement the project strategies outlined in Table 1. Their operational structure in the project involved a decentralized network of district coordinators, block coordinators, community supervisors, and vaccine ambassadors, or dedicated village volunteers. They also collaborated with grassroots community groups to further enhance their reach in Tribal communities.

C. Data collection

2.1. Tribal Populations

The IDIs and FGDs with Tribal populations aimed to identify factors influencing COVID-19 vaccine uptake for these populations and if and how the project's strategies contributed to it. We conducted separate FGDs with men and women, and IDIs with Tribal population members when one-on-one translators were needed. We attempted to conduct interviews with both vaccinated and unvaccinated individuals but given the advanced stage of the COVID-19 vaccination program in the states, most of our respondents were at least partially vaccinated. Across both states, 17 focus group discussions (FGDs) and 21 IDIs were conducted with Tribal community members.

2.2. Community Based Organizations

We conducted 5 FGDs with CBO staff at the district, block, and community levels in both states to understand the designs of project interventions, reach, effectiveness, and implementation experiences, including the barriers to and facilitators of their implementation, and adaptations made along the way to increase COVID-19 vaccine uptake in Tribal populations. We conducted 6 IDIs with additional community-based CBO staff to gain deeper insights into project implementation experiences.

2.3. Key Stakeholders

Across the two states, we interviewed 12 community-level stakeholders, such as village heads, vaccine ambassadors, and community health workers, at the block and district levels to better understand their roles and responsibilities in implementing the project strategies. We also sought their perspectives on the reach and effectiveness of the strategies and their experiences interacting with the project. Additionally, we interviewed a total of 29 district- and state-level stakeholders who were asked to reflect on the same issues and were further questioned about potential mechanisms for sustaining the project's strategies. District-level government stakeholders included members of the district-level COVID-19 task force, and district health officials. State-level respondents included representatives from United Nations organizations, government officials, and National Health Mission staff.

In total, we conducted 68 IDIs and 22 FGDs across the 2 states (Table 3).

Table 3. FGD and IDIs, by respondent and state.

Respondent	Jharkhand	Chhattisgarh	Total
Tribal population			
FGD	10	7	17
IDI with particularly vulnerable Tribal group	10	11	21
CBO			
IDI with community-based CBO staff at the district, block, and community levels	3	3	6
FGD with district-, block-, and community-level CBO staff	2	3	5
Key stakeholder			
IDI with community-level stakeholder	5	7	12
IDI with district-level government stakeholder	9	11	20
IDI with state-level stakeholder	3	6	9
Total	42	48	90

All of the qualitative data were collected in person from December 2022 to April 2023 in Jharkhand and Chhattisgarh. IDIs usually lasted 30–45 min, and FGDs 45–105 min. All participants were at least 18 years old. Oral informed consent was obtained from all the participants and conversations were audio recorded with permission. An agency transcribed all the conversations verbatim, and the research team reviewed the transcriptions for quality.

D. Data analysis and validation

We conducted a thematic analysis using the five dimensions of the RE-AIM framework [19]. We extracted textual data from the IDIs and FGDs into a spreadsheet with the categories from the analytical framework. Following this, we developed memos that summarized the information by category and compared and contrasted findings by district and state. While writing the memos, we triangulated data between FGDs and IDIs according to the three respondent categories highlighted in Table 3. We debriefed following each step to deepen our understanding of the data and conducted a meeting with a few respondents to validate study findings. We also conducted a learning workshop in October 2023, through which nearly 70 project participants were brought together, including CBOs, government partners, and state-level project staff, to review and validate the findings and conclusions. In the workshop, we also discussed how the learnings might be applied to other health programs. We also triangulate the qualitative findings of this study, where possible, with quantitative project data, which is routinely collected by the CBOs working at the district level in both states.

3. Results

Since there were no major differences in project strategies between the two states or by district, our findings are presented collectively across the RE-AIM domains of reach, effectiveness, adoption, implementation, and maintenance.

3.1. Reach

Most of the qualitative data suggest that the project's strategy to collaborate with trusted community stakeholders such as village heads, the project's village ambassadors, and community health workers succeeded in reaching Tribal populations in the project intervention districts in Chhattisgarh and Jharkhand and creating general awareness about vaccination sessions. Specifically, CBO project implementers said that the project strategy helped them gain trust and build rapport with Tribal populations and increased community-member participation in activities.

Tribal members whom we interviewed consistently said they viewed village heads, who make announcements in the evenings when everyone has returned from work, as the primary source of information about awareness activities and vaccination sessions. One district-level government staff worker agreed that the nominated village heads had a strong role in creating awareness of the COVID-19 vaccines, stating that "most effective were the words of *munda* [village head] only" [IDI-07, district-level stakeholder, Jharkhand]. In Chhattisgarh, some Tribal population members described learning about vaccination sessions through WhatsApp group messages sent by the members of the *panchayati raj*, an assembly of the village government. According to CBO staff, involving trusted community stakeholders who speak the local language helped them convey the benefits of vaccination more clearly.

Community health workers, particularly those in Jharkhand, were also considered critical information sources by the Tribal community. A community health worker described how she helped CBOs connect with Tribal populations, who generally tend to be wary of outsiders:

"When someone from the village stays in the meeting, then the villagers feel comfortable, otherwise the outsiders have to face some trouble. So, if we are present in any meeting either I [auxiliary nurse midwife] or a *sahiya* [accredited social health activist, a community health worker]... the meeting goes smoothly".

[IDI-02, community health worker, Jharkhand].

CBO staff similarly found that collaborating with community health workers helped them reach the Tribal community.

In addition, CBO staff perceived their efforts to partner with local organizations, including SHGs and *yuva mitan* (youth groups) clubs, to be important for increasing the Tribal community's awareness about vaccination initiatives. These groups encouraged participation in *ratri chaupals* (evening community gatherings), and appeared to increase community awareness of vaccination sessions through word-of-mouth.

For example, in Chhattisgarh, 24 SHG members motivated people within their Tribal community to get vaccinated. They formed groups of 3–4 and visited people in their fields and farms during work hours to increase awareness about the COVID-19 vaccination session. During these visits, SHG members described their personal experiences of receiving the vaccine and highlighted remaining in good health after vaccination to reassure others about the vaccine's safety. One SHG member said she tried to lead by example when encouraging others to receive the vaccine: "I had to first get vaccinated before I tell others to go for vaccination." [FGD-03, key stakeholder, Male Tribal population member, Chhattisgarh].

Youth groups helped organize *ratri chaupals*, and became regular facilitators at these events in Chhattisgarh. A total of 70 *ratri chaupals* were implemented in the two districts of Chhattisgarh. CBO staff said that involving youth and children in *nukkad natak* (street plays) during these gatherings injected new energy into the vaccination messages. More broadly, Tribal and CBO respondents said that the timing and structure of *ratri chaupals* increased the project's reach and that these gatherings were well attended.

Based on program data, overall, the project interventions reached 212,679 individuals in Giridih, Jharkhand, and 80,478 individuals in West Singhbhum, Jharkhand, during the project period. Similarly, the project reached 153,498 individuals in Gariabandh, Chhattisgarh, and 210,696 individuals in Kanker, Chhattisgarh.

3.2. Effectiveness

Considering the project's strong collaborations with the government, local organizations, and community health workers, and the implementation of a "whole-of-government strategy" during the COVID-19 vaccination rollout [20], assessing the effectiveness of the project's strategies alone was challenging. In this section, we evaluate the effectiveness of the project's strategies in increasing demand for, access to, and uptake of the COVID-19 vaccines among Tribal populations, but acknowledge that it was influenced by broader government policies and practices across the two states.

Overall, our interviews indicate that the project's four strategies appeared to enhance Tribal populations' access to, demand for, and uptake of COVID-19 vaccines. We found that the project's strategy of collaborating with trusted community stakeholders not only expanded its reach among Tribal populations, as described in the section above, but also generated demand and uptake among them. One CBO respondent mentioned that announcements from village leaders and their messengers (a project intervention) established the trust necessary to enhance vaccine demand and uptake:

"We have appointed a community supervisor which is a munda [an unelected community/village head]... and belongs to the same Tribal community, same society so whenever he communicates then the people do agree and get vaccinated".

[IDI-10, district coordinator, CBO, Jharkhand].

Tribal community members also acknowledged that the village head's recommendation to get vaccinated was perceived as a directive, which increased their intention to get vaccinated, with one individual saying, "The *sarpanch* [elected village head] said that my name has been identified for vaccination... It's a government order." [FGD-01, key stakeholder, Tribal population member, Chhattisgarh].

Another Tribal population member described how village heads were informed by community health workers about individuals who were or were not vaccinated, creating a sense of urgency:

"Sahiya [community health worker] tells *dakua* [a village leader] if someone goes to *Panchayat Bhavan* [village center] and is not taking the injection. Then, dakua in morning time does the announcement [about the next vaccination session]".

[FGD-01, key stakeholder, Female Tribal population member, Jharkhand].

Similarly, the CBOs and community members said that hiring vaccine ambassadors or volunteers from within the community (a project intervention) facilitated Tribal populations' access to vaccination. The project trained and engaged a total of 655 volunteers in the two districts of Jharkhand and 1017 in the two districts of Chhattisgarh. Tribal community members highlighted how project volunteers and government community health workers accompanied them to the vaccination sites using a project vehicle. One Tribal community member commented on the effectiveness of this intervention, stating:

"The project made it easy to access the vaccine. However, there were long vaccine queues, but everyone was there so we lined up, too".

[FGD-07, key stakeholder, Male Tribal population member, Jharkhand].

Engaging organizations rooted in the Tribal community was critical to mobilization. The community trusted them, especially when they assured people as to the absence of potential adverse effects resulting from the vaccine:

"So, we had to take the help from the head of the *gram panchayats* [village council] and lead members of the SHGs to convince people to take the COVID vaccine. We organized camps in villages to roll out the COVID vaccines among people. I convinced people to take the COVID vaccine by giving them my example and telling them that nothing would happen to them if they took the vaccine. So, I was able to convince 10 people to change their mind and take the COVID vaccine. I made a list containing the details of those 10 people and gave them to one of our nurses".

[IDI-05, local CBO, Chhattisgarh].

The use of interpersonal communication activities like door-to-door visits by the project's community volunteers/vaccine ambassadors and community health workers (project intervention) appeared to raise awareness about the importance of vaccination and motivate vaccination, especially among Tribal community members who were very hesitant. One couple described fear of vaccination and said that a neighbor's visit and door-to-door visits by the project staff and a government community health worker were motivating:

"So, after listening to them [community health worker and project staff] only they agreed. Like it happens that they will listen to only their caste people, they will do if they say or else they will not... In terms of this vaccine, it was the same way. They did listen to what the *sevika and sahiya* [community health workers] said".

[IDI-01, key stakeholder, PVTG Tribal population member, Jharkhand].

Another Tribal community respondent, initially hesitant about vaccination due to safety concerns, also said that the door-to-door visit motivated vaccination: "People from an organization came to tell us that taking the corona vaccine is necessary, and it doesn't cause fever, so we got vaccinated." [FGD-05, key stakeholder, Female Tribal population member, Jharkhand]. This respondent also acknowledged that hearing about vaccination from different sources, including community health workers, village leaders, government officials, and the project, helped them trust the vaccine and be more comfortable with vaccination. In some cases, the project's interpersonal communication activities seemed to contribute to vaccine uptake, although data from the interviews indicating whether uptake was a direct result of the project strategy or other reasons are limited.

While one-on-one interactions were effective in some settings, other respondents described receiving the vaccination without much explanation. One Tribal respondent indicated that the project staff met with her and other women and a community health worker, but "we did not get an explanation of why we need to get it. We got it because the *sahiya* [community health worker] was upset." [FGD-01, key stakeholder, Female Tribal population member, Jharkhand]. This suggests that despite the project's strategy to actively listen and respond to Tribal population member concerns, social pressure may have influenced vaccination, too.

The project's use of government health and non-health sector platforms to enhance the awareness of COVID-19 vaccines seemed effective. As one Tribal respondent stated:

"Everyone around was telling us to get vaccinated. The sarpanch, the *kotwar* [village announcer], everyone was recommending vaccination. The government was also ordering everyone to get the vaccine. If they said to do it, you have to do it".

(05, Tribal population community member, Chhattisgarh).

CBO respondents also felt that this strategy may have contributed to increased vaccine uptake among Tribal members who attended those events, but there is a limited amount of data as to whether or how this strategy directly influenced uptake.

3.3. Adoption

Our interviews with district-level CBOs and government officials suggested that there were no major barriers to adopting the project strategy, given that it was developed at that level, and collaboratively. However, interviews with government health workers and CBO staff at the block and community levels indicated delayed adoption and implementation of certain interventions, particularly door-to-door visits and vaccination sessions, due to community health workers' initial reluctance to assist.

At first, many community health workers who were expected to support CBOs in the implementation refused to participate because they did not receive the government-promised financial incentives for conducting COVID-19 vaccine-related activities during the initial rollout. Over time, most community health workers supported and developed trusted partnerships with the CBOs because they saw value in them, particularly as CBO staff provided transportation to conduct vaccination activities and supported them with routine tasks such as data entry and microplanning. One CBO staff member acknowledged this support, saying, "Community health workers have not been paid anything for 2–3 years, but they are still working with us." [FGD-02, CBOs, Jharkhand]

More broadly, some project stakeholders acknowledged that district-level CBO project staff appeared to motivate and energize the government community health workforce.

3.4. Implementation

Though the overarching project strategies were implemented in both states, flexibility was essential to allow adaptations to overcome Tribal populations' most prominent barriers to vaccine demand, access, and uptake at any given time.

That said, internal project factors such as staff attrition and external contextual factors, including health system strength, affected the project's ability to implement the strategies as intended. This section describes the facilitators of and barriers to implementation, and the adaptations to improve effectiveness. Table 4 provides a summary.

Table 4. Summary of internal and external barriers to and facilitators of project implementation.

Barrier and Facilitators	Description of Actions Taken
Internal barriers	
Staff attrition	• Quick hiring processes, when feasible; • Learning opportunities from colleagues at various levels of experience facilitated knowledge sharing; • Support and guidance from state-level project leadership.
Internal facilitators	
Regular meetings with state project leadership	• Provided support to teams facing challenges through frequent meetings; • Learning-by-doing approach guided program implementation and on-the-spot problem solving.
Hiring local staff	• Helped to increase trust and accelerated implementation.
External barriers	
Government's vaccine wastage policy	• Sensitizing community members in advance of the vaccination session; • Coordinating with other blocks or districts to identify additional eligible candidates helped ensure at least 10 individuals were present for vaccination.
Vaccine shortages	• Transfer if excess supply to blocks or districts with low or no inventory.
Backlog of COVID-19 vaccine data entry into Co-WIN	• CBOs supported data entry; • CBOs hired temporary data entry staff at the block and district levels.
Inadequate transportation funds available to community health workers	• CBOs provided transportation funds to frontline community health workers.
External facilitators	
"Whole of government" approach	• Strong political will led to increased collaboration with all of the departments, which helped with the project's implementation.
Strong partnerships with government and community and block health workers	• The project's relationships with Tribal populations, key leaders, and the health system offered valuable insights into program development and implementation; • These relationships also facilitated ongoing feedback about the effectiveness of program strategies and highlighted areas where adaptations were needed.

3.4.1. Internal Factors

As to the barriers to implementation, staff attrition hindered the implementation of the project's strategy. Staff turnover, which was primarily due to poor performance, resulted in frequent recruitment of new block-level coordinators. Attrition was also noted to be higher in areas that were considered sensitive due to the presence of certain militant groups commonly referred to as Naxalites. To address this gap, quick hiring processes were implemented, but recruitment times were often lengthy. One CBO also implemented an "all hands-on deck approach" during which the entire district-wide project workforce conducted vaccine mobilization activities in every village of the district (described further in Section 3.4.3, Adaptations to Project Interventions). In addition, some CBO staff noted varying levels of experience among their coworkers, ranging from former university professors to those learning on the job. These varying backgrounds at times facilitated knowledge sharing and learning. Despite these barriers, teams across both states acknowledged that working within supportive teams at the block and district levels facilitated quick implementation.

Facilitators

Two internal factors facilitated project implementation. First, strong support from the project's state leadership, which conducted regular meetings with CBO staff and teams that had trouble increasing vaccine uptake, helped troubleshoot problems quickly and effectively. One district-level CBO staff member described this approach, saying, "The state coordinator holds daily meetings in areas where teams were facing difficulties and creates microplans." (FGD-02, CBOs, Chhattisgarh)

CBO staff said that this learning-by-doing approach guided program implementation and problem-solving, and improved their understanding of what did and did not work. Beyond these meetings, the state and district coordinators visited local teams to overcome challenges and co-develop solutions. Together they conducted FGDs with community members, held conversations with panchayati raj and village leaders, and sought feedback from district government leaders, which helped them understand how their strategies were working.

The second facilitator was hiring local individuals with networks and experience, which CBO staff stated accelerated implementation and activities, particularly at the block and community levels. They were viewed as trusted insiders who knew how to navigate cultural sensitivities and adapt their communication to be culturally responsive.

3.4.2. External Factors

Barriers

A few external barriers affected the quality of project strategy implementation in the two states. First, the government's vaccine wastage policy significantly influenced the timing and locations in which vaccines were offered and administered to Tribal populations. Because districts enforced strong policies to minimize wastage, CBO and government community health workers explained that gathering enough vaccine recipients from Tribal communities was a logistical problem. Though vaccination sessions were organized for 10 people, if fewer arrived, health workers refrained from opening the vaccine vial until the tenth person arrived. As one Tribal community member said, "they [health worker] don't open it unless 10 candidates are present. Not even if 9 are present, they would wait for one more person to come." [FGD-03, Tribal population, Chhattisgarh].

CBOs staff explained that this policy led to situations in which some Tribal population members, despite attending a session, were turned away without getting vaccinated. In some cases, there was immediate coordination with another district or block to identify more eligible people for vaccination. However, this meant that people already at the vaccination session had to wait until more people arrived before vaccination could begin, which lowered the overall quality of service experience.

Second, CBO staff and health workers described broader vaccine shortages in the state, which were seen as a major barrier to vaccine mobilization and uptake. As one staff member said:

"We are facing an issue with the vaccine availability. This impacts our mobilizing activity because people would say that a team came telling us about the vaccine but when we reached, there was no vaccine available. We are feeling bad to mobilize now because even if we mobilize, they won't get vaccinated at the end. People are missing out doses during vaccination camps because of unavailability of vaccine taken at first dose".

[FGD-02, CBO, Jharkhand].

Some CBO respondents indicated that they helped transfer excess supply of vaccines to blocks or districts with low or no inventory:

"There was an instance of a vaccine camp where... there was no medicine and in the other village no one came to administer the vaccine. We immediately arranged for vehicles to transport the vaccines from one location to the other".
[IDI-04, CBO, Chhattisgarh].

Third, unpaid government data entry operators at the block and district levels resulted in a backlog of individuals awaiting data entry into Co-WIN, the national COVID-19 vaccine registration and reporting platform, in both states. This backlog hindered the generation of vaccination certificates (a key motivator of vaccination); the timing of the second vaccine dose for many individuals; and the preparation of lists of individuals who were due for vaccination. The CBOs and government community health workers used these data to determine the locations of their door-to-door visits, *ratri chaupal*, and, subsequently, the vaccination sessions. To alleviate the problem, CBOs supported data entry and hired temporary data entry staff at the block and district levels.

Fourth, resource constraints hindered intervention implementation. Transportation funds provided by the government to community health workers to conduct awareness and mobilization activities were quickly exhausted during the initial COVID-19 vaccine rollout. The absence of these funds made it difficult for health workers to accompany CBO staff on door-to-door activities, especially in distant and politically sensitive blocks, which generally have a higher density of Tribal population. The project stepped in to provide transportation to frontline community health workers, which was a key motivator for collaborating with CBO staff.

Facilitators

The "whole of government" approach to COVID-19 vaccination helped the project to benefit from high levels of political will within the health department and increased access to the various departments that were all working to increase vaccine uptake.

Specifically, strong political will and the demand to increase vaccination coverage increased the intensity of project implementation activities in the districts. The district magistrates held meetings to review and monitor vaccine data closely, creating a high level of accountability that was critical to achieving vaccination targets; as one CBO staff member stated, "If the district magistrate is strict, then the district' coverage is higher." [IDI-16, district-level stakeholder, Chhattisgarh].

The heightened accountability facilitated coordination and collaboration across various departments, and allowed the project team to access names and contact information of Tribal members eligible for the government's supportive services. CBOs cross-referenced the names of members listed in other departmental programs to develop a more comprehensive list of people due for vaccination and prioritize Tribal villages with low vaccination coverage for community awareness activities.

Second, as stated previously, partnerships with the government, particularly community- and block-level health workers, was critical for project implementation because of their relationships with Tribal populations and key leaders and their connection to the health system:

"We couldn't have visited these PVTG [Tribal] villages without the *mitanins* [community health workers]... who proved to be quite helpful for us because they are local people who know what goes on in their village. They provided us with staff and adequate vaccines to give to people. They informed the RHO and CHO [health officers] working in those PVTG villages beforehand so that we would be going there to give COVID vaccines to people".
[FGD-06, CBOs, Chhattisgarh].

3.4.3. Adaptations to Project Interventions

While project interventions were largely implemented as planned in both states, adaptations were made to improve effectiveness. Initially, the CBOs supported the governments by holding vaccination sessions at fixed times during the day, but these had low levels of turnout. After seeking community feedback and learning about how seasonal work affects people's availability, CBOs and district health officials changed the times and locations of the sessions. They continued to ask for feedback on when to schedule vaccination sessions, which led to flexible timings and higher turnout. As a district officer who collaborated with the project said:

> "Initially our team used to go for a session as per the official timings from 10 am to 4 pm. However, Tribal populations used to leave for their work early in the morning to the forest and come back after 5 pm, which usually meant that we would only be able to meet 1–2 people. Then it was discussed with the *patel* [village head] and *gayta pujari* [village priest] that the vaccination has to be arranged either early in the morning or after people come from work. Because the Tribal population would leave at 5 am, our teams used to be ready at 4:30 am to meet them and then again after 5 pm".

[IDI-01, District health official, Chhattisgarh].

The CBOs established a call center to follow up with individuals who were due for their second dose, including those who had not received a vaccine certificate, and in Chhattisgarh, conducted door-to-door awareness activities on blocks with the lowest vaccination rates.

To manage staff attrition and accelerate vaccine uptake in low-coverage blocks, one district-level CBO team changed how it conducted community awareness activities. Rather than having teams conduct their own area-specific activities, the CBO implemented an "all hands-on deck approach." The entire district-wide project workforce, including village ambassadors and block and district coordinators, conducted vaccine mobilization activities and sessions in every village across all blocks. To implement this adapted strategy, the CBO also provided government community health workers with transportation to and from vaccination sites and supported the delivery of vaccine boxes to the sessions in the villages.

As the focus shifted to increasing the uptake of the third or booster dose among Tribal populations, CBOs adapted their messages. Community health workers and CBOs organizing the *ratri chaupals* emphasized the urgency and advantage of receiving the third dose before it became a paid service. Many Tribal community members in both states acknowledged receiving this message. One stated:

> "Regarding the third dose, health workers told us, 'It's government-provided and free now [like the first and second doses]. Later, you'll have to go to Block Charma, and it will cost money".

[FGD-03, Tribal population, Chhattisgarh].

In some districts, routine immunization days in the villages were an additional platform for promoting the third dose of the COVID-19 vaccine to caregivers. When there was high demand, an additional vaccination camp was organized the day after the *ratri chaupal*.

3.5. Maintenance

Based on interviews with project staff and district government officials, there were indications that the project's interventions, especially its partnerships with community-based CBOs and leaders, had broad applicability in strengthening routine immunization and maternal health programs for Tribal populations. Funding was identified as a factor that sustained CBO support for COVID-19-related and other health-related programs at the district level, but there was broader acknowledgment that the involvement of communities and CBOs that worked with them was critical. Most immediately, continuous engagement with communities is crucial for identifying and adapting the most valuable and feasible project strategies.

Some government staff, particularly during the learning workshop, suggested focusing on adapting the project's endeavors for other health programs, such as scheduling *ratri chaupal*, implementing vaccination sessions with flexible timings, and seeking collaboration across departments to develop line-lists of Tribal population members who needed services. They also recommended creating and sharing a directory of CBOs and emphasized the importance of engagement between CBOs and the government in district-level meetings to continue sharing feedback and information about Tribal populations and other high-priority groups.

4. Discussion

Our assessment suggests the project strategies were successful in reaching Tribal populations, creating vaccine awareness, and generating demand that led to uptake. While attributing all vaccination uptake solely to these strategies is challenging due to broader COVID-19 initiatives being implemented at the same time, the project had a crucial role in catalyzing COVID-19 vaccination efforts in the two states.

It is evident that collaboration with trusted community stakeholders increased vaccine awareness and demand. Organizations like SHGs that are deeply embedded within the Tribal community appeared to reinforce the benefits of vaccination and increase uptake. Furthermore, the integration of community members into project activities, particularly as village ambassadors, expanded the project's reach in Tribal communities and conveyed information in culturally and linguistically familiar ways. These experiences underscore the significance of mitigating inequities by developing culturally responsive strategies and strengthening health systems so that they can be culturally responsive.

Recent studies conducted in India have similarly reflected on the importance of involving village leaders and partnering with local organizations to increase community engagement [24]. In particular, formal partnerships have been seen as facilitating community engagement [24] and shown to improve health practices and behaviors within the community [25]. For instance, partnerships with SHGs have been recognized as a promising strategy for reaching large numbers of women, including Tribal women, in India [26]. Research indicates that women residing in villages with active SHGs are more likely to access family planning methods, compared to those that lack such groups, highlighting the benefits of these partnerships [27]. Additionally, a recent social network analysis in rural India found that coordination between women's self-help groups and local health systems improved when the village leader and the community health worker played central roles in the network [10]. This finding suggests that their involvement can be critical in facilitating information exchange between local health systems and community groups [10].

Our findings reinforced this, as collaboration with SHGs through village leaders and community health workers contributed to increasing vaccine awareness, access, and uptake.

Our study also highlights the importance of recognizing that community engagement efforts should not solely focus on conveying information, but also on soliciting input from communities about their needs and incorporating their feedback into the project. For example, platforms like *ratri chaupals*, where community members can provide feedback, express concerns, and actively participate, helped ensure that the project's activities were culturally appropriate, community-driven, and responsive to specific needs and preferences. Integrating such community feedback mechanisms into programs can increase the reach of and demand for health services, specifically when aiming to improve routine immunization coverage among Tribal populations.

More broadly, there is a growing emphasis on prioritizing the involvement and collaboration of indigenous and tribal communities in designing solutions that can transform healthcare systems to become more responsive to their needs [28]. For example, in Canada, indigenous communities are beginning to actively participating in health policy-making processes [29]. Similarly, in the United States, initiatives have been launched to recruit health providers and community workers from Alaska Native and American Indian communities to better address their specific needs, and doing so has led to promising outcomes in increasing access to culturally responsive care and reducing the potential stigma associated with seeking care [30].

Equally important as involving and empowering Tribal community leaders in actively participating in health programs is creating a project environment that supports adaptability and flexibility. Key learnings from the project included collaborating with partners within Tribal communities and government, and using the information gathered through these collaborations to make better adaptations and decisions during program implementation, such as providing transportation for community health workers; improving data quality processes to ensure better reach; managing vaccine shortages by hiring additional vehicles; and supporting vaccine reallocation efforts.

While leveraging government program events such as *Aaapki Sarkar Aapki Dwar* (Your Scheme, Your Government at Your Doorstep) integrated vaccination with broader efforts, which reinforced the importance of vaccination to all populations, it was clear that vaccine ambassadors and village volunteers, along with community health workers, played a key role in rebuilding trust and communicating in a culturally appropriate manner among Tribal populations. Creating culturally appropriate and effective materials requires a deep understanding of cultural traditions and practices relating to health, wellness, and healing, which may differ from tribe to tribe with respect to such elements as using the herbs and remedies Tribal populations receive from their traditional healers in India [6] or connecting with one's land to support healing processes as in American Indian/Alaskan Native communities [31], among others.

Several Tribal health programs and policies in India could be entry points for integrating the learnings from this case study. For instance, the National Health Policy [32], which recognizes the need to address inequities experienced by vulnerable populations such as Tribal groups, could incorporate interventions to promote Tribal community engagement in the design and implementation of healthcare programs and policies. Similarly, the hiring of community health workers and medical providers from within those communities can help to overcome language barriers and address the potential bias and discrimination experienced when seeking healthcare. The National Health Mission could also adopt such approaches to tailor health services and communications to promote cultural sensitivity and empathy when interacting with Tribal communities [24].

Community feedback mechanisms could be integrated into the Integrated Child Development Services, which works to improve the health and nutrition of women and children, and other health programs. As programs integrate these mechanisms, documenting the lessons will be critical for strengthening the evidence-base for what works and why, so others can learn and adapt and sustain such initiatives. Most of all, sustaining processes that involve communities in decision-making, respecting their needs, and collaborating with these communities will be imperative for ultimately increasing uptake and use of vaccination and health services among Tribal populations.

Limitations

Key limitations to our study should be acknowledged. First, when we were unable to directly communicate with Tribal populations in their local languages, we relied on translators in a few instances, which may have hindered rapport building and caused us to miss nuances in their responses. Relatedly, we also recognize the role of interpreter bias in these situations, which may have influenced how certain comments were translated. Second, during our interviews, a few CBO staff members were new to their positions and may have lacked a comprehensive understanding of the project; we compensated for these gaps by speaking to other CBO supervisors based at the state level to gain a fuller understanding. Third, we had difficulty securing appointments with Tribal agency counterparts at the district level, so we sought insight through conversations with community leaders who interact with them. We attempted to increase the credibility of our findings by employing a triangulation approach, using multiple data sources to corroborate information (for example, speaking with multiple types of respondents), and engaging in respondent validation (member checking) by sharing our findings with individuals who were knowledgeable about the project and its context. A future quantitative assessment could provide additional data to complement this qualitative evaluation.

5. Conclusions

In conclusion, the project strategies appeared to be successful in effectively increasing vaccine awareness and demand among Tribal populations, and contributed to higher vaccine uptake. Although it is difficult to attribute all vaccination uptake solely to the project, due to concurrent COVID-19 vaccine initiatives, the project's collaboration with trusted community stakeholders, particularly through village leaders, community health workers, and vaccine ambassadors, facilitated culturally appropriate communication and reinforced the benefits of vaccination within the community. The study also highlights the importance of community engagement and feedback mechanisms in designing and implementing healthcare programs that cater to the specific needs of Tribal communities. These mechanisms led to program adaptations that enabled the project to work towards its goals despite implementation challenges. These findings underscore the value of flexible, adaptable, and culturally sensitive approaches in healthcare programs. Partnerships with CBOs and community engagement strategies developed through this project can serve as a model for future health initiatives among Tribal populations. Sustaining such community-centered processes is key to enhancing the uptake of health services.

Author Contributions: Conceptualization, A.M., N.K., A.G., A.B., J.C.S., V.D., K.S. and G.K.S.; methodology, A.M., N.K., S.G.D., V.D., K.S. and G.K.S.; validation, A.M., T.S., A.G., A.B., S.G.D., V.D., K.S. and G.K.S.; formal analysis, A.M., M.S., T.S. and N.K.; investigation, M.S. and S.G.D.; resources, G.K.S.; data curation, A.M., M.S. and T.S.; writing—original draft preparation, A.M., M.S. and T.S.; writing—review and editing, A.M., M.S., T.S., V.D., N.K., A.G., A.B., K.S., J.C.S. and G.K.S.; visualization, A.M., M.S. and T.S.; supervision, A.M. and G.K.S.; project administration, A.M., A.B., T.S. and G.K.S.; funding acquisition, G.K.S. All authors have read and agreed to the published version of the manuscript.

Funding: MOMENTUM Routine Immunization Transformation and Equity, as well as this research, were funded by the U.S. Agency for International Development (USAID) as part of the MOMENTUM suite of awards, and implemented by the JSI Research & Training Institute, Inc. with partners PATH, Accenture Development Partnerships, Results for Development, CORE Group, and The Manoff Group under USAID cooperative agreement #7200AA20CA00017. For more information about MOMENTUM, visit www.usaidmomentum.org (accessed on 15 January 2023). The contents of this journal article are the sole responsibility of the JSI Research & Training Institute, Inc., and do not necessarily reflect the views of USAID or the United States Government.

Institutional Review Board Statement: The study was conducted in accordance with the Declaration of Helsinki, and approved by the institutional review boards of SIGMA Research and Consulting, New Delhi (Protocol code U74140DL2008PTC182567 and 5 November 2022) and John Snow, Inc. (22-35E PH2 and 16 September 2022).

Informed Consent Statement: Informed consent was obtained from all subjects involved in the study.

Data Availability Statement: The data presented in this study are available on request from the corresponding author. The data are not publicly available due to the privacy concerns of the respondents.

Acknowledgments: We would like to acknowledge the following key contributors to our work: Apurva Rastogi, Andi Sutter, Raju Tamang, Katelyn Bryant-Comstock, Grace Chee, Rebecca Fields, and Vanessa Richart, as well as the finance, travel, and management teams at John Snow India Pvt. Ltd. We are also immensely grateful to all the community members, community-based NGOs, and state-level project teams who generously devoted their time and shared their experiences with us. Without them, this study would not have been possible.

Conflicts of Interest: All the authors declare that the research was conducted in the absence of any commercial or financial relationships that could be construed as a potential conflict of interest.

References

1. Samvaad, D.; Ministry of Tribal Affairs, Government of India. Available online: https://tribal.nic.in/downloads/Statistics/Statistics8518.pdf (accessed on 17 February 2023).
2. Chandramouli, D.C. Scheduled Tribes in India as Revealed in Census 2011. 2013. Available online: https://ruralindiaonline.org/en/library/resource/scheduled-tribes-in-india-as-revealed-in-census-2011/ (accessed on 12 July 2023).
3. Kumar, M.M.; Pathak, V.K.; Ruikar, M. Tribal Population in India: A Public Health Challenge and Road to Future. *J. Family Med. Prim. Care* **2020**, *9*, 508–512. [CrossRef] [PubMed]
4. Mahapatro, M.; Kalla, A.K. Health Seeking Behaviour in a Tribal Setting. *Health Popul. Perspect. Issues* **2000**, *23*, 160–169.
5. Islary, J. Health and Health Seeking Behaviour among Tribal Communities in India: A Socio-Cultural Perspective. *J. Tribal Intellect. Collect. India* **2014**, *2*, 1–16. [CrossRef]
6. Deb Roy, A.; Das, D.; Mondal, H. The Tribal Health System in India: Challenges in Healthcare Delivery in Comparison to the Global Healthcare Systems. *Cureus* **2023**, *15*, e39867. [CrossRef] [PubMed]
7. The Link between Indigenous Culture and Wellbeing: Qualitative Evidence for Australian Aboriginal Peoples. Available online: https://nla.gov.au/nla.obj-2496469627/view (accessed on 12 July 2023).
8. CDC. Tribal Practices for Wellness in Indian Country (TPWIC). Available online: https://www.cdc.gov/healthytribes/tribalpractices.htm (accessed on 12 April 2024).
9. Rahman, S.A.; Kielmann, T.; McPake, B.; Normand, C. Healthcare-Seeking Behaviour among the Tribal People of Bangladesh: Can the Current Health System Really Meet Their Needs? *J. Health Popul. Nutr.* **2012**, *30*, 353–365. [CrossRef] [PubMed]
10. Rudacha, J.; Hariharan, D.; Potter, J.; Ahmad, D.; Kumar, S.; Mohanan, P.S.; Irani, L.; Long, K.N.G. Measuring Coordination between Women's Self-Help Groups and Local Health Systems in Rural India: A Social Network Analysis. *BMJ Open* **2019**, *9*, e028943. [CrossRef] [PubMed]
11. Immunization among Tribal Population in India.Pdf. Available online: https://www.unicef.org/india/media/6716/file/Immunization%20among%20Tribal%20Population%20in%20India.pdf (accessed on 15 July 2023).
12. International Institute for Population Sciences Deonar, Mumbai-400088. International Institute for Population Sciences National Family Health Survey (NFHS-5), 2019–2021; India Report. Available online: https://dhsprogram.com/pubs/pdf/FR375/FR375.pdf (accessed on 15 July 2023).
13. India Marks One Year of COVID Vaccination. Available online: https://www.who.int/india/news/feature-stories/detail/india-marks-one-year-of-covid-vaccination (accessed on 1 January 2024).
14. Ministry of Health and Family. COVID Vaccination in Rural Areas—Myths vs. Facts. Available online: https://pib.gov.in/PressReleasePage.aspx?PRID=1727193 (accessed on 1 January 2024).
15. Barnagarwala, T. Why COVID-19 Vaccination Coverage Lags behind in Several of India's Tribal-Majority Districts. Available online: https://scroll.in/article/1010621/why-covid-19-vaccination-coverage-lags-behind-in-several-of-indias-tribal-majority-districts (accessed on 3 May 2023).
16. Esteves, L.A.; Iqbal, N. Gender and Social Disparities: What India's Acheivement of 1 Billion Vaccine Doses Doesn't Reveal. Available online: https://scroll.in/article/1009693/gender-and-social-disparities-what-indias-achivement-of-1-billion-vaccine-doses-doesnt-reveal (accessed on 2 January 2024).
17. Mehmood, Q.; Tebha, S.S.; Aborode, A.T. Aayush COVID-19 Vaccine Hesitancy among Indigenous People in India: An Incipient Crisis. *Ethics Med. Public Health* **2021**, *19*, 100727. [CrossRef] [PubMed]
18. COVID-19 and Tribal Communities: How State Neglect Increased Marginalisation during the Pandemic. *Economic and Political Weekly*. 8 September 2021. Available online: https://www.epw.in/engage/article/covid-19-and-tribal-communities-how-state-neglect (accessed on 1 January 2024).
19. Ministry of Tribal Affairs, Government of India. Report of the High Level Committee on Socio-Economic, Health and Educational Status of Tribal Communities of India. Available online: https://ruralindiaonline.org/en/library/resource/report-of-the-high-level-committee-on-socio-economic-health-and-educational-status-of-the-tribals-of-india/ (accessed on 12 July 2023).
20. What Is RE-AIM?—RE-AIM. Available online: https://re-aim.org/learn/what-is-re-aim/ (accessed on 2 January 2024).
21. Glasgow, R.E.; Vogt, T.M.; Boles, S.M. Evaluating the Public Health Impact of Health Promotion Interventions: The RE-AIM Framework. *Am. J. Public Health* **1999**, *89*, 1322–1327. [CrossRef] [PubMed]
22. Yin, R.K. Case Study Methods. In *APA Handbook of Research Methods in Psychology, Volume 2: Research Designs: Quantitative, Qualitative, Neuropsychological, and Biological*; APA Handbooks in Psychology®; American Psychological Association: Washington, DC, USA, 2012; pp. 141–155. ISBN 978-1-4338-1005-3.
23. Sahu, S. Demographic Trends and Occupational Structure of Particularly Vulnerable Tribal Groups of Jharkhand. *Int. J. Rev. Res. Soc. Sci.* **2019**, *7*, 316–322.
24. Dutta, T.; Agley, J.; Meyerson, B.E.; Barnes, P.A.; Sherwood-Laughlin, C.; Nicholson-Crotty, J. Perceived Enablers and Barriers of Community Engagement for Vaccination in India: Using Socioecological Analysis. *PLoS ONE* **2021**, *16*, e0253318. [CrossRef]
25. Saggurti, N.; Atmavilas, Y.; Porwal, A.; Schooley, J.; Das, R.; Kande, N.; Irani, L.; Hay, K. Effect of Health Intervention Integration within Women's Self-Help Groups on Collectivization and Healthy Practices around Reproductive, Maternal, Neonatal and Child

Health in Rural India. *PLoS ONE* **2018**, *13*, e0202562. Available online: https://journals.plos.org/plosone/article?id=10.1371/journal.pone.0202562 (accessed on 2 January 2024). [CrossRef] [PubMed]
26. Sethi, V.; Bhanot, A.; Bhalla, S.; Bhattacharjee, S.; Daniel, A.; Sharma, D.M.; Gope, R.; Mebrahtu, S. Partnering with Women Collectives for Delivering Essential Women's Nutrition Interventions in Tribal Areas of Eastern India: A Scoping Study. *J. Health Popul. Nutr.* **2017**, *36*, 20. [CrossRef] [PubMed]
27. The HUNGaMA Survey Report—2011. Available online: https://www.cse.iitb.ac.in/~sohoni/TD604/HungamaBKDec11LR.pdf (accessed on 2 January 2024).
28. Lasker, R.D.; Weiss, E.S. Broadening Participation in Community Problem Solving: A Multidisciplinary Model to Support Collaborative Practice and Research. *J. Urban Health* **2003**, *80*, 14–47. [CrossRef] [PubMed]
29. Nguyen, N.H.; Subhan, F.B.; Williams, K.; Chan, C.B. Barriers and Mitigating Strategies to Healthcare Access in Indigenous Communities of Canada: A Narrative Review. *Healthcare* **2020**, *8*, 112. [CrossRef] [PubMed]
30. O'Keefe, V.M.; Cwik, M.F.; Haroz, E.E.; Barlow, A. Increasing Culturally Responsive Care and Mental Health Equity with Indigenous Community Mental Health Workers. *Psychol. Serv.* **2021**, *18*, 84–92. [CrossRef] [PubMed]
31. Goodkind, J.R.; Gorman, B.; Hess, J.M.; Parker, D.P.; Hough, R.L. Reconsidering Culturally Competent Approaches to American Indian Healing and Well-Being. *Qual. Health Res.* **2015**, *25*, 486–499. [CrossRef] [PubMed]
32. Government of India, Ministry of Health and Family Welfare. National Health Policy 2017. Available online: https://main.mohfw.gov.in/sites/default/files/9147562941489753121.pdf (accessed on 2 January 2024).

Disclaimer/Publisher's Note: The statements, opinions and data contained in all publications are solely those of the individual author(s) and contributor(s) and not of MDPI and/or the editor(s). MDPI and/or the editor(s) disclaim responsibility for any injury to people or property resulting from any ideas, methods, instructions or products referred to in the content.

MDPI AG
Grosspeteranlage 5
4052 Basel
Switzerland
Tel.: +41 61 683 77 34

Vaccines Editorial Office
E-mail: vaccines@mdpi.com
www.mdpi.com/journal/vaccines

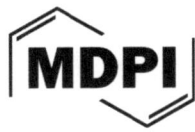

Disclaimer/Publisher's Note: The statements, opinions and data contained in all publications are solely those of the individual author(s) and contributor(s) and not of MDPI and/or the editor(s). MDPI and/or the editor(s) disclaim responsibility for any injury to people or property resulting from any ideas, methods, instructions or products referred to in the content.